D0557506

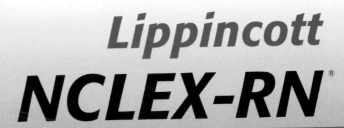

Lippincott
NCLEX-RN®
Alternate-Format
Questions
Sixth Edition

Diana Rupert, PhD, RN, CNE

Administrator
Indiana County Technology Center
School of Practical Nursing
Assistant Professor
Indiana University of Pennsylvania
Indiana, Pennsylvania

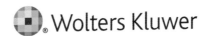

Philadelphia • Baltimore • New York • London
Buenos Aires • Hong Kong • Sydney • Tokyo

Senior Digital Product Manager: Renee Gagliardi
Associate Content Strategist: Bernadette Enneg
Senior Production Project Manager: Cynthia Rudy
Art Director: Jennifer Clements
Design Coordinator: Stephen Druding
Manufacturing Coordinator: Kathleen Brown
Prepress Vendor: SPi Global

Sixth edition

Library of Congress Cataloging-in-Publication Data

Names: Rupert, Diana L., author.
Title: Lippincott NCLEX-RN alternate format questions / Diana L. Rupert.
Other titles: NCLEX-RN alternate format questions
Description: Sixth edition. | Philadelphia : Wolters Kluwer, [2017] | Includes bibliographical references.
Identifiers: LCCN 2015049571 | ISBN 9781496325310 (paperback)
Subjects: | MESH: Nursing Care | Nursing Process | Licensure, Nursing | Examination Questions
Classification: LCC RT55 | NLM WY 18.2 | DDC 610.73076—dc23 LC record available at http://lccn.loc.gov/2015049571

Faculty Reviewers

Danielle Artis, MSN, RN, CPN
Instructor
Trinity Washington University
Washington, District of Columbia

Patti Cantamessa, MS, RN
Assistant Professor
Farmingdale State College
Farmingdale, New York

Ruth Chen, RN, PHD
Department Education Coordinator
School of Nursing, McMaster University
Hamilton, Ontario, Canada

Mohamed Toufic El Hussein, RN, MSN, PHD
Associate Professor
Mount Royal University
Calgary, Alberta, Canada

Nancy Fleming, RN, HBSCN, MAED
Professor
Confederation College
Thunder Bay, Ontario, Canada

Jessica M. Flores, RN, BSN
Arizona State University
Tempe, Arizona

Kimbra Gabhart, MSN-BC, RN
Assistant Professor
Elizabethtown Community & Technical College
Elizabethtown, Kentucky

Sue Gabriel, EDD, MSN, MFS, RN, SANE-A, CFN,
FACFEI, DABFN
Associate Professor
Nebraska Wesleyan University
Lincoln, Nebraska

Barbara Huggins, DNP, RN, PMHCNS-BC, CNE
Professor of Nursing
Saddleback College HSHS Division
Mission Viejo, California

Eileen Kane
Instructor
Worcester State College
Worcester, Massachusetts

Nicole de Bosch Kemper, RN, MSN
Instructor
University of British Columbia, Okanagan
Kelowna, British Columbia

Christine L. Krause, MSN, CPNP
Faculty
Aria Health School of Nursing
Penn State University Abington
Bensalem, Pennsylvania

Chrystal Lewis, MSN, RN
Instructor
University of Alabama
Tuscaloosa, Alabama

Tatayana Maltseva, MSN, ARNP, PMHNP-BC
Clinical Assistant Professor
Florida International University
North Miami, Florida

Jane Moore, RN, PHD, CCRN, APN
Assistance Professor
Brock University
Saint Catharines, Ontario, Canada

Lisa Moralejo, RN, MSN
Instructor
University of British Columbia, Okanagan
Kelowna, British Columbia

Mary T. Moseley, EDD, MN, BSN
Professor of Nursing
Northern Virginia Community College,
Medical Education Campus
Springfield, Virginia

Student/Recent Graduate Reviewers

Helen C. Ballestas, RN, MS, CRRN

Carol Blakeman, MSN, ARNP

Cheryl L. Brady, RN, MSN

Barbara Broome, RN, PHD

Marsha L. Conroy, RN, MSN, APN

Kim Cooper, RN, MSN

Linda Carman Copel, PHD, APRN, BC, CGP, NCC, DAPA

Susan Denman, RN, PHD, APRN-BC, FNP

Marsha Gerdeman, RN, MS

Karla Jones, RN, MS

Kathy J. Keister, RN, PHD

Elayne J. Sugar-Karrel, RN, MSN

Allison J. Terry, RN, MSN, PHD

Acknowledgments

Many thanks to Renee Gagliardi, Bernadette Enneg, and the staff at Wolters Kluwer, who have helped in the development of this book. I appreciate all of your expertise in making this a valuable resource for pre-licensure students. Also, thank you to the Canadian and United States faculty reviewers. I appreciate all of your guidance and expertise. Thank you to the graduate nurses for their input bringing the student perspective. I wish you the best in your nursing career.

To my growing family:

Cliff, my husband and best friend, thank you for all that you do for me. I have been blessed to have you as my husband.

My children: Jeff and Amy, Mike, Pat, and Taylor. I am so proud of each one of you.

My grandson Connor: You are so much fun!

My parents: Donald and Dorothy Hill. You are both an inspiration to me.

Thanks to you all. I love you!

About the Author

Dr. Diana Rupert is an alumnus of Indiana University of Pennsylvania. She began her nursing career 25 years ago as a pediatric nurse before moving to home health and then education. She has almost 20 years of teaching experience, including practical nursing programs, a diploma nursing program, baccalaureate, and masters nursing programs.

Dr. Rupert is the administrator at the Indiana County Technology Center, School of Practical Nursing, Indiana, Pennsylvania, and an assistant professor at Indiana University of Pennsylvania. She has presented on NCLEX topics via webinar, workshops, and small group sessions and is the author of three books for NCLEX preparation.

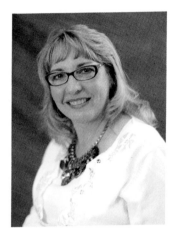

Contents

Preparing for the NCLEX®

Welcome to the most comprehensive registered nurse (RN) alternate-format question preparation book! You have made a good decision to spend some concentrated time feeling comfortable with answering alternate-format style questions. Because these types of questions can be more difficult, answering them correctly can provide a boost to your score due to the adaptive nature of the NCLEX-RN.

NCLEX basics

Passing the National Council Licensure Examination (NCLEX®) is an important landmark in your career as a nurse. The first step on your way to passing the NCLEX is to understand what it is and how it is administered.

NCLEX structure

The NCLEX is a test written by nurses who, like most of your nursing instructors, have an advanced degree and clinical expertise in a particular area. Only one small difference distinguishes nurses who write NCLEX questions: they are trained to write questions in a style particular to the NCLEX.

If you have completed an accredited nursing program, you have already taken numerous tests written by nurses with backgrounds and experiences similar to those of the nurses who write for the NCLEX. The test-taking experience you have already gained will help you pass the NCLEX. So your NCLEX review should be just that—a review.

The NCLEX is designed for one purpose: to determine whether it is appropriate for you to receive a license to practice as a nurse. By passing the NCLEX, you demonstrate that you possess the minimum level of knowledge necessary for a competent entry-level-practitioner to practice nursing safely.

Clarification on Measurements, Terminology, and Medications

This book is prepared for student nurses in both the United States and Canada. Since there are some differences in terminology and techniques, this book offers a variety of methods and expressions so that either group of nursing students can understand the question presented and then the steps needed to correctly answer. Examples of some common variations are shown below.

Please be advised that reviewers from both the United States and Canada have screened each question for alignment with the most current NCLEX test plan and current standards of practice in each country.

Topic	United States	Canada
Weight	Pounds, ounces	Kilograms
Laboratory measurements	Metric	SI units
Nursing career ladder	■ Registered nurse ■ Licensed practical/vocational nurse ■ Nursing assistant, certified nurse aide, home health aide, patient care technician (PCT)	■ Registered nurse ■ Registered practical nurse ■ Residential care worker, support worker, home health aide, unregulated health care worker (UHW)
Medications	Slight differences in medications prescribed for disease processes Documented in generic names	
Laboratory tests	Slight difference in components of lab tests	

If you have completed your nursing education in a foreign country, you must follow certain guidelines to be eligible to work as a registered nurse (RN) in the United States. (See *Guidelines for international nurses,* page 4.)

In nursing school, you probably took separate courses, such as pharmacology, nursing leadership, and health assessment, as well as courses that addressed adult health, pediatric, maternal–neonatal, and psychiatric nursing. In contrast, the NCLEX is integrated, meaning that different subjects are mixed together.

As you answer NCLEX questions, you may encounter patients in any stage of life, from neonatal to geriatric. These patients—clients, in NCLEX terminology—may be of any background, may be completely well or extremely ill, and may have any of a variety of disorders.

Client Needs

The NCLEX draws questions from four categories of *client needs* that were developed by the National Council of State Boards of Nursing (NCSBN), the organization that sponsors and manages the NCLEX. Client needs categories ensure that a wide variety of topics appears on every NCLEX.

The NCSBN developed client needs categories after conducting a practice analysis of new nurses. All aspects of nursing care observed in the study were broken down into four main categories, some of which were broken down further into subcategories. (See *Client needs categories,* page 5.)

Integrated Processes

Integrated throughout the client needs categories and subcategories are five key processes that are fundamental to the practice of nursing:

- **Nursing process**—a scientific, clinical reasoning approach to client care that includes assessment, analysis, planning, implementation, and evaluation
- **Caring**—an atmosphere of mutual respect and trust that exists between the nurse and the client in which the nurse provides encouragement, support, hope, and compassion to help the client achieve desired outcomes
- **Communication and documentation**—nonverbal and verbal exchanges or interactions among the nurse and the client, the client's significant other, and the health care team and the validation of client care in written and electronic records that reflect standards of practice and accountability in the provision of care
- **Teaching and learning**—making possible the gaining of knowledge, attitudes, and skills to promote a change in behavior

 Culture and spirituality—each client that a nurse interacts with brings a unique perspective which is, in many cases, related to the client's cultural background or spirituality. This new addition to the integrated process category tests a nurse's ability to integrate both of these influences appropriately in a client's, family's, or population's care.

NCLEX Test Plan

The four client needs categories and their corresponding subcategories provide the basic framework for the NCLEX test plan. Question writers and the other people who compile the examination use the NCLEX test plan to ensure that the content and distribution of test questions cover the full spectrum of nursing activities and competencies across all client care settings.

Critical Thinking

You will notice that the revised Bloom's taxonomy is used to document the cognitive level of the question. The revised taxonomy includes the levels Remembering, Understanding, Applying, Analyzing, Evaluating, and Creating. Most test questions are written at the applying or higher cognitive levels, which require critical thinking. Critical thinking relies on the nurse's knowledge, skills, and ability to solve the problem. Critical thinking is highlighted in the test-taking strategy and for all rationales in this book to help you focus on where or how to find the correct answer.

Testing by computer

Like many standardized tests today, the NCLEX is administered by computer. That means you will not be filling in empty circles, sharpening pencils, or erasing frantically. It also means that you must become familiar with computer tests, if you are not already. Fortunately, the skills required to take the NCLEX on a computer are simple enough to allow you to focus on the questions, not the keyboard.

When you take the test, depending on the question format, you will be presented with a question and four or more possible answers, a blank space in which you have to enter your answer, a figure on which you will click the mouse to select the correct area of the figure, a series of charts or exhibits to view in order to select the correct response, items you must prioritize by dragging and dropping them in place, an audio recording to listen to in order to select the correct response, or a question and four graphic options.

The NCLEX is a *computer-adaptive test,* meaning that the computer reacts to the answers you give, supplying more difficult questions if you answer correctly and slightly easier questions if you answer incorrectly. Each test is thus uniquely adapted to the individual test-taker.

In order to become eligible to work as an RN in the United States, you will need to complete several steps. In addition to passing the NCLEX-RN, you may need to obtain a certificate and credentials evaluation from the Commission on Graduates of Foreign Nursing Schools (CGFNS®) and acquire a visa. Since requirements differ from state to state, it is important that you first contact the board of nursing in the state where you want to practice nursing.

CGFNS certification program

Most states require that you obtain CGFNS certification. This certification requires the following:

- A review and authentication of your credentials, including your nursing education, registration, and licensure

- A passing score on the CGFNS Qualifying Examination of nursing knowledge

- A passing score on an English language proficiency test

In order to be eligible to take the CGFNS Qualifying Examination, you must complete a minimum number of classroom and clinical practice hours in medical–surgical nursing, maternal–neonatal nursing, pediatric nursing, and psychiatric and mental health nursing from a government-approved nursing school. You must also be registered as a first-level nurse in your country of education and currently hold a license as an RN in some jurisdiction.

The CGFNS Qualifying Examination is a paper-and-pencil test that includes 260 multiple-choice questions. It is administered under controlled testing conditions. Because the test is designed to predict your likelihood of successfully passing the NCLEX-RN examination, it is based on the NCLEX-RN test plan.

You may select from three English proficiency examinations: Test of English as a Foreign Language (TOEFL®), Test of English for International Communication (TOEIC®), or International English Language Testing System (IELTS). Each test has different passing scores, and the scores are valid for up to 2 years.

CGFNS credentials evaluation service

This evaluation is a comprehensive report that analyzes and compares your education and licensure with U.S. standards. It is prepared by the CGFNS for a state board of nursing, an immigration office, an employer, or a university. It requires that you complete an application, submit appropriate documentation, and pay a fee.

More information about the CGFNS certification program and credentials evaluation service is available at www.cgfns.org.

Visa

You cannot legally immigrate to work in the United States without an occupational visa (temporary or permanent) from the United States Citizenship and Immigration Services (USCIS). The visa process is separate from the CGFNS certification process, although some of the same steps are involved. Some visas require prior CGFNS certification and a *VisaScreen®* Certificate from the International Commission on Healthcare Professions. The *VisaScreen* program involves the following:

- A credentials review of your nursing education and current registration or licensure

- Successful completion of either the CGFNS certification program or the NCLEX-RN

- A passing score on an approved English language proficiency examination

Once you successfully complete all parts of the *VisaScreen* program, you will receive a certificate to present to the USCIS. The visa-granting process can take up to a year.

You can obtain more detailed information about visa application at www.uscis.gov.

This book includes question difficulty data to help you gauge yourself as you answer the practice items. You will find an icon, identifying the difficulty level of the item, next to the question's rationale.

- **E** Easy
- **M** Moderate
- **D** Difficult
- **C** Challenge

The difficulty data is derived from *Lippincott NCLEX-RN PassPoint*, an adaptive quizzing program that simulates the computerized-adaptive testing experience. (As noted in the front cover of this book, you have a free 7-day trial to this product.)

You have a great deal of flexibility with the amount of time you spend on individual questions. The examination lasts a maximum of 6 hours, however, so do not waste time. If you fail to answer a set number of questions within 6 hours, the computer will determine that you lack minimum competency.

Most students have plenty of time to complete the test, so take as much time as you need to get the question right without wasting time. Keep moving at a decent pace to help maintain concentration.

Each question on the NCLEX is assigned a category based on client needs. This chart lists client needs categories and subcategories and the percentages of each type of question that appears on an NCLEX.

Category	Subcategories	Percentage of NCLEX questions
Safe and effective care environment	■ Management of care	17%–23%
	■ Safety and infection control	9%–15%
Health promotion and maintenance	n/a	6%–12%
Psychosocial integrity	n/a	6%–12%
Physiological integrity	■ Basic care and comfort	6%–12%
	■ Pharmacological and parenteral therapies	12%–18%
	■ Reduction of risk potential	9%–15%
	■ Physiological adaptation	11%–17%

If you find as you progress through the test that the questions seem to be increasingly difficult, it is a good sign. The more questions you answer correctly, the more difficult the questions become.

Some students, though, knowing that questions get progressively harder, focus on the degree of difficulty of subsequent questions to try to figure out if they are answering questions correctly. Avoid the temptation to do this, as this may get you off track. Stay focused on selecting the best answer for each question put before you.

The computer test finishes when one of these events occurs:

■ You demonstrate minimum competency, according to the computer program.

■ You demonstrate a lack of minimum competency, according to the computer program.

■ You have answered the maximum number of questions (265 total questions).

■ You have used the maximum time allowed (6 hours).

Alternate-format questions

In April 2004, the NCSBN added alternate-format items to the examination. These currently include seven types:

■ Multiple response–multiple choice

■ Fill in the blank

■ Hotspot

■ Chart/exhibit

■ Ordered response

■ Audio

■ Graphic options

However, most of the questions on the NCLEX are four-option, multiple-choice items with only one correct answer. Certain strategies can help you understand and answer any type of NCLEX question.

The NCSBN has not yet established a percentage of alternate-format items to be administered to each candidate. Since the NCLEX is a computer-adaptive test based on the candidate's ability, there are alternate-format question types in all areas of the test plan, across all difficulty levels.

Multiple-response, multiple-choice question

The first type of alternate-format item is the *multiple-response, multiple-choice question*. Unlike a traditional multiple-choice question, each multiple-response, multiple-choice question has two or more correct answers for every question, and it will contain five to six answer options. You will recognize this type of question because it will ask you to *select all that apply*—not just the best answer (as may be requested in the more traditional multiple-choice questions).

Keep in mind that for each multiple-response, multiple-choice question, you must select at least two answers, and you must select all correct answers for the item to be counted as correct. Never are all of the answers correct. On the NCLEX, there is no partial credit in the scoring of these items.

Fill-in-the-blank question

The second type of alternate-format item is the *fill in the blank*. These questions require you to provide the answer yourself, rather than select it from a list of options. You will perform a calculation and then type your answer (a number without any words, units of measurement, commas, or spaces) in the blank space provided after the question. Rules for rounding are included in the question stem if appropriate. A calculator button is provided so you can easily do your calculations electronically.

Hotspot question

The third type of alternate-format item is a question that asks you to identify an area on an illustration or graphic. For these so-called *hotspot questions*, the computerized examination will ask you to place your cursor and click over the correct area on an illustration. Try to be as precise as possible when marking the location. As with the fill in the blanks, the identification questions on the computerized examination may require extremely precise answers to be considered correct.

Chart/exhibit question

The fourth type of alternate-format item is the *chart/ exhibit* format. Here you will be given a problem and an exhibit that contains additional information you will need in order to answer the question. By clicking on the EXHIBIT button, you can access a series of three screens to review. Your answer can then be chosen from four multiple-choice answer options.

Ordered response question

The fifth type of alternate-format item involves prioritizing, or placing in correct order, a series of statements using a *drag-and-drop* technique. You will decide which of the given options is first, click and hold it with the mouse, then drag it into the first box given beneath, and drop it into place. You will repeat this process until you have placed all the available options in the lower boxes.

Audio question

The sixth type of alternate-format item involves listening with a set of headphones to an *audio* clip in order to answer the question. Your answer is chosen from four multiple-choice answer options.

Graphic option question

The final type of alternate-format item is the *graphic option* question. You will be presented with a question and options that are graphics instead of text.

Understanding the question

NCLEX questions are usually long. As a result, it is easy to feel overwhelmed with information. To focus on the question, apply proven strategies for answering NCLEX questions, including the following:

- Determining what the question is asking
- Determining relevant facts about the client
- Rephrasing the question in your mind
- Choosing the best option(s) before entering your answer

Determine what the question is asking

Read the question twice. If the answer is not apparent, rephrase the question in simpler, more personal terms. Breaking down the question into easier, less

intimidating terms may help you to focus more accurately on the correct answer.

For example, a question might read: "A client with a history of heart failure is admitted to the coronary care unit with pulmonary edema. The client is intubated and placed on a mechanical ventilator. Which parameter would the nurse monitor closely to assess the client's response to a bolus dose of furosemide intravenously?"

The options for this question—numbered from 1 to 4—may be:

☐ **1.** Daily weight

☐ **2.** 24-Hour intake and output

☐ **3.** Serum sodium levels

☐ **4.** Hourly urine output

Sometimes, getting used to the test format is as important as knowing the material covered. Try your hand at these sample questions, and you will have a leg up when you take the real test!

Sample four-option, multiple-choice question

The oncoming registered nurse (RN) is receiving shift report from the departing RN. When discussing the care of a client, the following arterial blood gas (ABG) results are noted: pH 7.16; $PaCO_2$, 80 mm Hg (80 mmol/L); PaO_2, 46 mm Hg (6.1 kPa); HCO_3^-, 24 mEq/L (24 mmol/L); SaO_2, 81%. For which condition would the nurses' plan care?

☐ **1.** Metabolic acidosis

☐ **2.** Metabolic alkalosis

☐ **3.** Respiratory acidosis

☐ **4.** Respiratory alkalosis

Answer: 3

Sample multiple-response, multiple-choice question

The nurse is caring for a 45-year-old married client who has undergone hemicolectomy for colon cancer. The client has two children. Which concepts about families would the nurse consider when providing care? Select all that apply.

☐ **1.** Illness in one family member can affect all members.

☐ **2.** Family roles do not change because of illness.

☐ **3.** A family member may have more than one role in the family.

☐ **4.** Children typically are not affected by adult illness.

☐ **5.** The effects of an illness on a family depend on the stage of the family's life cycle.

☐ **6.** Changes in sleeping and eating patterns may be signs of stress in a family.

Answer: 1, 3, 5, 6

Sample fill-in-the-blank calculation question

An infant who weighs 8 kg is to receive ampicillin 25 mg/kg intravenous every 6 hours. How many milligrams would the nurse administer per dose? Record your answer using a whole number.

_____ mg

Answer: 200

Sample hotspot question

An elderly client has a history of aortic stenosis. Identify the area where the nurse would place the stethoscope to **best** hear the murmur.

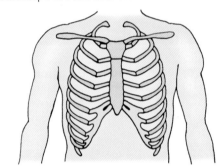

Answer:

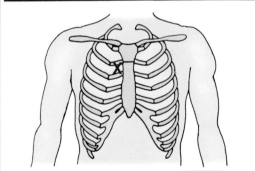

Sample chart/exhibit question

A 3-year-old client is being treated for severe status asthmaticus. After reviewing the progress notes (shown below), the nurse would determine that this client is being treated for which condition?

Progress notes	
4/5/16 0600	Client was acutely restless, diaphoretic, and with SOB at 0530. Dr. T. Smith notified and ordered ABG analysis. ABG drawn from R radial artery. Stat results as follows: pH 7.28, PaCO₂ 55 mm Hg (7.3 kPa), HCO₃⁻ 26 mEq/L (26 mmol/L). Dr. Smith with client now. ——— J. Collins, RN.

☐ **1.** Metabolic acidosis

☐ **2.** Respiratory alkalosis

☐ **3.** Respiratory acidosis

☐ **4.** Metabolic alkalosis

Answer: 3

Sample ordered response question

When teaching an antepartal client about the passage of the fetus through the birth canal during labor, the nurse describes the cardinal mechanisms of labor. Place these events in the sequence in which they occur. All options must be used.

1. Flexion
2. External rotation
3. Descent
4. Expulsion
5. Internal rotation
6. Extension

Answer: 3, 1, 5, 6, 2, 4

Sample audio question

Listen to the audio clip. What sound would the nurse document in the lung bases of this client with heart failure?

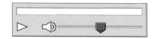

☐ **1.** Crackles

☐ **2.** Rhonchi

☐ **3.** Wheezes

☐ **4.** Pleural friction rub

Answer: 1

Sample graphic option question

Which electrocardiogram strip would the nurse document as atrial flutter?

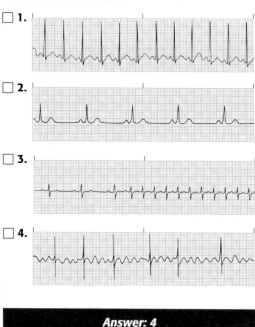

Answer: 4

Read the question again, ignoring all details except what is being asked. Focus on the last line of the question. It asks you to select the appropriate assessment for monitoring a client who received a bolus of furosemide intravenously.

Determine which facts about the client are relevant

Next, sort out the relevant client information. Start by asking whether any of the information provided about the client is not relevant to the facts needed to answer the question. For instance, do you need to know that the client has been admitted to the coronary care unit? Probably not; the reaction to furosemide will not be affected by the location in the hospital.

Determine what you do know about the client. In the example, you know that

■ the client has just received an intravenous bolus of furosemide, a crucial fact

■ the client has pulmonary edema, the most fundamental aspect of the client's underlying condition

- the client is intubated and placed on a mechanical ventilator, suggesting that the pulmonary edema is serious
- the client has a history of heart failure, a fact that may or may not be relevant

After you have determined relevant information about the client and the question being asked, consider rephrasing the question to make it clearer. Eliminate jargon and put the question in simpler, more personal terms. Here is how you might rephrase the question in the example: "My client has pulmonary edema. The client requires intubation and mechanical ventilation. The client has a history of heart failure. The client received an intravenous bolus of furosemide. What assessment parameter would I monitor?"

Choose the best option

Armed with all the information you now have, it is time to select an option. You know that the client received a bolus of furosemide, a diuretic. You know that monitoring fluid intake and output is a key nursing intervention for a client taking a diuretic, a fact that eliminates options 1 and 3 (daily weight and serum sodium levels), narrowing the answer down to option 2 or 4 (24-hour intake and output or hourly urine output).

You also know that the drug was administered by intravenous bolus, suggesting a rapid effect. (In fact, furosemide administered by intravenous bolus takes effect almost immediately.) Monitoring the client's 24-hour intake and output would be appropriate for assessing the effects of repeated doses of furosemide. Hourly urine output, however, is most appropriate in this situation because it monitors the immediate effect of this rapid-acting drug.

Key strategies

Regardless of the type of question, four key strategies will help you determine the correct answer for each question. (See *Strategies for success*, below.) These strategies are as follows:
- Considering the nursing process
- Referring to Maslow's hierarchy of needs
- Reviewing client safety
- Reflecting on principles of therapeutic communication
- Considering the standards of care

Strategies for success

Keeping a few main strategies in mind as you answer each NCLEX question can help ensure greater success. These five strategies are critical for answering NCLEX questions correctly:
- If the question asks what the nurse would do in a situation, use the nursing process to determine which step in the process would be next.
- If the question asks what the client needs, use Maslow's hierarchy to determine which need to address first.
- If the question indicates that the client does not have an urgent physiologic need, focus on the client's safety.
- If the question involves communicating with a client, use the principles of therapeutic communication.
- If the question involves a nursing procedure, consider the standards of care.
- If the question asks for an action, stay within your nursing scope of practice.

Nursing process

One of the ways to answer a question is to apply the nursing process. Steps in the nursing process include
- assessment;
- diagnosis;
- planning;
- implementation;
- evaluation.

The nursing process may provide insights that help you analyze a question. According to the nursing process, assessment comes before diagnosis, which comes before planning, which comes before implementation, which comes before evaluation.

You are halfway to the correct answer when you encounter a four-option, multiple-choice question that asks you to assess the situation and then provides two assessment options and two implementation options. You can immediately eliminate the implementation options, which then gives you, at worst, a 50–50 chance of selecting the correct answer. Use the following sample question to apply the nursing process.

A client returns from an endoscopic procedure during which the client was sedated. Before offering the client food, which action would the nurse take?

☐ **1.** Assess the client's respiratory status.

☐ **2.** Check the client's gag reflex.

☐ **3.** Place the client in a side-lying position.

☐ **4.** Have the client drink a few sips of water.

According to the nursing process, the nurse must assess a client before performing an intervention. Does the question indicate that the client has been properly assessed? No, it does not. Therefore, you can eliminate options 3 and 4 because they are both interventions.

That leaves options 1 and 2, both of which are assessments. Your nursing knowledge would tell you the correct answer—in this case, option 2. The sedation required for an endoscopic procedure may impair the client's gag reflex, so you would assess the gag reflex before giving food to the client to reduce the risk of aspiration and airway obstruction.

Why not select option 1, assessing the client's respiratory status? You might select this option, but the question is specifically asking about offering the client food, an action that would not be taken if the client's respiratory status were at all compromised. In this case, you are making a judgment based on the phrase "Before offering the client food." If the question were trying to test your knowledge of respiratory depression following an endoscopic procedure, it probably would not mention a function—such as giving food to a client—that clearly occurs only after the client's respiratory status has been stabilized.

Maslow's hierarchy

Knowledge of Maslow's hierarchy of needs can be a vital tool for establishing priorities on the NCLEX. Maslow's theory states that physiologic needs are the most basic human needs of all. Only after physiologic needs have been met can safety concerns be addressed. Only after safety concerns are met can concerns involving love and belonging be addressed, and so forth. Apply the principles of Maslow's hierarchy of needs to the following sample question.

A client reports severe pain 2 days after surgery. Which action would the nurse perform **first?**

☐ **1.** Offer reassurance of less pain to the client.

☐ **2.** Allow the client time to verbalize feelings.

☐ **3.** Check the client's vital signs.

☐ **4.** Administer an analgesic.

In this example, two of the options—3 and 4—address physiologic needs. Options 1 and 2 address psychosocial concerns. According to Maslow, physiologic needs must be met before psychosocial needs, so you can eliminate options 1 and 2.

Now, use your nursing knowledge to choose the best answer from the two remaining options. In this case, option 3 is correct because the client's vital signs would be checked before administering an analgesic (assessment before intervention). When prioritizing according to Maslow's hierarchy, remember your ABCs—airway, breathing, and circulation—to help you further prioritize. Check for a patent airway before addressing breathing. Check breathing before checking the health of the cardiovascular system.

Just because an option appears on the NCLEX does not mean it is a viable choice for the client referred to in the question. Always examine your choice in light of your knowledge and experience. Ask yourself, "Does this choice make sense for this client?" Allow yourself to eliminate choices—even those that might normally take priority—if they do not make sense for a particular client's situation.

Client safety

As you might expect, client safety takes high priority on the NCLEX. You will encounter many questions that can be answered by asking yourself, "Which answer will best ensure the safety of this client?" Use client safety criteria for situations involving laboratory values, drug administration, or nursing care procedures.

You may encounter a question in which some options address the client and others address the equipment. When in doubt, select an option relating to the client; never place equipment before a client.

For instance, suppose a question asks what the nurse would do first when entering a client's room where an infusion pump alarm is sounding. If two options deal with the infusion pump, one with the infusion tubing, and another with the client's catheter insertion site, select the one relating to the client's catheter insertion site. Always check the client first; the equipment can wait.

Therapeutic communication

Some NCLEX questions focus on the nurse's ability to communicate effectively with the client. Therapeutic communication incorporates verbal or nonverbal responses and involves

- listening to the client;
- understanding the client's needs;
- promoting clarification and insight about the client's condition.

Like other NCLEX questions, those dealing with therapeutic communication require choosing the best response. First, eliminate options that indicate the use of poor therapeutic communication techniques, such as those in which the nurse

- tells the client what to do without regard to the client's feelings or desires (the "do this" response);
- asks a question that can be answered "yes" or "no," or with another one-syllable response;
- seeks reasons for the client's behavior;
- implies disapproval of the client's behavior;
- offers false reassurances;
- attempts to interpret the client's behavior rather than allowing the client to verbalize his own feelings;

- offers a response that focuses on the nurse, not the client.

When answering NCLEX questions, look for responses that

- allow the client time to think and reflect;
- encourage the client to talk;
- encourage the client to describe a particular experience;
- reflect that the nurse has listened to the client, such as through paraphrasing the client's response.

Avoiding pitfalls

Even the most knowledgeable students can get tripped up on certain NCLEX questions. (See *A tricky question*, below.) Students commonly cite three areas that can be difficult for unwary test-takers:

- Knowing the difference between the NCLEX and the "real world"
- Delegating care
- Knowing laboratory values

A tricky question

The NCLEX occasionally asks a particular kind of question called the "further teaching" question, which involves client-teaching situations. These questions can be tricky. You will have to choose the response that suggests that the client has *not* learned the correct information. Here is an example:

A client undergoes a total hip replacement. Which statement by the client indicates that he/she requires further teaching?

- ☐ **1.** "I'll need to keep several pillows between my legs at night."
- ☐ **2.** "I'll need to remember not to cross my legs. It's such a bad habit."
- ☐ **3.** "The occupational therapist is showing me how to use a 'sock puller' to help me get dressed."
- ☐ **4.** "I don't know if I'll be able to get off that low toilet seat at home by myself."

The answer you should choose here is option 4 because it indicates that the client has a poor understanding of the precautions required after a total hip replacement and that he or she needs further teaching. *Remember:* If you see the phrase *further teaching* or *further instruction*, you are looking for a wrong answer by the client.

NCLEX versus the real world

Some students who take the NCLEX have extensive practical experience in health care. For example, many test-takers have worked as licensed practical nurses or nursing assistants. In one of those capacities, test-takers might have been exposed to less than optimum clinical practice and may carry those experiences over to the NCLEX.

Take the NCLEX with the understanding that what happens in the real world may differ from what the NCLEX and your nursing instructors say should happen.

If you have had practical experience in health care, you may know a quicker way to perform a procedure or tricks to get by when you do not have the right equipment. Situations such as staff shortages may force you to improvise. On the NCLEX, such scenarios can lead to trouble. Always check your practical experiences against textbook evidence-based nursing care, taking care to select the response that follows the textbook.

Delegating care

On the NCLEX, you may encounter questions that assess your ability to delegate care. Delegating care involves coordinating the efforts of other health care workers to provide effective care for your client. On the NCLEX, you may be asked to assign duties to

- licensed practical nurses or licensed vocational nurses, registered practical nurses;
- direct care workers, such as nursing assistants and personal care aides, unregulated health care workers;
- other support staff, such as nutrition assistants and housekeepers.

In addition, you will be asked to decide when to notify a physician (health care provider), a social worker, or another hospital staff member. In each case, you will have to decide when, where, and how to delegate.

As a general rule, it is acceptable to delegate actions that involve stable clients or standard, unchanging procedures. Bathing, feeding, dressing, and transferring clients are examples of procedures that can be delegated.

Be careful not to delegate complicated or complex activities. In addition, do not delegate activities that involve assessment, evaluation, or your own nursing judgment. On the NCLEX and in the real world, these duties fall squarely on your shoulders. Make sure that you take primary responsibility for assessing and evaluating the client and for making decisions about the client's care. Never hand off those responsibilities to someone with less training.

Deciding when to notify a health care provider/physician, a social worker, or another hospital staff member is an important element of nursing care. On the NCLEX, however, choices that involve notifying the health care provider are usually incorrect. Remember that the NCLEX wants to see you, the nurse, at work.

If you are sure the correct answer is to notify the health care provider/physician, it is essential to make sure that the client's safety has been addressed before notifying a health care provider/physician or another staff member. On the NCLEX, the client's safety has a higher priority than notifying other health care providers.

Study preparations

If you are like most people preparing to take the test, you are probably feeling nervous, anxious, or concerned. Keep in mind that most test-takers pass the NCLEX the first time around.

Passing the test will not happen by accident, though; you will need to prepare carefully and efficiently. To help jump-start your preparations:

- Determine your strengths and weaknesses.
- Create a study schedule.
- Set realistic goals.
- Find an effective study space.
- Think positively.
- Start studying sooner rather than later.

Strengths and weaknesses

Most students recognize that, even at the end of their nursing studies, they know more about some topics than others. Because the NCLEX covers a broad range of material, you should make some decisions about how intensively you will review each topic. Many nursing schools use standardized testing from nursing education companies. The feedback received on these standardized tests can also be helpful in assessing your knowledge level and content areas for further study.

Organize your decisions on a list. Divide a sheet of paper in half vertically. On one side, list topics you think you know well. On the other side, list topics you need to review. Pay no attention if one side is longer than the other. When you are done studying, you will feel strong in every area.

To make sure your list reflects a comprehensive view of all the areas you studied in school, look at the contents page in the front of this book. For each topic listed, place it in the "know well" column or "needs review" column. Separating content areas this way shows immediately which topics need less study time and which topics need more time.

Scheduling study time

Study when you are most alert. Most people can identify a period of the day when they feel most alert. If you feel most alert and energized in the morning, for example, set aside sections of time in the morning for topics that need a lot of review. Then you can use the evening, a time of lesser alertness, for topics that need some refreshing. The opposite is true as well; if you are more alert in the evening, study difficult topics at that time.

Set up a basic schedule for studying. Using a calendar or organizer, determine how much time remains before you will take the NCLEX. (See *2 to 3 months before the NCLEX*, right.) Fill in the remaining days with specific times and topics to be studied. For example, you might schedule the respiratory system on a Tuesday morning and the gastrointestinal system that afternoon. Remember to schedule difficult topics during your most alert times.

Keep in mind that you should not fill each day with studying. Be realistic and set aside time for normal activities. Try to create ample study time before the NCLEX and then stick to the schedule.

Part of creating a schedule means setting goals you can accomplish. You no doubt studied a great deal in nursing school, and by now you have a sense of your own capabilities. Ask yourself, "How much can I cover in a day?" Set that amount of time aside and then stay on task. You will feel better about yourself—and your chances of passing the NCLEX—when you meet your goals regularly.

2 to 3 months before the NCLEX

With 2 to 3 months remaining before you plan to take the examination, take these steps:

- Establish a study schedule. Set aside ample time to study and also leave time for social activities, exercise, family or personal responsibilities, and other matters.
- Become knowledgeable about the NCLEX-RN examination, its content, the types of questions it asks, and the testing format.
- Begin studying your notes, texts, and other study materials.
- Take some NCLEX practice questions to help you diagnose strengths and weaknesses as well as to become familiar with NCLEX-style questions.

Study space

Find a space conducive to effective learning and then study there. Whatever you do, do not study with a television on in the room. Instead, find a quiet, inviting study space that

- is located in a quiet, convenient place, away from normal traffic patterns;
- contains a solid chair that encourages good posture (avoid studying in bed; you will be more likely to fall asleep and not accomplish your goals);
- uses comfortable, soft lighting with which you can see clearly without eye strain;
- has a temperature between 65°F and 70°F (18°C and 21°C);
- contains flowers or green plants, familiar photos or paintings, and easy access to soft, instrumental background music.

Consider taping positive messages around your study space. Make signs with words of encouragement, such as "You can do it!" "Keep studying!" and "Remember the goal!" These upbeat messages can help keep you going when your attention begins to waver.

Maintaining concentration

When you are faced with reviewing the amount of information covered by the NCLEX, it is easy to become distracted and lose your concentration. When you lose concentration, you make less effective use of valuable study time. To help stay focused, keep these tips in mind:

- Alternate the order of the subjects you study during the day to add variety to your study. Try alternating between topics you find most interesting and those you find least interesting.
- Approach your studying with enthusiasm, sincerity, and determination.

- Once you have decided to study, begin imme-diately. Do not let anything interfere with your thought processes once you have begun.
- Concentrate on accomplishing one task at a time, to the exclusion of everything else.
- Do not try to do two things at once, such as study-ing and watching television or conversing with friends.
- Work continuously without interruption for a while, but do not study for such a long period that the whole experience becomes grueling or boring.
- Allow time for periodic breaks to give yourself a change of pace. Use these breaks to ease your transition into studying a new topic.
- When studying in the evening, wind down from your studies slowly. Do not progress directly from studying to sleeping.

Taking care of yourself

Never neglect your physical and mental well-being in favor of longer study hours. Maintaining physical and mental health is critical for success in taking the NCLEX. (See *4 to 6 weeks before the NCLEX*, right.)

You can increase your likelihood of passing the test by following these simple health rules:

- Get plenty of rest. You cannot think deeply or con-centrate for long periods when you are tired.
- Drink enough noncaffeinated beverages. Mild dehydration increases the effort required to concentrate and reason while distracting attention through feelings of fatigue and thirst.

4 to 6 weeks before the NCLEX

With 4 to 6 weeks remaining before you plan to take the examination, take these steps:

- Focus on your areas of weakness. That way, you will have time to review these areas again before the test date.
- Find a study partner or form a study group.
- Take a practice test to gauge your skill level early.
- Take time to eat, sleep, exercise, and socialize to avoid burnout.

- Eat nutritious meals. Maintaining your energy level is impossible when you are undernourished.
- Exercise regularly. Regular exercise helps you work harder and think more clearly. As a result, you will study more efficiently and increase the likelihood of success.

If you are having trouble concentrating but would rather push through than take a break, try making your studying more active by reading out loud. Active study-ing can renew your powers of concentration. By reading review material out loud to yourself, you are engaging your ears as well as your eyes—and making your study-ing a more active process. Hearing the material out loud also fosters memory and subsequent recall.

You can also rewrite in your own words a few of the more difficult concepts you are reviewing. Explaining these concepts in writing forces you to think through the material and can jump-start your memory.

Study schedule

When you were creating your schedule, you might have asked yourself, "How long should I study? One hour at a stretch? Two hours? Three?" To make the best use of your study time, you will need to answer those questions.

Optimum study time

Experts are divided about the optimum length of study time. Some say you should study no more than 1 hour at a time several times a day. Their reasoning: you remember the material you study at the beginning and end of a session best and tend to remember less material studied in the middle of the session.

Other experts say you should hold longer study sessions because you lose time in the beginning, when you are just getting warmed up, and again at the end, when you are cooling down. Therefore, say those experts, a long, concentrated study period will allow you to cover more material.

So what is the answer? It does not matter as long as you determine what is best for *you*. At the begin-ning of your NCLEX study schedule, try study periods of varying lengths. Pay close attention to those that seem more successful.

Remember that you are a trained nurse who is competent at assessment. Think of yourself as a cli-ent, and assess your own progress. Then implement the strategy that works best for you.

So does that mean that short sections of time are useless? Not at all. We all have spaces in our day that might otherwise be dead time. (See *1 week before the NCLEX*, right.) These are perfect times to review for the NCLEX but not to cover new material because by the time you get deep into new material, your time will be over. Always keep some flash cards or a small notebook handy for situations when you have a few extra minutes.

You will be amazed how many short sessions you can find in a day and how much reviewing you can do in 5 minutes. The following places offer short stretches of time you can use:

- Eating breakfast
- Waiting for, or riding on, a train or bus

With 1 week remaining before the NCLEX, take these steps:

- Take a review test to measure your progress.
- Record key ideas and principles on note cards or audiotapes.
- Rest, eat well, and avoid thinking about the examination during nonstudy times.
- Treat yourself to one special event. You have been working hard, and you deserve it!

- Waiting in line at the bank, post office, bookstore, or other places

Creative studying

Even when you study in a perfect study space and concentrate better than ever, studying for the NCLEX can get a little, well, dull. Even people with terrific study habits occasionally feel bored or sluggish. That is why it is important to have some creative tricks in your study bag to liven up your studying during those downtimes.

Creative studying does not have to be hard work. It involves making efforts to alter your study habits a bit. Some techniques that might help include studying with a partner or group and creating flash cards or other audiovisual study tools.

Study partners

Studying with a partner or group of students can be an excellent way to energize your studying. Working with a partner allows you to test each other on the material you have reviewed. Your partner can give you encouragement and motivation. Perhaps most important, working with a partner can provide a welcome break from solitary studying.

Exercise some care when choosing a study partner or assembling a study group. A partner who does not fit your needs will not help you make the most of your study time. Look for a partner who

- possesses similar goals to yours. For example, someone taking the NCLEX at approximately the same date who feels the same sense of urgency as you do might make an excellent partner.
- possesses about the same level of knowledge as you. Tutoring someone can sometimes help you learn, but partnering should be give-and-take so both partners can gain knowledge.

can study without excess chatting or interruptions. Socializing is an important part of creative study, but remember, you have still got to pass the NCLEX—so stay serious!

Audiovisual tools

Flash cards and other audiovisual tools foster retention and make learning and reviewing fun.

Flash cards can provide you with an excellent study tool. The process of writing material on a flash card will help you remember it. In addition, flash cards are small and easily portable, perfect for those 5-minute slivers of time that show up during the day.

Creating a flash card should be fun. Use magic markers, highlighters, and other colorful tools to

With 1 day before the NCLEX, take these steps:

- Drive to the test site, review traffic patterns, and find out where to park. If your route to the test site occurs during heavy traffic or if you are expecting bad weather, set aside extra time to ensure prompt arrival.
- Do something relaxing during the day.
- Avoid concentrating on the test.
- Rest, eat, and drink well, and avoid dwelling on the NCLEX during nonstudy periods.
- Call a supportive friend or relative for some last-minute words of encouragement.

make them visually stimulating. The more effort you put into creating your flash cards, the better you will remember the material contained on the cards.

Flowcharts, drawings, diagrams, and other image-oriented study aids can also help you learn material more effectively. Substituting images for text can be a great way to give your eyes a break and recharge your brain. Remember to use vivid colors to make your creations visually engaging.

If you learn more effectively when you hear information rather than see it, consider recording key ideas using a handheld tape recorder. Recording information helps promote memory because you say the information aloud when taping and then listen to it when playing it back. Like flash cards, tapes are portable and perfect for those short study periods during the day. (See *The day before the NCLEX*, page 15.)

Practice tests

Practice questions should constitute an important part of your NCLEX study strategy. Practice questions can improve your studying by helping you review material and familiarizing yourself with the exact style of questions you will encounter on the NCLEX.

Consider working through some practice questions as soon as you begin studying for the NCLEX. For example, you might try a half-dozen questions from each chapter in this book.

If you score well, you probably know the material contained in that chapter fairly well and can spend less time reviewing that particular topic. If you have trouble with the questions, spend extra study time on that topic.

Practice questions can also provide an excellent means of marking your progress. Do not worry if you have trouble answering the first few practice questions you take; you will need time to adjust to the way the questions are asked. Eventually, you will become accustomed to the question format and begin to focus more on the questions themselves.

If you make practice questions a regular part of your study regimen, you will be able to notice areas in which you are improving. You can then adjust your study time accordingly.

As you near the examination date, continue to answer practice questions, and also set aside time to take an entire NCLEX practice test. (We have included

The day of the NCLEX

On the day of the NCLEX, take these steps:
- Get up early.
- Wear comfortable clothes, preferably with layers you can adjust to fit the room temperature.
- Drink a glass of water and eat a small nutritious breakfast.
- Make sure you have proper identification and your authorization to test.
- Leave your house early.
- Arrive at the test site at least 30 minutes prior to the scheduled time.
- Listen carefully to the instructions given before entering the test room.
- Succeed, succeed, *succeed!*

comprehensive tests at the back of this book.) That way, you will know exactly what to expect. (See *The day of the NCLEX*, above.) The more you know ahead of time, the better you are likely to do on the NCLEX.

Taking an entire practice test is also a way to gauge your progress. When you find yourself answering questions correctly, it will give you the confidence you need to conquer the real NCLEX.

PART TWO

Fundamentals of nursing

Basic physical care

1. The nurse at an outpatient surgical clinic witnesses client signatures. When obtaining signatures, which clients are able to sign their own consent for a procedure/surgery? Select all that apply.

- [ ] **1.** A 7-year-old who needs an open reduction internal fixation (ORIF) of the right arm
- [ ] **2.** A 62-year-old with macular degeneration who is ordered a routine colonoscopy
- [ ] **3.** A married 17-year-old who requires a chole-cystectomy for relief of nausea and pain
- [ ] **4.** A 72-year-old widow with dementia who needs a mastectomy for cancer removal
- [ ] **5.** A 16-year-old who is obtaining an elective breast reduction for back pain relief

Ⓜ Rationale: There are many factors for the nurse to consider when evaluating whether a client can consent to surgery. These include being mentally ill or disabled; a minor; under the influence of alcohol, drugs, or medication; in labor; under great stress or in pain at the time of consent; and in a semiconscious state. The 7- and 16-year-old are minors, while the 17-year-old is married and an emancipated minor and able to give consent. Having difficulty seeing because of macular degeneration does not preclude the ability to have the consent read and then provide consent. Depending upon the severity of the dementia, the client will need to be evaluated for competence before independently providing consent.

Test-taking strategy: Analyze to determine what the question asks for, which is identifying individuals who are able to consent for a procedure/surgery. Consider the information related to informed consent and the ability to understand and make a decision. Review informed consent and the guidelines for obtaining a medical consent if you had difficulty answering this question.

Client needs category: Safe and effective care environment

Client needs subcategory: Management of care

Cognitive level: Applying

2. A nurse is developing a care plan for a client with an injury to the frontal lobe of the brain. Which nursing actions would be included as part of the care plan? Select all that apply.

- [ ] **1.** Keep instructions simple and brief because the client will have difficulty concentrating.
- [ ] **2.** Speak clearly and slowly because the client will have difficulty hearing.
- [ ] **3.** Assist with bathing and toileting because the client will have vision disturbances.
- [ ] **4.** Orient the client to person, place, and time as needed because the client will have memory problems.
- [ ] **5.** Assess vital signs frequently throughout the nursing shift because vital bodily functions will be affected.

Ⓓ Rationale: Damage to the frontal lobe of the brain affects personality, memory, reasoning, concentration, and motor control of speech. Damage to the temporal lobe, not the frontal lobe, causes hearing and speech problems. Damage to the occipital lobe causes vision disturbances. Damage to the brain stem affects vital functions.

Test-taking strategy: Analyze to determine what the question asks for, which is the nursing actions needed when caring for a client with an injury to the frontal lobe of the brain. Recall the physiologic functions of the different areas of the brain to understand what type of damage has occurred. "Select all that apply" questions require considering each option to decide its merit. Compare each option in relation to the functions of the frontal lobe and deficits that arise following injury. Review the functions of specific sections of the brain if you had difficulty answering this question.

Client needs category: Physiological integrity

Client needs subcategory: Basic care and comfort

Cognitive level: Applying

3. A nurse, assigned to a client with emphysema, is providing shift report. Which nursing interventions would be appropriate to include? Select all that apply.

☐ **1.** Reduce fluid intake to less than 850 ml per shift.

☐ **2.** Teach diaphragmatic, pursed-lip breathing.

☐ **3.** Administer low-flow oxygen as needed.

☐ **4.** Maintain the client in a supine position as much as possible.

☐ **5.** Encourage alternating client activity with rest periods.

☐ **6.** Teach the use of postural drainage and chest physiotherapy.

Answer: 2, 3, 5, 6

Ⓜ Rationale: Diaphragmatic, pursed-lip breathing strengthens respiratory muscles and enhances oxygenation in clients with emphysema. Low-flow oxygen would be administered because a client with emphysema has chronic hypercapnia and a hypoxic respiratory drive. Alternating activity with rest allows clients to perform activities without distress. If the client has difficulty mobilizing copious secretions, the nurse would teach the client and family members how to perform postural drainage and chest physiotherapy. Fluid intake would be increased to 3,000 ml/day, if not contraindicated, to liquefy secretions and facilitate their removal. The client would be placed in high Fowler's position to improve ventilation.

Test-taking strategy: Analyze to determine what the question asks for, which is the essential nursing interventions to include when nurses discuss care in the shift report. Recall the pathophysiology of emphysema and the client's physical needs created by the disease process. "Select all that apply" questions require considering each option to decide its merit. Consider each nursing intervention against the ability to improve the respiratory status of a client with emphysema. Review the care of a client with emphysema if you had difficulty answering this question.

Client needs category: Safe and effective care environment

Client needs subcategory: Management of care

Cognitive level: Applying

---

4. A neonatal nurse is assessing a 2-week-old's pain level following open heart surgery. To assess the pain level using an age-appropriate scale, which scales would be appropriate? Select all that apply.

☐ **1.** Numerical 0 to 10 scale

☐ **2.** FLACC scale

☐ **3.** Wong-Baker FACES Pain Rating Scale

☐ **4.** Visual analog scale

☐ **5.** NIPS

Answer: 2, 5

Ⓜ Rationale: All of the scales measure pain; however, only the Face, Legs, Activity, Cry, Consolability (FLACC) scale and the Neonatal Infant Pain Scale (NIPS) are behavioral scales appropriate for a neonate. Behavior scales look at the neonate's behavior and then use a rating scale to objectively determine a numerical score. A 3- to 8-year-old child typically uses the Wong-Baker FACES pain scale to identify his or her level of pain. Visual analog scales and numerical scales are typically used for children over 8 years old.

Test-taking strategy: Analyze to determine what the question asks for, which is pain scale appropriate for a neonate. Consider how a neonate expresses pain and eliminate options. Eliminate options 1, 3, and 4 as the neonate is not able to respond to questions.

Client needs category: Physiological integrity

Client needs subcategory: Basic care and comfort

Cognitive Level: Analyzing

5. A nurse is caring for a client who underwent surgical repair of a detached retina in the right eye. Which nursing interventions would the nurse perform postoperatively? Select all that apply.

- ☐ **1.** Place the client in a prone position.
- ☐ **2.** Approach the client from the left side.
- ☐ **3.** Encourage deep breathing and coughing.
- ☐ **4.** Discourage the client from bending down.
- ☐ **5.** Orient the client to the environment.
- ☐ **6.** Administer a stool softener.

Answer: 2, 4, 5, 6

Ⓜ Rationale: A detached retina is repaired by surgical procedures such as a scleral buckle, pneumatic retinopexy, or a vitrectomy, which places the retina back in its proper position. Postoperatively, the nurse would approach the client from the left side—the unaffected side—to avoid startling. The nurse would also discourage the client from bending down, deep breathing, hard coughing and sneezing, and other activities that can increase intraocular pressure during the postoperative period. The client would be oriented to the environment to reduce the risk of injury. Stool softeners would be administered to discourage straining during defecation. The client would lie on the back or on the unaffected side to reduce intraocular pressure in the affected eye.

Test-taking strategy: Analyze to determine what information the question asks for, which is the postoperative care following repair of a detached retina. "Select all that apply" questions require considering each option to decide its merit. Recall the pathophysiology of a detached retina and the surgical intervention needed to allow the retina to remain in place and heal. Consider potential complications and nursing interventions essential in preventing those complications. Review postoperative care of a client with a detached retina if you had difficulty answering this question.

Client needs category: Physiological integrity

Client needs subcategory: Reduction of risk potential

Cognitive level: Applying

6. A nurse is planning care for a client with hyperthyroidism. Which nursing interventions are appropriate? Select all that apply.

- ☐ **1.** Instill isotonic eyedrops as necessary.
- ☐ **2.** Provide several small, well-balanced meals.
- ☐ **3.** Provide regular rest periods.
- ☐ **4.** Keep the environment warm.
- ☐ **5.** Encourage frequent visitors.
- ☐ **6.** Weigh the client daily.

Answer: 1, 2, 3, 6

Ⓒ Rationale: Hyperthyroidism is the condition where the thyroid is overactive and produces excessive amounts of thyroid hormone, which controls body metabolism. If the client has exophthalmos (a sign of hyperthyroidism), the conjunctivae would be moistened often with isotonic eyedrops. Hyperthyroidism results in increased appetite, which can be satisfied by frequent, small, well-balanced meals. The nurse would provide the client with rest periods to reduce metabolic demands. The client would be weighed daily to check for weight loss, a possible consequence of hyperthyroidism. Because metabolism is increased in hyperthyroidism, heat intolerance and excitability result. Therefore, the nurse would provide a cool and quiet environment, not a warm and busy one, to promote client comfort.

Test-taking strategy: Analyze to determine what the question asks for, which is the nursing interventions necessary in the care of a client with hyperthyroidism.

Recall the signs and symptoms and pathophysiology of hyperthyroidism. Relate hyperthyroidism to an abnormal increase in metabolism. "Select all that apply" questions require considering each option to decide its merit. Consider each nursing intervention against its ability to reduce the potential side effects from the body's metabolism increase. Review nursing care of a client with hyperthyroidism if you had difficulty answering this question.

Client needs category: Physiological integrity

Client needs subcategory: Basic care and comfort

Cognitive level: Applying

7. A client has a tumor of the posterior pituitary gland. A nurse planning care would include which nursing interventions? Select all that apply.

☐ **1.** Weigh the client daily.

☐ **2.** Restrict fluids.

☐ **3.** Measure urine specific gravity.

☐ **4.** Encourage intake of coffee or tea.

☐ **5.** Monitor intake and output.

Answer: 1, 3, 5

Ⓜ Rationale: The pituitary gland is divided into the anterior and posterior sections with each section secreting specific hormones. Tumors of the posterior pituitary gland can lead to diabetes insipidus because of deficiency of vasopressin, also called antidiuretic hormone (ADH). Decreased ADH reduces the kidneys' ability to concentrate urine, resulting in excessive urination, thirst, and fluid intake. To monitor fluid balance, the nurse would weigh the client daily, measure urine specific gravity, and monitor intake and output. The nurse would also encourage fluids to keep intake equal to output and prevent dehydration. Coffee, tea, and other fluids that have a diuretic effect would be avoided.

Test-taking strategy: Analyze to determine what the question asks for, which is nursing interventions in the care of a client with a posterior pituitary tumor. Focus on the pathophysiology and implications of a tumor of the posterior pituitary gland. Recall that the posterior pituitary secretes oxytocin and vasopressin (ADH). Vasopressin stimulates water retention and raises blood pressure. Review the role of the posterior pituitary and manifestations caused by a tumor if you had difficulty answering this question.

Client needs category: Physiological integrity

Client needs subcategory: Basic care and comfort

Cognitive level: Applying

8. A nurse is preparing to administer an intra-muscular injection in the deltoid muscle. In which anatomical location would the nurse administer this injection?

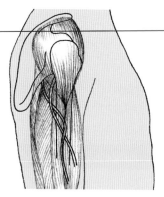

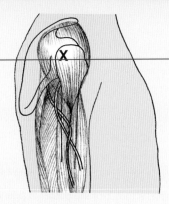

ⓜ **Rationale:** To locate the deltoid muscle, find the lower edge of the acromion process and the point on the lateral arm in line with the axilla. The needle would be inserted 1" to 2" (usually two or three fingerbreadths) below the acromion process and at a 90° angle, or slightly angled, toward the process.

Test-taking strategy: Analyze to determine what information the question asks for, which is the location for an intramuscular injection in the deltoid muscle. Focus on the anatomy of the upper arm and the location of the deltoid muscle, and recall the process for administering an intramuscular injection. Recall that the deltoid intramuscular injection site is triangular in shape, with the base of the triangle on the lower edge of the acromion process. Visualize the process for completing the injection. Review the skill of completing an intramuscular injection in the deltoid site if you had difficulty answering this question.

Client needs category: Physiological integrity

Client needs subcategory: Pharmacological and parenteral therapies

Cognitive level: Applying

9. A nurse is performing a fecal occult blood test using a Hemoccult slide for a client with a possible lower gastrointestinal bleed. Place the steps for performing the fecal occult blood test in the correct order. All options must be used.

1. Allow the specimens to penetrate the test paper.

2. Put on gloves.

3. Apply a drop of Hemoccult developing solution to boxes A and B on the slide's reverse side.

4. Place a stool smear on box A of the slide.

5. Apply a stool smear from another part of the specimen to box B on the slide.

6. Put a drop of Hemoccult developing solution on each control dot on the slide's reverse side.

Answer: 2, 4, 5, 1, 6, 3

Ⓒ Rationale: After receiving the stool specimen from the client, the nurse would put on gloves and then follow the other steps in the order listed above. Two separate samples of stool from the bowel movement would be placed on the slide. Before using the developer on the stool smear samples, the nurse would allow approximately 3 to 5 minutes to allow adequate time for the sample to penetrate the test paper. The nurse would also check the expiration date; the nurse would discard the developer if the date has expired. A blue reaction at the stool smear indicates a positive result.

Test-taking strategy: Analyze to determine what information the question asks for, which is the correct sequence for performing a fecal occult blood test using a Hemoccult slide. Recall the process of standard precautions when in contact with body secretions that may contain blood, and visualize the sequence of steps of the procedure to be performed. Consider that application of the sample is required before the developing solution can be applied. Review the skill of performing a fecal occult blood test using a Hemoccult slide if you had difficulty answering this question.

Client needs category: Health promotion and maintenance
Client needs subcategory: None
Cognitive level: Applying

---

10. A nurse is caring for a client with a hiatal hernia who states abdominal and sternal pain after eating and when lying down. Which instructions would the nurse recommend when teaching this client? Select all that apply.

☐ **1.** Avoid constrictive clothing.

☐ **2.** Lie down for 30 minutes after eating.

☐ **3.** Decrease the intake of caffeine and spicy foods.

☐ **4.** Eat three meals per day.

☐ **5.** Sleep with the upper body elevated.

☐ **6.** Maintain a normal body weight.

Answer: 1, 3, 5, 6

Ⓜ Rationale: A hiatal hernia occurs when a portion of the stomach pushes through the diaphragm. A hiatal hernia may cause abdominal and sternal pain after eating. The discomfort is associated with reflux of gastric contents. To reduce gastric reflux, the nurse would instruct the client to avoid constrictive clothing, caffeine, and spicy foods; sleep with the upper body elevated; lose weight, if obese; remain upright for 2 hours after eating; and eat small, frequent meals.

Test-taking strategy: Analyze to determine what information the question asks for, which is selecting instructions to provide a client experiencing pain after eating. Focus on the pathophysiology of hiatal hernia and recall the clinical manifestations of this disorder. Relate the cause of the disorder to instructions that would reduce the symptoms by preventing the reflux of gastric contents. Review methods to decrease the symptoms of hiatal hernia if you had difficulty answering this question.

Client needs category: Physiological integrity
Client needs subcategory: Basic care and comfort
Cognitive level: Applying

11. A nurse, caring for a client with heart failure, is assessing peripheral blood flow. In which area would the left dorsalis pedis pulse be palpated?

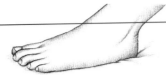

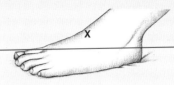

Rationale: Many peripheral pulse sites may be used to assess pulse and circulatory status by palpation. The dorsalis pedis pulse can be palpated on the medial dorsal surface of the foot when the client's toes are pointed down. This pulse can be difficult to palpate and may seem to be absent in healthy clients.

Test-taking strategy: Use knowledge of medical terminology to determine the site for palpation. If unsure of the location of dorsalis pedis, break the word apart. Dorsalis means dorsal aspect. Focus on the location of the dorsalis pedis pulse and recall the correct finger placement when performing the assessment. Review peripheral pulse sites if you had difficulty answering this question.

Client needs category: Physiological integrity

Client needs subcategory: Physiological adaptation

Cognitive level: Understanding

12. A client with renal failure is placed on a potassium-restricted diet. For lunch, the client consumed 6 oz of hamburger on a bun, one cup of cooked broccoli, a raw pear, and iced tea. Using the chart provided, calculate how many milliequivalents of potassium were in this meal.

Intake and output

DIETARY SOURCES OF POTASSIUM

Foods and Beverages	Serving Size	Amount of Potassium (mEq/ mmol)
Meats		
Beef	4 oz (112 g)	11.2
Chicken	4 oz (112 g)	12.0
Scallops	5 large	30.0
Vegetables		
Broccoli (cooked)	1/2 cup	7.0
Carrots (raw)	1 large	8.8
Potatoes (baked)	1 small	15.4
Tomatoes (raw)	1 medium	10.4
Fruits		
Bananas	1 medium	12.8
Cantaloupe	6 oz (168 g)	13.0
Pears (raw)	1 medium	6.2
Beverages		
Orange juice	1 cup (240 ml)	11.4
Prune juice	1 cup (240 ml)	14.4
Tomato juice	1 cup (240 ml)	11.6
Milk (whole or skim)	1 cup (240 ml)	8.8

☐ **1.** 24.4   ☐ **3.** 31.4

☐ **2.** 30   ☐ **4.** 37

---

13. A nurse is teaching a client with left leg weakness to walk with a cane. The nurse would include which nursing points about safe cane use in the client teaching? Select all that apply.

☐ **1.** Place the cane 8 to 10 inches (20.3 to 25.4 cm) from the base of the little toe.

☐ **2.** Hold the cane on the uninvolved side of the body.

☐ **3.** Adjust the cane so that the handle is level with the hip bone.

☐ **4.** Walk by moving the involved leg, then the cane, and then the uninvolved leg.

☐ **5.** Shorten the stride length on the involved side.

☐ **6.** Avoid leaning on the cane to get in and out of a chair.

Answer: 4

Ⓜ Rationale: According to the chart, 4 oz (112 g) of beef contains 11.2 mEq (mmol) of potassium. Add 5.6 mEq (mmol) for the additional 2 oz (56 g) for a total of 16.8 mEq (mmol) of potassium in the beef. The amount of potassium in one cup of broccoli is 14 mEq (mmol). A pear has 6.2 mEq (mmol). Thus, the total amount of potassium in this meal is 37 mEq (mmol). The iced tea and bun do not contain significant amounts of potassium and, therefore, are not listed on the chart.

Test-taking strategy: Analyze to determine what information the question asks for, which is the amount of potassium in the following meal. Use basic math skills to calculate the totals requested. Pay particular attention to using prudent strategies for addition such as making sure to maintain number alignment, maintain placement of decimals, and proofread work. Double-check to make sure that you included all of the mEq (mmol) of potassium noted in the chart with no error in transcription.

Client needs category: Physiological integrity
Client needs subcategory: Physiological adaptation
Cognitive level: Analyzing

Answer: 2, 3, 6

Ⓜ Rationale: To ambulate safely, a client with leg weakness would hold the cane in the hand opposite the involved leg with the handle level adjacent to the hip bone. The client would not lean on the cane to get in or out of a chair because of the risk of falls. The cane base would be placed 4 to 6 inches (10.2 to 15.3 cm) from the base of the little toe. When walking, the client would move the cane and involved leg simultaneously, alternating with the uninvolved leg in equal length strides and timing.

Test-taking strategy: Analyze to determine what information the question asks for, which is nursing points necessary for the safe use of a cane. Recall the placement of the cane in relation to the involved side and the importance of ensuring client safety. Consider the potential for losing balance, which is important for anyone needing a cane. Review ambulation with an assistive device if you had difficulty answering this question.

Client needs category: Physiological integrity
Client needs subcategory: Reduction of risk potential
Cognitive level: Applying

14. A nurse is caring for a client who is recovering from an illness requiring prolonged bed rest. Based on the nursing documentation below, which procedure would the nurse implement next?

Progress notes	
2/10/16 1015	Client instructed in contraction of back extensors, hip extensors, knee extensors, and ankle flexors and extensors. Client able to demonstrate correct technique without joint motion or muscle lengthening. c/o being "a little tired" after holding each contraction 5 seconds and repeating three times. Instructed to repeat exercises three times daily; client verbalized understanding of all information given. ———F. Brown, RN

☐ **1.** Performing active range-of-motion exercises of the legs

☐ **2.** Performing isometric exercises of the legs

☐ **3.** Providing assistance walking the client to the bathroom

☐ **4.** Performing passive range-of-motion exercises of the legs

---

Answer: 1

Ⓜ **Rationale:** Active range-of-motion exercises involve moving the client's joints through their full range of motion; they require some muscle strength and endurance. The client would have received passive range-of-motion exercises since admission to maintain joint flexibility and would have been taught isometric exercises to build strength and endurance for transfers and ambulation. Walking to the bathroom would be unsafe without the ability to first dangle the legs over the bedside and transfer from bed to chair.

Test-taking strategy: Look at the key word "next" indicating that the client has reached a point when there is a clear next step in progress. Focus on the types of exercise being discussed with the client and review the correct sequence of activities when advancing the client's mobility status. Recall the dangers of progressing too quickly or regressing in ability. Review the range-of-motion exercises and isometric exercises if you had difficulty answering this question.

Client needs category: Physiological integrity

Client needs subcategory: Reduction of risk potential

Cognitive level: Applying

---

15. The nurse is providing care for a client who has had a stroke. Since the onset of symptoms, the client has been experiencing left-sided hemianopsia. Which nursing interventions are appropriate? Select all that apply.

☐ **1.** Place the client's belongings on the right side of the bed.

☐ **2.** Approach the client from the left side.

☐ **3.** Refuse to acknowledge the condition to promote the client's independence.

☐ **4.** Stand on the right side of the bed when providing care.

☐ **5.** Provide the client with an eye patch for the right eye.

☐ **6.** Dim the lights in the room to prevent eye strain.

Answer: 1, 4

Ⓜ **Rationale:** Hemianopsia is a condition in which the client has lost half of the visual field. It is most often associated with a stroke. In this case, the stroke has affected the client's left side; therefore, placing belongings on the right side of the bed will enable the client to best see them. Standing on the right side of the bed when providing care will ensure the client is able to see the nurse. Approaching the client from the left side is counterproductive because the client would not be able to adequately see the nurse. Using an eye patch or dimming the lights will not help with treating or managing the condition.

Test-taking strategy: Analyze to determine what information the question asks for, which is nursing interventions for a client with left-sided hemianopsia. Begin by thinking of the visual deficits and how these impact the client's ability to complete activities. Recall the clinical effects of hemianopsia, and consider the client's basic need to have meaningful interactions with the nursing staff and environment. Also, differentiate between a deficit on the right side and one on the left side. Review the care of a client with hemianopsia if you had difficulty answering this question.

Client needs category: Physiological integrity

Client needs subcategory: Basic needs and comfort

Cognitive level: Applying

---

16. The nurse is evaluating infection control practices performed by a spouse on a loved one who has methicillin-resistant *Staphylococcus aureus* (MRSA) in a right leg wound. Which actions indicate that the spouse requires further teaching? Select all that apply.

☐ **1.** The spouse places soiled dressing supplies in the kitchen garbage can.

☐ **2.** Disinfectant spray is used on the table where dressing supplies are prepared.

☐ **3.** Clean gloves are used for wound dressing removal.

☐ **4.** Sheets with wound drainage are washed in lukewarm water.

☐ **5.** Dressing supplies are placed in a clean, dry location.

☐ **6.** Routine hand hygiene is performed before and after care.

E Rationale: Methicillin-resistant *Staphylococcus aureus* (MRSA) is a bacterium that causes infections in different parts of the body and is resistant to some commonly used antibiotics. Infection control practices prevent the spread of the infection. Further teaching is needed if a nurse notes that soiled dressing supplies are placed in a community garbage can such as one located in the kitchen. Soiled sheets need to be washed in hot water and dried in a clothes dryer. It is correct to clean and disinfect the area where dressing supplies are prepared. Routine hand hygiene followed by wearing clean gloves is appropriate when removing the dressing. Sterile gloves may be needed when completing dressing care.

Test-taking strategy: Analyze to determine what information the question asks for, which is incorrect action when caring for a wound with MRSA. Consider actions that may spread a contagious infection such as improper or lack of handwashing, improper disinfecting or washing of soiled materials, or improper elimination of waste. Review infection control practices if you had difficulty answering this question.

Client needs category: Safe and effective care environment

Client needs subcategory: Safety and infection control

Cognitive level: Evaluating

17. The health care provider writes an order that a client may have 12 oz (360 ml) of clear liquids at each meal and may supplement this with an additional 10 oz (300 ml) at each shift (7 to 3, 3 to 11, and 11 to 7). How many milliliters would the nurse document for the day shift (7 to 3) if the client took in all of the ordered volumes? Record your answer using a whole number.

_____ milliliters

18. The nurse is recording the intake and output for a client with the following: D_5NS 1,000 ml, urine 450 ml, emesis 125 ml, Jackson-Pratt drain #1 35 ml, Jackson-Pratt drain #2 32 ml, and Jackson-Pratt drain #3 12 ml. How many milliliters would the nurse document as the client's output? Record your answer using a whole number.

_____ milliliters

19. The nurse is preparing the room for a client diagnosed with varicella. Which sign would the nurse place on the room door?

☐ **1.**

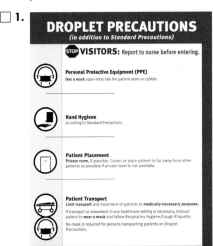

☐ **2.**

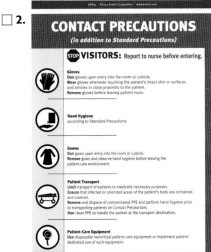

☐ **3.**

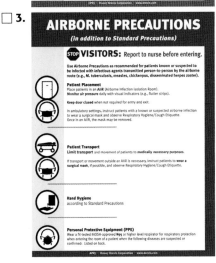

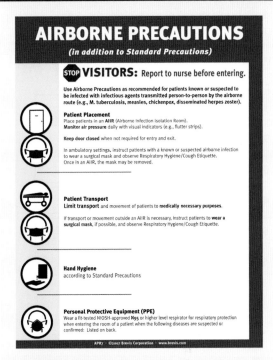

Ⓜ Rationale: In addition to contact precautions, the nurse would place the client diagnosed with varicella in airborne precautions. Airborne precautions include a face mask for the client/respirator for the nurse and personal protective equipment including gown and gloves. Droplet precautions are indicated for viruses, *B. ordetella pertussis*, and group A streptococcus. Contact precautions are indicated anytime a nurse may come in contact with any body fluids.

Test-taking strategy: Analyze to determine what the question asks for, which is transmission-based precautions indicated for a client diagnosed with varicella. Recall that varicella is a contagious herpes zoster (VZV) virus. The disease spreads through coughs and sneezes; thus, airborne precautions are required. Review Varicella and transmission-based precautions if you had difficulty answering this question.

Client needs category: Safe and effective care environment

Client needs subcategory: Safety and infection control

Cognitive level: Analyzing

20. The nurse received an order for a sputum sample to be obtained in the morning. Prior to the client's breakfast, the nurse explains the procedure to the client, obtains all equipment, washes hands, and dons clean gloves. Place the next nursing actions in proper sequence. All options must be used.

| 1. Instruct the client to cough. |
| 2. Remove gloves/hand hygiene. |
| 3. Label the container. |
| 4. Perform oral hygiene. |
| 5. Place the client in a Fowler position. |
| 6. Obtain the sample. |

Answer: 5, 1, 6, 4, 2, 3

D **Rationale:** Sputum samples are best to be obtained in the morning while respiratory secretions are more abundant and not diluted with fluids. To complete the procedure, the nurse would seat the client in a Fowler (upright) position and instruct the client to cough to expectorate a sputum sample. Once the sample is obtained, the nurse will assist with oral hygiene, perform hand hygiene, and label the container to send it to the lab.

Test-taking strategy: Analyze to determine what the question asks for, which is standard procedure for obtaining a sputum culture. Begin by considering the best way to promote sputum expectoration such as the upright position and encouraging a cough. Recall that oral hygiene would dilute or contaminate sputum, but oral hygiene following specimen retrieval would be acceptable to clear any remaining sputum from the mouth. Lastly, end with hand hygiene and then label the container.

Client needs category: Physiological integrity
Client needs subcategory: Reduction of risk potential
Cognitive level: Analyzing

Basic psychosocial needs

1. A nurse is caring for a newly admitted client who appears anxious and fearful. The client states, "I do not trust any of you. Stay away from me!" Which nursing actions would be beneficial? Select all that apply.

☐ **1.** The nurse would mirror the client's mannerisms and anxiety level.

☐ **2.** The nurse would agree with the client and ask the client for his/her trust.

☐ **3.** The nurse would calmly state, "I am here to help you. What can I do?"

☐ **4.** The nurse would state, "Tell me why you do not trust me."

☐ **5.** The nurse would sit quietly near the client and respond to questions.

☐ **6.** The nurse would notify the health care provider and ask for a sedative.

Answer: 3, 4, 5

M **Rationale:** When providing care to a new client with anxiety and fear issues, the nurse must first reduce client anxiety and develop a trusting relationship. Obtaining the client's perspective by asking an open-ended question allows the client to elaborate and reduce client anxiety. Also, offering a sense of self to the client with phrases such as "What can I do?" or sitting quietly near the client allows the client to see the calmness of the nurse and provides an opportunity to seek help when ready. Mirroring (reflecting) the anxiety of the client raises client anxiety. Agreeing with the client inappropriately validates the client's feeling of mistrust, which raises anxiety. Asking for a sedative (chemical restraints) prior to providing therapeutic nursing communication is not acceptable.

Test-taking strategy: Analyze to determine what the question asks for, which is nursing actions to reduce client anxiety and fear. "Select all that apply" questions require considering each option to decide its merit. Always look to therapeutic communication skills as a means of reducing anxiety and developing a trusting relationship. Note any open-ended questions that allow the client to verbalize feelings. Review therapeutic anxiety-reducing nursing actions if you had difficulty answering this question.

Client needs category: Psychosocial integrity

Client needs subcategory: None

Cognitive level: Analyzing

---

2. A nurse is caring for a client who is disoriented to time, place, and person and is attempting to get out of bed and pull out an intravenous line. The nurse receives orders from a health care provider to apply a vest restraint and bilateral soft wrist restraints. In carrying out this order, which nursing actions would be appropriate? Select all that apply.

☐ **1.** Perform a face-to-face behavior evaluation every hour.

☐ **2.** Tie the restraints in quick-release knots.

☐ **3.** Tie the restraints to the side rails of the bed.

☐ **4.** Document the client's condition.

☐ **5.** Document alternative methods used before the restraints were applied.

☐ **6.** Document the client's response to the intervention.

Answer: 1, 2, 4, 5, 6

Ⓓ Rationale: Preventing a client from falling or harming himself or herself is of utmost importance. Applying restraints is a last resort when all other alternative interventions have been attempted. A face-to-face evaluation must be performed every hour. Restraints are tied in knots that can be released quickly and easily. The nurse would document the client's condition, any alternative methods used before the restraints were applied, and the client's response to the interventions. Restraints would never be secured to side rails because doing so can cause injury if the side rail is lowered without untying the restraint.

Test-taking strategy: Analyze to determine what information the question asks for, which is initiation and care of a disoriented client placed in restraints. Consider the client's safety needs and review basic care and comfort procedures for clients who are confused and at increased risk for falls. Also, realize that health care facilities have policies on the use of restraints. Review standard practices and institutional policies for initiation and care of a disoriented client in a restraint if you had difficulty answering this question.

Client needs category: Safe and effective care environment

Client needs subcategory: Safety and infection control

Cognitive level: Applying

3. A client has just been diagnosed with terminal cancer and is being transferred to home hospice care. The client's daughter tells the nurse, "I don't know what to say to my mother if she asks me if she's going to die." Which responses by the nurse would be appropriate? Select all that apply.

☐ **1.** "You are unfamiliar with what to say to your mother if asked about her dying?"

☐ **2.** "Let's talk about your mother's illness and how it will progress."

☐ **3.** "You sound like you have some questions about your mother dying. How can I help?"

☐ **4.** "Don't worry, hospice will take care of your mother."

☐ **5.** "Tell me how you're feeling about your mother dying."

Ⓔ **Rationale:** Talking about death is an uncomfortable situation. Paraphrasing the daughter's question allows the daughter to elaborate on her thoughts and feelings. It is also important to assess the daughter's knowledge base so the daughter feels prepared to talk with her mother. Conveying information clearly and openly can alleviate fears and strengthen the individual's sense of control. Encouraging verbalization of feelings helps build a therapeutic relationship based on trust and reduces anxiety. Advising the daughter not to worry, or having her tell her mother that, ignores her feelings and discourages further communication.

Test-taking strategy: Begin by determining which responses promote open, therapeutic communication. Also, consider the psychosocial needs of the family of a dying client. Eliminate responses that do not answer the client's question or are condescending. Review therapeutic communication skills if you had difficulty answering this question.

Client needs category: Psychosocial integrity

Client needs subcategory: None

Cognitive level: Analyzing

4. While providing care to a client, the nurse notes multiple blue, purple, and yellow ecchymotic areas on the arms and trunk. When the nurse asks about these bruises, the client responds, "I tripped." What actions would the nurse take? Select all that apply.

☐ **1.** Document the client's statement and complete a body map indicating the size, color, shape, location, and type of injuries.

☐ **2.** Contact the local authorities to report suspicions of abuse.

☐ **3.** Assist the client in developing a safety plan for times of increased violence.

☐ **4.** Call the client's partner to arrange a meeting to discuss the situation.

☐ **5.** Instruct the client to leave the abusive situation as soon as possible.

☐ **6.** Provide the client with telephone numbers of local shelters and safe houses.

Ⓒ **Rationale:** The nurse would objectively document the assessment findings. A detailed description of physical findings of abuse in the medical record is essential if legal action is pursued. All individuals, men or women, suspected of being abuse victims would be counseled on a safety plan, which consists of recognizing escalating violence within the family, formulating a plan to exit quickly, and knowing the telephone numbers of local shelters and safe houses. The nurse would not report this suspicion of abuse because the client is a competent adult who has the right to self-determination. Contacting the client's spouse without consent violates confidentiality. The nurse would respond to the client in a nonthreatening manner that promotes trust, rather than ordering the client to break off the relationship.

Test-taking strategy: Analyze to determine what information the question asks for, which is nursing actions to take when a client is suspected of being an abuse victim. Consider actions reflecting objectivity and remain nonjudgmental while developing trust with the client. Review the nurse's responsibilities when caring for a potential abuse victim and consider the client's age to determine appropriate actions. Review the Nurse's Code of Ethics and Standards of Care if you had difficulty answering this question.

Client needs category: Psychosocial integrity
Client needs subcategory: None
Cognitive level: Analyzing

5. A nurse is caring for a terminally ill client. The nurse assesses the client for identification of the psychosocial stage of acceptance. Place the following five stages of death and dying in the order in which Elisabeth Kübler-Ross noted that they most often occur. All options must be used.

| **1.** Bargaining |
| **2.** Denial and isolation |
| **3.** Acceptance |
| **4.** Anger |
| **5.** Depression |

Answer: 2, 4, 1, 5, 3

Ⓜ Rationale: Elisabeth Kübler-Ross outlined similarities to psychosocial responses to impending death or loss. Duration during each stage may vary or even overlap from individual to individual. According to Kübler-Ross, the five stages of death and dying are denial and isolation, anger, bargaining, depression, and acceptance.

Test-taking strategy: The key words are "in order" assuming that there is a progression or sequence. Critically think through the options to place each in a particular order. Begin with denial being the first and ending with acceptance if you are arranging by simply the definition of the words. Review the stages of death and dying and work of Elisabeth Kübler-Ross if you had difficulty answering this question.

Client needs category: Psychosocial integrity
Client needs subcategory: None
Cognitive level: Applying

6. A client with chronic renal failure was recently told by the health care provider of being a poor candidate for a transplant because of chronic uncontrolled hypertension and diabetes mellitus. Now the client tells the nurse, "I want to go off dialysis. I'd rather not live than be on this treatment for the rest of my life." Which responses are appropriate? Select all that apply.

☐ **1.** Take a seat next to the client and sit quietly to reflect on what was said.

☐ **2.** Say to the client, "We all have days when we don't feel like going on."

☐ **3.** Leave the room to allow the client privacy to collect thoughts.

☐ **4.** Say to the client, "You're feeling upset about the news you got about the transplant."

☐ **5.** Say to the client, "The treatments are only 3 days a week. You can live with that."

Answer: 1, 4

Ⓜ Rationale: Silence is a therapeutic communication technique that allows the nurse and client to reflect on what has taken place or been said. By waiting quietly and attentively, the nurse encourages the client to initiate and maintain a conversation. By reflecting on the client's implied feelings, the nurse promotes communication. Using such platitudes as "We all have days when we don't feel like going on" fails to address the client's needs. The nurse would not leave the client alone abruptly stopping therapeutic communication. Reminding the client of the treatment frequency does not address the feelings.

Test-taking strategy: Analyze to determine what information the question asks for, which is responses to a statement to end life-sustaining treatment. Recall the principles of client advocacy and therapeutic communication. Review the care of the client under emotional stress and principles of therapeutic communication if you had difficulty answering this question.

Client needs category: Psychosocial integrity
Client needs subcategory: None
Cognitive level: Analyzing

7. A nurse is caring for a client with advanced cancer. After reading the nursing note below, determine the nurse's next intervention.

Progress notes	
1/7/16	Client states, "The doctor says my
1545	chemotherapy isn't working anymore. They can
	only treat my symptoms now. I don't want to
	die in the hospital, I want to be in my own
	bed." ————————————R. Daly, RN

☐ **1.** Reread the document on patient/client rights to the client.

☐ **2.** Call the client's spouse to discuss the client's statements.

☐ **3.** Tell the client that only in the hospital can there be adequate pain relief.

☐ **4.** Explain the use of an advance directive to express the client's wishes.

Answer: 4

Ⓔ **Rationale:** An advance directive is a legal document used as a guideline for life-sustaining medical care of a client with an advanced disease or disability who can no longer indicate his or her own wishes. This document can include a living will, which instructs the health care provider to administer no life-sustaining treatment, and a durable power of attorney for health care, which names another person to act on the client's behalf for medical decisions if the client cannot act for self. By explaining the use of an advanced directive to the client at this time, the client has the opportunity to document future wishes. The document on client rights does not specifically address the client's wishes regarding future care. Calling the spouse is a breach of the client's right to confidentiality. Stating that only a hospital can provide adequate pain relief in a terminal situation demonstrates inadequate knowledge of the resources available in the community through hospice and home care agencies in collaboration with the client's health care provider.

Test-taking strategy: Use the process of elimination to select the option that is the most important "next" step to be taken by the nurse. Focus on the needs of a client who is making difficult medical decisions, consider referrals available to the nurse, and review the use of advance directives. Eliminate options focused on the nurse and spouse or those that tell the client what should be done. Look for documents that provide client-guided care in the final period of life. Review the principles of advanced directives and Patient's Bill of Rights if you had difficulty answering this question.

Client needs category: Psychosocial integrity

Client needs subcategory: None

Cognitive level: Applying

---

8. The nurse is caring for a client whose cultural background is different than his or her own. Which nursing actions are appropriate? Select all that apply.

☐ **1.** Consider that nonverbal cues, such as eye contact, may have a different meaning in different cultures.

☐ **2.** Respect the client's cultural beliefs through word and actions.

☐ **3.** Ask the client if there are cultural or religious requirements that should be considered in the plan of care.

☐ **4.** Explain the nurse's beliefs so that the client will understand the differences.

☐ **5.** Understand that all cultures experience pain in the same way.

Answer: 1, 2, 3

Ⓔ **Rationale:** Nonverbal cues may have different meanings in different cultures. In one culture, eye contact may be a sign of disrespect; in another, eye contact may show respect and attentiveness. The nurse would always respect the client's cultural beliefs and ask if there are cultural or religious requirements. This may include food choices or restrictions, body coverings, or time for prayer. The nurse would attempt to understand the client's culture; it is not the client's responsibility to understand the nurse's culture. The nurse would never impose his or her own beliefs on clients. Culture influences a client's expression of pain. For example, pain may be openly expressed in one culture and quietly endured in another.

9. A nurse is caring for a middle-aged client who has undergone hemicolectomy for colon cancer. The client has two children. Which concepts about families would the nurse consider when providing care for this client? Select all that apply.

☐ **1.** Illness in one family member can affect all members.

☐ **2.** Family roles do not change because of illness.

☐ **3.** A family member may perform more than one role at a time.

☐ **4.** Children typically are not affected by adult illness.

☐ **5.** The effects of an illness on a family depend on the stage of the family's life cycle.

☐ **6.** Changes in sleeping and eating patterns may be signs of stress in a family.

Answer: 1, 3, 5, 6

Ⓜ **Rationale:** Illness in one family member can affect all family members, even children. Each member of a family may have several roles to perform. A middle-aged client, for example, may have the roles of father/mother, husband/wife, wage earner, child care provider, and housekeeper. When one family member cannot fulfill a role because of illness, the roles of the other family members are affected. Families move through certain predictable life cycles (such as birth of a baby, a growing family, adult children leaving home, and grandparenting). The impact of illness on the family depends on the stage of the life cycle as family members take on different roles and the family structure changes. Illness produces stress in families; changes in eating and sleeping patterns are signs of stress.

Test-taking strategy: Analyze to determine what information the question asks for, which is considerations regarding family that may influence the client's care. Select options that impact family dynamics and roles of the family members. Review the impact of stress and illness on the family and recall the manifestations that may result from stress if you had difficulty answering this question.

Client needs category: Health promotion and maintenance

Client needs subcategory: None

Cognitive level: Analyzing

10. A nurse is assessing a newly admitted client's support system. In documenting the family assessment, who should be considered as part of the client's family? Select all that apply.

☐ **1.** People related by blood or marriage

☐ **2.** People whom the client views as family

☐ **3.** People who live in the same house

☐ **4.** People whom the nurse thinks are important to the client

☐ **5.** People of the same racial background who live in the same house as the client

☐ **6.** People who provide for the physical and emotional needs of the client

Answer: 2, 6

C **Rationale:** During admission, it is important to identify a client's support system. When providing care and teaching to a client, the nurse should consider family members to be all the people whom the client views as family. Family members may also include those people who provide for the physical and emotional needs of the client. The traditional definition of a family has changed and may include people not related by blood or marriage, those of a different racial background, and those who may not live in the same house as the client. Family members are defined by the client, not by the nurse.

Test-taking strategy: Analyze to determine what information the question asks for, which is who is considered to be family to provide support. "Select all that apply" questions require considering each option to decide its merit. Recall the components of a family group and consider the changes that have taken place in society relating to family members. Review the definition of family if you had difficulty answering this question.

Client needs category: Health promotion and maintenance

Client needs subcategory: None

Cognitive level: Analyzing

---

11. A home health nurse is working with the family of a client who has Alzheimer's disease. The nurse notes that the client's spouse is too exhausted to provide care all alone. The adult children live too far away to provide relief on a weekly basis. Which nursing interventions would be helpful? Select all that apply.

☐ **1.** Calling a family meeting to tell the absent children that they must participate in caregiving

☐ **2.** Suggesting that the spouse seek psychological counseling to help cope with exhaustion

☐ **3.** Recommending community resources for adult day care and respite care

☐ **4.** Encouraging the spouse to talk about the difficulties involved in caring for a loved one

☐ **5.** Asking whether friends or church members can help with errands or provide short periods of relief

☐ **6.** Recommending that the client be placed in a long-term care facility

Answer: 3, 4, 5

D **Rationale:** Many community services exist for Alzheimer's clients and their families. Encouraging use of these resources may make it possible to keep the client at home and to alleviate the spouse's exhaustion. The nurse can also support the caregiver by urging him or her to talk about the difficulties faced in caring for a spouse. Friends and church members may be able to help provide care to the client, allowing the caregiver time for rest, exercise, or an enjoyable activity. Arranging a family meeting to tell the children to participate more would probably be ineffective and might evoke anger or guilt. Counseling might be helpful, but it would not alleviate the caregiver's physical exhaustion or address the client's immediate needs. A long-term care facility is not an option until the family is ready to make that decision.

Test-taking strategy: Analyze to determine what information the question asks for, which is determining nursing interventions helpful for a caregiving spouse. Think of the nurse's role when offering emotional support to individuals struggling with the stressors associated with caring for the chronically ill. Select the options that meet the needs identified as "relief" for exhaustion and help in providing "sole" care. Review roles of the nurse for client advocacy and ethical standards if you had difficulty answering this question.

Client needs category: Psychosocial integrity

Client needs subcategory: None

Cognitive level: Analyzing

12. The home health nurse is completing the admission paperwork for a new client diagnosed with osteomyelitis who will be receiving home service intravenous therapy for the next month. The client is 32 years old and happily married. Which of the following findings will warrant further investigation? Select all that apply.

☐ **1.** The client reports having many hobbies and interests outside of the home.

☐ **2.** The client voices concerns about recovering quickly to return to work in the next month.

☐ **3.** The client talks repeatedly about the inability to grow old with his/her spouse.

☐ **4.** The client spends a great deal of time reflecting back on teen years.

☐ **5.** The client is talkative about the spouse and children.

ⓒ Rationale: At age 32, the client is in the middle adult stage of life. The repeated discussions about the lack of a future or death and reflections back on life are not appropriate or expected for this stage of development and should be investigated further. An interest in civic responsibilities and the establishment of hobbies is expected. During this developmental period, the greatest concern typically relates to establishing gainful employment and significant relationships. This is being demonstrated by the client's willingness to discuss family, which includes spouse and children.

Test-taking strategy: The key phrase in this question is "warrant further investigation," indicating that there is a nursing concern. Consider each option for a statement that is inconsistent with the client's developmental stage. Review Erikson's developmental stages if you had difficulty answering this question.

Client needs category: Psychosocial integrity

Client needs subcategory: None

Cognitive level: Analyzing

---

13. The nurse is caring for a client who developed fluctuating moods related to a recent cerebral vascular accident. When discussing the client's mood in a family meeting, which statements confirm a family's understanding of how to support the client? Select all that apply.

☐ **1.** "I do not take what she says personally and try to address the issue of anger."

☐ **2.** "All the kids just leave the room if she gets emotional; that provides privacy."

☐ **3.** "I tell her how I feel and yell back if needed so not to keep all of my frustration inside."

☐ **4.** "I allow her to vent feelings and then find a different topic to discuss."

☐ **5.** "Sometimes, I sit down and cry too and then we pick ourselves up and move on."

ⓒ Rationale: Changes in the brain that occur following the cerebral vascular accident can lead to periods of an emotional outburst resulting in anger or depression. The family may experience changes in their loved one that include uncharacteristic verbal outbursts or crying within usual conversation. It is important to identify that these outbursts are a result of the illness and not take the outburst personally. Allowing the client to vent her feelings and experience the frustration with the client allows for the sharing of emotions and provides emotional support. Afterwards, moving on to a different topic or moving on within the day's activity does not allow the client to remain in the emotional state. Leaving the client or yelling at the client is not therapeutic to support the client through this time.

Test-taking strategy: The key words are "how to support the client." Read each option to consider how the action would improve the client's mood. Always consider the disease process that has changed the mood. Look for therapeutic interventions that the family uses. Review supportive care of a post–cerebral vascular attack client if you had difficulty answering this question.

Client needs category: Psychosocial integrity

Client needs subcategory: None

Cognitive level: Analyzing

Medication and I.V. administration

1. The nurse is caring for a female client with dysmenorrhea that interferes with activities of daily living. The client is prescribed ibuprofen 400 mg three times daily. Which nursing action is completed with medication administration? Select all that apply.

☐ **1.** Obtain pulse and blood pressure.

☐ **2.** Assess urine output.

☐ **3.** Offer a light snack.

☐ **4.** Assess pain level.

☐ **5.** Monitor client temperature.

☐ **6.** Offer an 8-oz (240 ml) glass of water.

Answer: 3, 4, 6

Ⓜ **Rationale:** Ibuprofen is a nonsteroidal anti-inflammatory that interrupts prostaglandin synthesis reducing cramping and pain associated with menstrual periods. When administering the medication, the nurse would assess the client's pain level and offer the medication with a light snack and glass of water to reduce gastrointestinal irritation. Obtaining a pulse and blood pressure is common with antihypertensive medication administration. Assessing urine output is common with corticosteroids or diuretics. Monitoring client temperature occurs with antibiotics.

Test-taking strategy: The key phrase is "completed with medication administration" indicating that the action is important to the action of the medication or minimizing side effects. Compare each nursing action to the intended action of the medication. Review nonsteroidal anti-inflammatory medications and administration if you had difficulty answering this question.

Client needs category: Physiological integrity

Client needs subcategory: Pharmacological and parenteral therapies

Cognitive level: Applying

---

2. A 10-year-old is returning to the surgical unit following an appendectomy. The client has a patient-controlled analgesia (PCA) pump with the button resting on the client's lap. The parents are very unsure of the client having the ability to administer a narcotic. Which statements, made by the nurse, reassure the parents of the client's appropriate understanding and use? Select all that apply.

☐ **1.** "Because of programmable pump limits, the client cannot overdose on narcotic medication."

☐ **2.** "A nursing monitor alerts the nurse to frequent pain medication requests."

☐ **3.** "A 10-year-old has the cognitive ability to understand pain control via PCA."

☐ **4.** "The nurse will assess the client's pain status and sedation scale hourly."

☐ **5.** "Do not worry about it. We have had clients even younger use a PCA pump."

Answer: 1, 3, 4

Ⓜ **Rationale:** Many parents are unsure about allowing their child access to narcotic pain medications via a pump even after a surgical procedure. Parents have fears that the child will use the medication inappropriately or hit the button too many times causing an overdose. Parents also feel more comfortable guiding decisions for a school-aged child. All PCA pumps have prescribed doses, calculated specifically to the client's weight, with lockout points to prevent an overdose. Nurses also assess clients with a PCA on an hourly basis. The nurse would use a pain scale to evaluate pain relief and also the sedation scale to monitor the effects of the narcotic. The nurse is correct to state that 10-year-olds have the ability to understand the correlation between using medication and pain control. The client will be instructed to push the button before the pain becomes severe. The PCA pump is not linked to a nursing monitor to relay information about use of the pump. By checking the pump setting though, the nurse can see how many times the client pushed the button and at what time. A nurse would not use a nontherapeutic technique of telling a parent "not to worry about it."

Test-taking strategy: Analyze to determine what the question asks, which is statements that reassures parents of therapeutic PCA use for a school-aged child. Consider therapeutic communication techniques with parents and the safeguards built into the PCA pumps. Review the use of the PCA pump for various age groups if you had difficulty answering this question.

Client needs category: Physiological integrity

Client needs subcategory: Basic care and comfort

Cognitive level: Analyzing

3. A health care provider prescribes intravenous normal saline solution to be infused at a rate of 150 ml/hour for a client. How many liter(s) of solution will the client receive during an 8-hour shift? Record your answer using one decimal place (e.g., 6.2).

_____ liters

Answer: 1.2

Ⓜ **Rationale:** The ordered infusion rate is 150 ml/hour. The nurse would multiply 150 ml by 8 hours to determine the total volume in milliliters the client will receive during an 8-hour shift (1,200 ml). Then the nurse would convert milliliters to liters by dividing by 1,000. The total volume in liters that the client will receive in 8 hours is 1.2 L.

Test-taking strategy: Analyze to determine what information the question asks for, which is the volume of intravenous solution to be received in an 8-hour period. Consider the hourly information presented in the question to determine how to set up the math calculation for the 8-hour time frame. Use your knowledge of the metric system converting 1,000 ml = 1 L. Proofread your math calculation for accuracy. Review basic drug calculations and basic conversions if you had difficulty answering this question.

Client needs category: Physiological integrity

Client needs subcategory: Pharmacological and parenteral therapies

Cognitive level: Applying

4. The nurse is evaluating a parent's understanding of measuring one tablespoon of medication in a medicine cup. At which level on the medicine cup would the nurse confirm an appropriate dose?

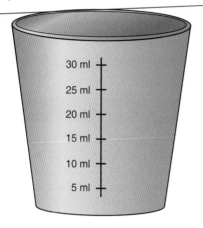

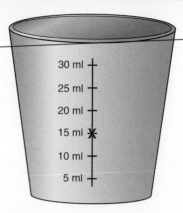

Ⓜ Rationale: One tablespoon equals 15 ml of medication.

Test-taking strategy: Analyze to determine what the question is asking, which is the one tablespoon level on the medicine cup. Recall that in household measurements, one tablespoon equals 15 ml. Also, recall that 3 teaspoons (5 ml) equals one tablespoon (15 ml). Review conversions and medication amounts if you had difficulty answering this question.

Client needs category: Safe and effective care environment

Client needs subcategory: Management of care

Cognitive level: Applying

---

5. A client is prescribed heparin 6,000 units subcutaneously every 12 hours for deep vein thrombosis prophylaxis. The pharmacy dispenses a vial containing 10,000 units/1 ml. How many milliliter(s) of heparin would the nurse administer? Record your answer using one decimal place (e.g., 6.2).

_____ milliliter(s)

Answer: 0.6

Ⓔ Rationale: The dose dispensed by the pharmacy is 10,000 units/1 ml, and the desired dose is 6,000 units. The nurse should use the following equations to determine the amount of heparin to administer:

Dose on hand/quantity on hand = dose desired/X

10,000 units/1 ml = 6,000 units/X

10,000 units × X = 6,000 units × 1 ml

X = 6,000 units × 1 ml/10,000 units

X = 0.6 ml.

Test-taking strategy: Analyze to determine what information the question asks for, which is the amount of milliliters for a dose of medication. One method of calculation is the ratio and proportion method to set up this problem. When using this method, ensure that units divided by milliliters of medication is maintained on both sides of the equation. Review basic drug calculations if you had difficulty answering this question.

---

6. A nurse is ordered to administer ampicillin 125 mg intramuscularly every 6 hours to a 10-kg child with a respiratory tract infection. The drug label reads, "The recommended dose for a client weighing less than 40 kg is 25 to 50 mg/kg/day intramuscularly or intravenously in equally divided doses at 6- to 8-hour intervals." The drug concentration is 125 mg/5 ml. Which nursing interventions are appropriate at this time? Select all that apply.

☐ **1.** Draw up 10 ml of ampicillin to administer.

☐ **2.** Administer the medication at 1000, 1400, 1800, and 2200.

☐ **3.** Assess the client for allergies to penicillin.

☐ **4.** Administer the medication because the dosage is within the recommended range.

☐ **5.** Question the prescriber about the order exceeding the recommended dosage.

☐ **6.** Obtain a sputum culture, as ordered, before administering the medication.

Answer: 3, 4, 6

Rationale: Because ampicillin is a penicillin antibiotic, the nurse would assess the client for penicillin allergies before administering this drug. The ampicillin dose is within the recommended range for a 10-kg client: 50 mg/kg × 10 kg = 500 mg. A dose of 500 mg divided by four (given every 6 hours) = 125 mg. Cultures should be obtained before antibiotics are given. The nurse should draw up 5 ml—not 10 ml—to administer the correct dose, according to the concentration on the label. The correct dosing schedule is every 6 to 8 hours, not every 4 hours.

Test-taking strategy: Analyze to determine what information the question asks for, which is appropriate interventions for a pediatric client to receive an antibiotic. To begin, a nurse must determine the safe dosage for the 10-kg pediatric client and review medication administration (antibiotic) safety practices as well. Review pediatric drug calculations and dosage guidelines for pediatric antibiotics if you had difficulty answering this question.

Client needs category: Physiological integrity

Client needs subcategory: Pharmacological and parenteral therapies

Cognitive level: Analyzing

7. A cardiologist prescribes digoxin 125 mcg by mouth every morning for a client diagnosed with heart failure. The pharmacy dispenses tablets that contain 0.25 mg each. How many tablet(s) would the nurse administer in each dose? Record your answer using one decimal place (e.g., 6.2).

_____ tablet(s)

Answer: 0.5

Ⓔ Rationale: The nurse would begin by converting 125 mcg to milligrams:

125 mcg/1,000 = 0.125 mg.

Then the nurse would use the following formula to calculate the drug dosage:

Dose on hand/quantity on hand = dose desired/X

0.25 mg/1 tablet = 0.125 mg/X

$0.25 \times X = 0.125 \times 1$ tablet

$X = 0.5$ tablet

Test-taking strategy: Analyze to determine what information the question asks for, which is the number of tablets in each dose. Use knowledge of drug calculations and the calculation method of ratio and proportion to set up this problem. Ensure that conversions to milligrams are completed first before inserting into the milligram per tablet proportion. Proofread your math calculation for accuracy. Review basic drug calculations and basic conversions if you had difficulty answering this question.

Client needs category: Physiological integrity

Client needs subcategory: Pharmacological and parenteral therapies

Cognitive level: Applying

---

8. A 75-year-old client is admitted to the hospital with lower gastrointestinal bleeding. The client's hemoglobin on admission to the emergency department is 7.3 g/dl (73 g/L). The health care provider prescribes 2 units of packed red blood cells to infuse over 2 hours each. Each unit of packed red blood cells contains 250 ml. The blood administration set has a drip factor of 10 gtt/ml. What is the flow rate in drops per minute? Round your answer to the nearest whole number (e.g., 62).

_____ gtt/minute

Answer: 21

Ⓜ Rationale: Each unit of packed red blood cells contains 250 ml, which should infuse over 2 hours (120 minutes). Therefore, the rate per minute is:

250 ml/120 minutes = 2.08 ml/minute.

Multiply by the drip factor to determine the flow rate:

2.08 ml $\times$ 10 gtt = 20.8 gtt/minute
(round up to 21 gtt/minute).

Test-taking strategy: Analyze to determine what information the question asks for, which is the drop rate per minute of blood. Recall that this is a two-step calculation as the nurse must calculate the milliliter per minute before placing into the drip rate formula. Proofread your math calculation for accuracy. Review intravenous drug calculations and basic conversions if you had difficulty answering this question.

Client needs category: Physiological integrity

Client needs subcategory: Pharmacological and parenteral therapies

Cognitive level: Analyzing

---

9. A nurse is preparing a teaching plan for a client who was prescribed enalapril maleate for the treatment of hypertension. Which instructions would the nurse include in the teaching plan? Select all that apply.

- ☐ **1.** Instruct the client to avoid salt substitutes.
- ☐ **2.** Tell the client that light-headedness is a common adverse effect that does not need to be reported.
- ☐ **3.** Inform the client of a potential sore throat for the first few days of therapy.
- ☐ **4.** Advise the client to report facial swelling or difficulty breathing immediately.
- ☐ **5.** Tell the client that blood tests will be necessary every 3 weeks for 2 months and periodically after that.
- ☐ **6.** Advise the client not to change the position suddenly to minimize the risk of orthostatic hypotension.

Ⓓ **Rationale:** The nurse would tell the client to avoid salt substitutes because they may contain potassium, which can cause light-headedness and syncope. Facial swelling or difficulty breathing would be reported immediately because they may be signs of angioedema, which would require discontinuation of the drug. The client would also be advised to change positions slowly to minimize the risk of orthostatic hypotension. The nurse would tell the client to report light-headedness, especially during the first few days of therapy, so dosage adjustments can be made. The client would also report signs of infection, such as sore throat and fever, because the drug may decrease the white blood cell (WBC) count. Because this effect is generally seen within 3 months, the WBC count and differential should be monitored periodically.

Test-taking strategy: Analyze to determine what information the question asks for, which is instructions for the teaching plan of a client beginning enalapril maleate. Recall the classes of antihypertensives and, specifically, angiotensin-converting enzyme (ACE) inhibitors and relate the type of adverse reactions to expect. This information, along with the dosage, would formulate the basis for a teaching plan. Review the drug classification of ACE inhibitors if you had difficulty answering this question.

Client needs category: Physiological integrity

Client needs subcategory: Pharmacological and parenteral therapies

Cognitive level: Applying

10. After sustaining a closed head injury, a client is prescribed phenytoin 100 mg intravenously every 8 hours for seizure prophylaxis. Which nursing interventions are necessary when administering phenytoin? Select all that apply.

☐ **1.** Administer phenytoin through any peripheral intravenous site.

☐ **2.** Mix intravenous doses in solutions containing dextrose 5% in water.

☐ **3.** Administer an intravenous bolus no faster than 50 mg/minute.

☐ **4.** Monitor electrocardiogram (ECG), blood pressure, and respiratory status continuously when administering phenytoin intravenously.

☐ **5.** Do not use an in-line filter when administering the drug.

☐ **6.** Monitor the client for signs of early toxicity, such as drowsiness, nystagmus, ataxia, dysarthria, tremor, and slurred speech.

Answer: 3, 4, 6

Ⓓ **Rationale:** Administer an intravenous bolus by slow (50 mg/minute) intravenous push method; too rapid an injection may cause hypotension and circulatory collapse. Continuous monitoring of ECG, blood pressure, and respiratory status is essential when administering phenytoin intravenously. Early toxicity may cause drowsiness, nausea, vomiting, nystagmus, ataxia, dysarthria, tremor, and slurred speech. Later effects may include hypotension, arrhythmias, respiratory depression, and coma. Death may result from respiratory and circulatory depression. Phenytoin would not be administered by intravenous push in veins on the back of the hand; larger veins are needed to prevent discoloration associated with purple glove syndrome. Mix intravenous doses in normal saline solution and use the solution within 30 minutes; doses mixed in dextrose 5% in water will precipitate. Use of an in-line filter is recommended.

Test-taking strategy: Analyze to determine what information the question asks for, which is nursing interventions of a client-prescribed intravenous phenytoin. Recall specific parameters of medication administration because of uniqueness of the medication and relate side effects specifically to the action of medication. Review the therapeutic class of anticonvulsants, concentrating on the nursing interventions, if you had difficulty answering this question.

Client needs category: Physiological integrity

Client needs subcategory: Pharmacological and parenteral therapies

Cognitive level: Applying

---

11. A client returns to the room from the postanesthesia care unit after undergoing a right hemicolectomy. The health care provider orders 1 L of dextrose 5% in half-normal saline solution to infuse at 125 ml/hour. The drop factor of the available intravenous tubing is 15 gtt/ml. What is the drip rate in drops per minute? Round your answer to the nearest whole number (e.g., 62).

_____ gtt/minute

Answer: 31

Ⓜ **Rationale:** The flow rate is 125 ml/hour, or 125 ml/60 minutes. Use the following equation to determine the drip rate:

125 ml/60 minutes × 15 gtt/1 ml = 31.25 gtt/minute (round down to 31 gtt/minute).

Test-taking strategy: Analyze to determine what information the question asks for, which is the drip rate per minute of I.V. fluid. Recall how to calculate intravenous drip rates and proofread the math calculation. Rounding is completed to the nearest complete drop. Review intravenous drip rate calculations if you had difficulty answering this question.

Client needs category: Physiological integrity

Client needs subcategory: Pharmacological and parenteral therapies

Cognitive level: Applying

---

12. A physician prescribes intravenous heparin 25,000 units in 250 ml of normal saline solution to infuse at 600 units/hour for a client who suffered an acute myocardial infarction (MI). After 6 hours of heparin therapy, the client's partial thromboplastin time is subtherapeutic. The health care provider orders the infusion to be increased to 800 units/hour. The nurse would set the infusion pump to deliver how many milliliters per hour? Record your answer using a whole number.

_____ milliliters/
     hour

Ⓜ Rationale: The nurse would calculate the infusion rate using the following formula:

$$\text{Dose on hand/quantity on hand} = \text{dose desired}/X$$
$$25{,}000 \text{ units}/250 \text{ ml} = 800 \text{ units/hour} \div X$$
$$25{,}000 \text{ units} \times X = 250 \text{ ml} \times 800 \text{ units/hour}$$
$$25{,}000 \times X = 200{,}000 \text{ ml/hour}$$
$$X = 8 \text{ ml/hour}$$

Test-taking strategy: Analyze to determine what information the question asks for, which is calculating an increased dosage of heparin to be infused. Recall your knowledge of ratio proportion calculations that help solve for X amounts. This allows for calculation of the new rate at milliliters per hour. Proofread your math calculation for accuracy. Review setting an intravenous infusion device that delivers milliliters per hour, and the calculation method of ratio and proportion to obtain the specific dosage if you had difficulty answering this question.

Client needs category: Physiological integrity

Client needs subcategory: Pharmacological and parenteral therapies

Cognitive level: Applying

---

13. After undergoing small-bowel resection, a client is prescribed metronidazole 500 mg intravenously. The mixed solution is 100 ml. The nurse is to administer the drug over 30 minutes. The drop factor of the available intravenous tubing is 15 gtt/ml. What is the drip rate in drops per minute? Record your answer using a whole number (e.g., 62).

_____ drops/minute

Ⓔ Rationale: The nurse would use the following equation to calculate the drip rate:

$$\text{Total volume (ml)/administration time (in minutes)}$$
$$\times \text{drip factor (gtt/ml)} = X$$
$$100 \text{ mL}/30 \text{ minutes} \times 15 \text{ gtt/ml} = X$$
$$X = \frac{1500 \text{ gtt}}{30 \text{ minutes}}$$
$$X = 50 \text{ gtt/minute}$$

Test-taking strategy: Analyze to determine what information the question asks for, which is the drip rate per minute of a secondary infusion. Recall the standard formula. Proofread the math calculation. Review the calculation of intravenous drip rates if you had difficulty answering this question.

Client needs category: Physiological integrity

Client needs subcategory: Pharmacological and parenteral therapies

Cognitive level: Applying

14. A client with an intravenous line in place states having pain at the insertion site. Assessment of the site reveals a vein that is red, warm, and hard. Which actions would the nurse take? Select all that apply.

- ☐ **1.** Slow the infusion rate while notifying the prescriber.
- ☐ **2.** Discontinue the infusion at the affected site.
- ☐ **3.** Restart the infusion distal to the discontinued intravenous site.
- ☐ **4.** Assess the client for skin sloughing.
- ☐ **5.** Apply warm soaks to the intravenous site.
- ☐ **6.** Document the assessment, nursing actions taken, and the client's response.

Answer: 2, 5, 6

Ⓓ **Rationale:** Redness, warmth, pain, and a hard, cordlike vein at the intravenous catheter insertion site suggest that the client has phlebitis. The nurse would discontinue the intravenous infusion and insert a new catheter proximal to or above the discontinued site or in the other arm. Applying warm soaks to the site reduces inflammation. The nurse would document the assessment of the intravenous site, the actions taken, and the client's response to the situation. Slowing the infusion rate would not reduce the phlebitis. Restarting the infusion at a site distal to the phlebitis may contribute to the inflammation. Skin sloughing is not a symptom of phlebitis; it is associated with extravasation of certain toxic medications.

Test-taking strategy: Analyze to determine what information the question asks for, which is the nursing actions needed when a client reports symptoms at the intravenous catheter site. "Select all that apply" questions require considering each option to decide its merit. Recall the assessment findings associated with intravenous sites and the interventions for an abnormal assessment. Note that the symptoms stated are also symptoms of irritation and phlebitis, requiring nursing intervention. Review intravenous site management if you had difficulty answering this question.

Client needs category: Physiological integrity

Client needs subcategory: Pharmacological and parenteral therapies

Cognitive level: Applying

15. After suffering an acute myocardial infarction (MI), a client with a history of type 1 diabetes is prescribed metoprolol intravenously. Which nursing interventions are associated with intravenous administration of metoprolol? Select all that apply.

☐ **1.** Monitor glucose levels closely.

☐ **2.** Monitor for heart block and bradycardia.

☐ **3.** Monitor blood pressure closely.

☐ **4.** Mix the drug in 50 ml of dextrose 5% in water and infuse over 30 minutes.

☐ **5.** Be aware that the drug is not compatible with morphine.

Answer: 1, 2, 3

Ⓜ **Rationale:** Metoprolol masks the common signs of hypoglycemia; therefore, glucose levels would be monitored closely in diabetic clients. When used to treat an MI, metoprolol is contraindicated in clients with heart rates less than 45 beats/minute and any degree of heart block, so the nurse would monitor the client for bradycardia and heart block. Metoprolol masks common signs and symptoms of shock, such as decreased blood pressure, so blood pressure would also be monitored closely. The nurse would give the drug undiluted by direct injection. Although metoprolol would not be mixed with other drugs, studies have shown that it is compatible when mixed with morphine sulfate or when administered with alteplase infusion at a Y-site connection.

Test-taking strategy: Analyze to determine what information the question asks for, which is nursing interventions when administering intravenous metoprolol. Recall the pharmacological classification of antihypertensives, specifically β-blockers, and concentrate on intravenous administration. Look to the exaggerated actions of β-blockers for potential side effects. Review the intravenous administration of the β-blocker metoprolol if you had difficulty answering this question.

Client needs category: Physiological integrity

Client needs subcategory: Pharmacological and parenteral therapies

Cognitive level: Applying

16. When administering medication, the nurse ensures client safety by following the rights of medication administration. Identify the "rights of medication administration." Select all that apply.

☐ **1.** Right room

☐ **2.** Right client

☐ **3.** Right dose

☐ **4.** Right medication

☐ **5.** Right time

☐ **6.** Right route

Answer: 2, 3, 4, 5, 6

Ⓔ **Rationale:** A nurse must always implement safe nursing practices when administering medications. Following the rights of medication administration helps protect the client from medication errors. Safe procedure includes confirming the right client, dose, medication, time, and route. Confirming the room number does not guarantee that the right client will receive the correct medication.

Test-taking strategy: Analyze to determine what information the question asks for, which is safety guidelines for medication administration. Recall the standards of practice guidelines for medication administration. Logically consider what would ensure safe medication administration. Review the rights of medication administration if you had difficulty answering this question.

Client needs category: Physiological integrity

Client needs subcategory: Pharmacological and parenteral therapies

Cognitive level: Remembering

17. A client is to be started on a furosemide. Which interventions would be included in the teaching plan? Select all that apply.

☐ **1.** Advise the client to reduce dietary sodium intake.

☐ **2.** Encourage the use of salt substitutes.

☐ **3.** Tell the client to alert the health care provider about any visible edema.

☐ **4.** Instruct the client to take the medication as directed.

☐ **5.** Suggest taking the medication just before bedtime to establish a routine.

Answer: 1, 3, 4

Ⓒ Rationale: Furosemide is a loop diuretic. Client teaching focuses on actions related to the fluid gradient and electrolyte balance. Reducing dietary sodium intake will help increase the effectiveness of diuretic medication and may allow smaller doses to be ordered. Diuretics are commonly prescribed to control fluid accumulation in the body; therefore, the presence of edema may indicate the need for the health care provider to adjust the therapy. Compliance is very important with diuretics. In order to effectively monitor therapy, the nurse would encourage the client to take the medication exactly as prescribed. Salt substitutes are not recommended because they contain potassium instead of sodium and may cause serious cardiovascular effects. Diuretics cause an increased urine output, which may interfere with the client's sleep if taken at bedtime.

Test-taking strategy: Analyze to determine what information the question asks for, which is pharmacologic actions and use of diuretics and the educational needs of clients taking these drugs. Recall the nature of diuretics (to remove fluid from the system) and consider potential side effects (dehydration, electrolyte imbalance) to guide the teaching content. Review diuretic therapy and client teaching if you had difficulty answering this question.

Client needs category: Health promotion and maintenance

Client needs subcategory: None

Cognitive level: Applying

18. A client receives a short-acting insulin and an intermediate-acting insulin before breakfast at 0800. Using the chart below, when might the nurse expect the onset of the intermediate-acting insulin to take effect?

Medication administration record			
Insulin type	**Onset**	**Peak**	**Duration**
Lispro (Humalog)	15–30 minutes	1–2 hours	4–5 hours
Humulin Regular	20–60 minutes	2–4 hours	8–10 hours
Humulin NPH	1–2 hours	4–8 hours	10–20 hours
Glargine (Lantus)	1–2 hours	Relatively flat	20–24 hours

☐ **1.** 1500

☐ **2.** 1300

☐ **3.** 1000

☐ **4.** 0830

Answer: 3

Ⓜ Rationale: The timing of insulin's effects varies according to the type. Referring to the chart, the nurse would note that the onset of action for the intermediate-acting insulin (Humulin NPH) is 1 to 2 hours. Because the administration time was 0800, the effects should begin 1 to 2 hours after administration, at approximately 1000.

Test-taking strategy: Analyze to determine what information the question asks for, which is identifying the onset of intermediate-acting insulin. Begin by identifying which insulin in the table is classified as an intermediate-acting insulin. Note that rapid-acting, short-acting, intermediate-acting, and long-acting insulins are documented, respectively. It is important for the nurse to recognize the onset of action to determine when blood sugar levels decline. Once the intermediate-acting insulin is selected, read the chart to confirm the onset of action and calculate the time using military time. Review administration of various types of insulin if you had difficulty answering this question.

Client needs category: Physiological integrity

Client needs subcategory: Pharmacological and parenteral therapies

Cognitive level: Analyzing

19. A client has an intravenous line in place for 3 days and begins to state discomfort at the insertion site. Based on the nurse's progress note below, what condition has **most** likely occurred?

Progress notes	
02/15/16 0730	Intravenous site assessed and found to have blanching around the site, swelling, and coolness to the touch. Laboratory results include a white blood cell count within normal limits.———————— ————————Sue Thompson, RN

☐ **1.** Infiltration

☐ **2.** Phlebitis

☐ **3.** Infection

☐ **4.** Infection and infiltration

Answer: 1

Rationale: The assessment findings of pallor, swelling, skin that is cool to the touch at the intravenous insertion site, and a normal WBC count all indicate infiltration. The infusion would be discontinued and restarted in a different site. Phlebitis would be evidenced by redness at the cannula tip and along the length of the vein. Infection would be evidenced by an elevated WBC count.

Test-taking strategy: Analyze to determine what information the question asks for, which is potential diagnosis of intravenous site complications. Focus on the symptoms noted in the question and nurse's documentation for clues that either validate or eliminate options. Use the process of elimination to make the correct selection. Review the signs and symptoms of intravenous site complications if you had difficulty answering this question.

Client needs category: Physiological integrity

Client needs subcategory: Pharmacological and parenteral therapies

Cognitive level: Applying

---

20. A client is prescribed an intravenous solution of 1,000 ml to be infused from 0800 to 2000. The nurse will use an infusion pump that delivers the solution in milliliters per hour. At what rate would the nurse set the pump to deliver the solution? Record your answer using a whole number (e.g., 62).

_____ milliliters/
hour

Answer: 83

Rationale: First, determine how many hours the infusion needs to run. 0800 to 2000 is 12 hours. Use the following equation to determine the milliliters per hour:

$$\frac{\text{Volume to infuse}}{\text{Infusion time}} = \text{Flow rate per hour}$$

$$\frac{1{,}000 \text{ ml}}{12 \text{ hours}} = 83.3 \text{ ml/hour (rounded to 83 ml/hour)}$$

The pump would be set to deliver 83 ml/hour.

Test-taking strategy: Analyze to determine what information the question asks for, which is the milliliters per hour that the infusion device is to be set. Use the standard formula calculating the milliliters per hour. Review calculations of intravenous infusion rates if you had difficulty answering this question.

Client needs category: Physiological integrity

Client needs subcategory: Pharmacological and parenteral therapies

Cognitive level: Analyzing

---

21. A nurse enters a client's semiprivate room and prepares to administer the 0900 medications. Place the following steps in chronological sequence indicating the measures to take in order to safely administer these medications. All options must be used.

1. Administer the medications.

2. Obtain the correct unit dose medications.

3. Confirm the client's identity.

4. Check the client's medication administration record (MAR) for the 0900 medications.

5. Open the unit dose packages.

Answer: 4, 2, 3, 5, 1

Ⓜ **Rationale:** Following sequential steps helps ensure safe medication administration. The nurse would first check to see which medications the client is due to receive at 0900 and then obtain them. Next, the nurse would confirm the client's identity in the semiprivate room according to facility protocol. Once the client is properly identified, the nurse would open the drug packages at the bedside, administer the medications to the client, and document administration.

Test-taking strategy: Analyze to determine what information the question asks for, which is medication administration safety practices. Consider the step-by-step process to obtain the medication through documenting the medication for a logical flow of events. Recall the most logical process to note any errors in administration. Review medication administration techniques if you had difficulty answering this question.

Client needs category: Physiological integrity

Client needs subcategory: Pharmacological and parenteral therapies

Cognitive level: Applying

22. The nurse prepares to administer medications into a client's jejunostomy tube. Identify the area where the nurse would expect the jejunostomy tube to be located.

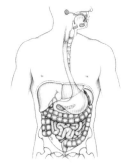

Answer:

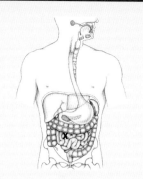

Ⓓ **Rationale:** A jejunostomy tube is often placed for long-term nutritional support. The tubes are inserted surgically in the jejunum and are not easily dislodged. The jejunum is the immediate portion of the small intestine that connects proximally with the duodenum and distally with the ileum.

Test-taking strategy: Analyze to determine what information the question asks for, which is the location of the jejunostomy tube. Use knowledge of medical terminology to identify that jejunostomy relates to jejunum, which is the small intestine. Review the anatomy of the gastrointestinal system and the correct placement for a jejunostomy tube if you had difficulty answering this.

Basic physical assessment

1. A client who was involved in a motor vehicle accident is admitted to the intensive care unit. The emergency department admission record indicates that the client was hit in the right temporal lobe. A nurse would expect the client to demonstrate which abnormalities? Select all that apply.

☐ **1.** Difficulty comprehending language

☐ **2.** Decreased hearing

☐ **3.** Aphasia

☐ **4.** Amnesia for recent events

☐ **5.** Ataxic gait

☐ **6.** Personality changes

Answer: 1, 2, 4

Ⓓ Rationale: The temporal lobe controls hearing, language comprehension, and the storage and recall of memories; therefore, the client would likely have difficulty comprehending language, diminished hearing, and amnesia for recent events. Aphasia and personality changes might be expected from injury to the frontal lobe. An ataxic gait would indicate injury primarily to the cerebellum.

Test-taking strategy: Analyze to determine what information the question asks for, which is deficits that may occur when there is damage to the temporal lobe of the brain. Recall the anatomy and physiology of the brain and the specific function of each section, focusing particularly on the temporal lobe. Review the temporal lobe functions if you had difficulty answering this question.

Client needs category: Physiological integrity

Client needs subcategory: Physiological adaptation

Cognitive level: Analyzing

2. The nurse is coassigned with a licensed practical/vocational nurse (LPN/VN) to care for 20 clients on a skilled, long-term care facility. When working as a team, which nursing duties would the nurse delegate to the LPN/VN? Select all that apply.

☐ **1.** Administer morphine sulfate 30 mg intramuscular every 4 hours as needed.

☐ **2.** Hang 2 units of packed red blood cells.

☐ **3.** Inject furosemide 40 mg intravenously daily.

☐ **4.** Place a nasogastric tube for gastric decompression.

☐ **5.** Calculate output every 8 hours and report to the health care provider.

☐ **6.** Insert a 20-French Foley catheter.

Answer: 1, 4, 5, 6

Ⓒ Rationale: It is important to understand the LPN/VN scope of practice when delegating nursing duties. Specific duties of the LPN/VN vary slightly from state to state or province to province; however, in most states/provinces, LPN/VNs are unable to hang blood and blood products and unable to push intravenous medications. LPN/VNs are able to administer intramuscular medications, administer narcotic medications, place a nasogastric tube or Foley catheter, and report a client's output to the health care provider.

Test-taking strategies: Analyze to determine what information the questions asks for, which is the scope of practice for the LPN/VN. Review each option to analyze the level of nursing responsibility and where the action fits into the scope of practice. Review nursing standards and responsibilities in the scope of practice for LPN/VNs if you had difficulty answering this question.

Client needs category: Safe and effective care environment

Client needs subcategory: Management of care

Cognitive level: Analyzing

3. A nurse is assessing a client who reports burning on urination and a temperature of 99.8°F (37.7°C). On physical examination, the nurse notes right-sided costovertebral angle tenderness. On the anatomical position drawing, identify the area of client tenderness.

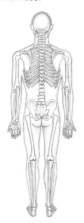

Answer:

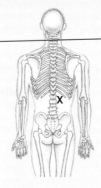

Ⓓ Rationale: To determine whether costovertebral angle tenderness (a sign of glomerulonephritis) is present, the nurse would percuss the costovertebral angle (the angle over each kidney that is formed by the lateral and downward curve of the lowest rib and the vertebral column). Since the kidney lies directly below this area, tapping disturbs the inflamed tissue causing pain. The costovertebral angle can be percussed by placing the palm of one hand over the costovertebral angle and striking it with the fist of the other hand.

Test-taking strategy: Analyze to determine what information the question asks for, which is to document right-sided costovertebral tenderness on the anatomical drawing. Note that the question infers burning on urination, suggesting a urinary/kidney problem narrowing the area for percussion. Review the assessment techniques for the renal system and the clinical manifestations of the findings if you had difficulty answering this question.

Client needs category: Physiological integrity
Client needs subcategory: Physiological adaptation
Cognitive level: Applying

4. A client presents to the emergency department with liver failure and obvious jaundice. When palpating a client's abdomen, identify the area that would provide the **most** essential information.

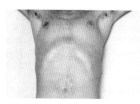

Answer:

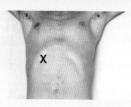

Ⓓ Rationale: Palpation of the liver in the right upper quadrant would provide essential information on the organ's status. Palpation in a systematic manner identifies masses, enlargement, and degree of tenderness. The nurse can best palpate the liver by standing on the client's right side and placing the nurse's right hand on the client's abdomen, along the right midclavicular line. The nurse would point the fingers of the right hand toward the client's head, just under the right rib margin.

Test-taking strategy: Analyze to determine what information the question asks for, which is identifying an abdominal area that would provide "essential" assessment information. With the stem of the question noting liver failure, assessing the status of the liver would provide the "essential" information. Recall the anatomy in the abdominal cavity and, specifically, techniques for assessing the liver. Review the anatomy of the abdominal cavity if you had difficulty answering this question.

Client needs category: Physiological integrity

Client needs subcategory: Physiological adaptation

Cognitive level: Analyzing

---

5. The nurse notices that the client's temperature over the past 24 hours has risen from 98.8°F (37.1°C) to 101.6°F (38.7° C). The nurse completes a head to toe assessment and documents the following nurse's note.

Progress notes	
6/26/15 1400	Temp 101.6°F (38.7°C), Pulse 88, Resp- 24, Blood pressure 132/78 Lungs clear. Harsh cough noted. No sputum. Denies chest pain. Abdomen soft. Positive bowel sounds. Voiding dark amber urine. Last bowel movement this morning. Gait steady on abulation. No lower extremity edema noted. —————————— ————————————————R. Brown, RN

What would be the nurse's next nursing action?

☐ **1.** Pass on the data to the next shift.

☐ **2.** Notify the health care provider.

☐ **3.** Apply oxygen at 2 L per nasal cannula.

☐ **4.** Obtain a urine culture.

Answer: 2

🅒 **Rationale:** When the nurse notes a significant rise in temperature to a febrile status, the nurse must first complete a head to toe assessment to obtain all client data and then notify the health care provider. The health care provider may then opt to assess the client or order diagnostic studies to determine a reason for the rise in client temperature. The nurse would pass the data on to the next shift; however, only the health care provider can order diagnostic testing. Early identification of a problem can lead to subsequent treatment. There are no data that the client is short of breath or oxygen compromised so that oxygen needs to be applied. The nurse would not complete a urine culture without a health care provider's order.

Test-taking strategy: The key word is "next" stating that one nursing action would be done before all others. Typically, the nurse uses the ABCs of airway, breathing, and circulation as a guide. In this situation, it is the client's significant rise in temperature. In lieu of further data to align nursing action, the best option is to notify the health care provider. Review priority actions with a rise in client temperature if you had difficulty answering this question.

Client needs category: Safe and effective care environment

Client needs subcategory: Management of care

Cognitive level: Analyzing

6. While examining the hands of a client with osteoarthritis, a nurse notes Heberden's nodes on the second (index) finger. Identify the area on the finger where the nurse observes the node.

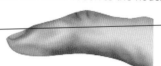

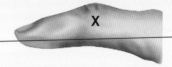

X

Ⓜ Rationale: Heberden's nodes appear on the distal interphalangeal joints. Bouchard's nodes appear on the proximal interphalangeal joints. These bony and cartilaginous enlargements are usually hard and painless and typically occur in middle-aged and elderly clients with osteoarthritis.

Test-taking strategy: Analyze to determine what information the question asks for, which is the location of Heberden's nodes on the finger. Recall that osteoarthritis affects the joints of the body narrowing the selected areas. Review the anatomy of the hand and the pathophysiology of osteoarthritis if you had difficulty answering this question.

Client needs category: Physiological integrity

Client needs subcategory: Physiological adaptation

Cognitive level: Applying

---

7. The nurse is notifying the health care provider via telephone of a change in condition of a client diagnosed with an exacerbation of asthma. Arrange the nursing statements in order as they would be communicated using the SBAR method. All options must be used.

1. Respirations are now 32 breaths/minute. The pulse oximeter is 89%. Lungs reveal wheezing in all lung fields. Slight nasal flaring is noted.

2. Mr. Smith was admitted yesterday with an exacerbation of asthma. He typically controls his asthma with oral medication and inhalers at home. He is ordered albuterol treatments twice daily. Oxygen is prescribed at 2 L.

3. Hello. My name is Nurse Jones from Unit D.

4. I recommend that we increase his oxygen dose and prescribe an extra albuterol treatment.

5. I am notifying you because Bob Smith has become increasingly more short of breath with audible wheezing this afternoon.

Answer: 3, 5, 2, 1, 4

Ⓜ Rationale: SBAR communication stands for Situation, Background, Assessment, and Recommendation. First, the nurse must identify self and where he/she is calling from. Next, the nurse would begin explaining the client situation (change in condition). The nurse would provide background information such as diagnosis, admission status, and date. The nurse would provide a focused assessment on the area of concern. Lastly, the nurse would offer a recommendation for client care.

Test-taking strategy: Analyze to determine what the question asks, which is order for SBAR communication between a nurse and a health care provider. Recall that SBAR communication provides a framework for communication between members of the health care team regarding a client's condition. SBAR is an easy-to-remember mnemonic that walks the nurse through the information needed in the exchange. Review SBAR communication and the information required if you had difficulty answering this question.

Client needs category: Safe and effective care environment

Client needs subcategory: Management of care

Cognitive level: Analyzing

8. The nurse is providing preoperative instructions on the use of an incentive spirometer and how to obtain the maximum benefit. Place an X at the location on the spirometer that **best** identifies proper use.

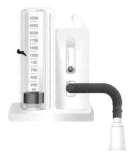

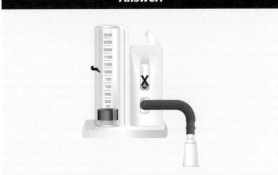

D Rationale: The incentive spirometer is a device that measures how deeply the client inhales. Deep inhalation wakes the lungs after surgery and helps to prevent atelectasis and pneumonia. The right chamber contains a floating ball, which is used to determine if the client is using proper inhaling technique. The other adjacent chamber has a piston that rises documenting the level achieved. A goal can be set on this side encouraging the client to strive for a higher level.

Test-taking strategy: Analyze to determine what information the question asks for, which is the location on the incentive spirometer that shows appropriate inhalation. Recall the instruction to the client that encourages maintaining the floating ball between the documented areas thus meeting the inhalation goal. Recall that maintaining within this range allows the piston to rise in the adjacent chamber. Review proper incentive spirometry instructions if you had difficulty answering this question.

Client needs category: Health promotion and maintenance

Client needs subcategory: None

Cognitive level: Applying

9. A nurse is caring for a client diagnosed with herpes zoster. Place in chronological order the pathophysiological changes that the nurse would anticipate in assessing the progression of the disease. All options must be used.

1. Fever, malaise, and red nodules appear in a dermatome distribution.

2. The virus multiplies in the ganglia, causing deep pain, itching, and paresthesia or hyperesthesia.

3. Vesicles crust and scab but no longer shed the virus.

4. Residual antibodies from the initial infection mobilize but are ineffective.

5. Vesicles appear, filled with either clear fluid or pus.

6. Varicella-zoster virus is reactivated.

Answer: 6, 4, 1, 2, 5, 3

Ⓓ **Rationale:** Herpes zoster (shingles) is an acute inflammation caused by infection with the herpes virus varicella-zoster (chickenpox virus). After acquiring chickenpox, the virus remains inactive (dormant) in certain nerves of the body. The reason the virus becomes active is not clear. The pathophysiologic changes associated with this disorder follow a typical viral path and occur in the order described above.

Test-taking strategy: Analyze to determine what information the question asks for, which is the progression of the herpes zoster disease process. Recall the steps from the reactivation of the virus to the crusting, which identifies the concluding stage of the disease. Review the pathophysiology of herpes zoster if you had difficulty answering this question.

Client needs category: Physiological integrity
Client needs subcategory: Physiological adaptation
Cognitive level: Applying

---

10. An elderly client has a history of aortic valve stenosis. Identify the area where the nurse would place the stethoscope to **best** hear the murmur.

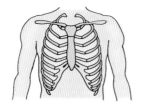

Answer:

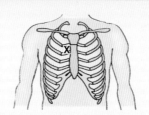

Ⓜ **Rationale:** Aortic stenosis occurs from a constriction that restricts blood flow through the heart and causes the left ventricle to enlarge. This enlargement can lead to heart failure and development of life-threatening irregular heartbeats. The murmur of aortic stenosis is low pitched, rough, and rasping. It is heard best in the second intercostal space, to the right of the sternum.

Test-taking strategy: Analyze to determine what information the question asks for, which is identifying the site to assess a murmur in a client with aortic valve stenosis. Review the anatomy of the cardiovascular system and consider the pressure changes within the heart when stenosis occurs. Critically think about the nature of a murmur being a backflow of blood and the location in the noted area. Review anatomical structures of the heart and techniques for assessment if you had difficulty answering this question.

Client needs category: Physiological integrity

Client needs subcategory: Physiological adaptation

Cognitive level: Analyzing

---

11. A nurse is assessing a client who has a rash on the chest and upper arms. Which questions would the nurse ask in order to gain further information about the client's rash? Select all that apply.

☐ **1.** "When did the rash start?"

☐ **2.** "Are you allergic to any medications, foods, or pollen?"

☐ **3.** "How old are you?"

☐ **4.** "What have you been using to treat the rash?"

☐ **5.** "Have you recently traveled outside the country?"

☐ **6.** "Do you smoke cigarettes or drink alcohol?"

Answer: 1, 2, 4, 5

Ⓜ Rationale: The nurse would first find out when the rash began; this can assist with the correct diagnosis. The nurse would also ask about allergies; rashes can occur when a person changes medications, eats new foods, or contacts pollen. It is also important to find out how the client has been treating the rash; some topical ointments or oral medications may worsen it. The nurse would ask about recent travel; exposure to foreign foods and environments can cause a rash. The client's age and smoking and drinking habits would not provide further insight into the rash or its cause.

Test-taking strategy: Analyze to determine what information the question asks for, which is specific assessment questions when a client presents with a rash. "Select all that apply" questions require considering each option to decide its merit. Begin selection by asking the benefit of the information received from the question and how it may relate to a rash. Review the anatomy and pathophysiology of the integumentary system and history-taking techniques if you had difficulty answering this question.

Client needs category: Physiological integrity

Client needs subcategory: Physiological adaptation

Cognitive level: Applying

12. While assessing a client's spine for abnormal curvatures, a nurse notes kyphosis. Using a picture diagram to instruct the client about kyphosis, in which location would the nurse note the structural abnormality?

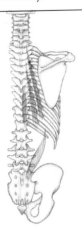

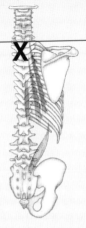

Ⓜ **Rationale:** Kyphosis is characterized by an accentuated forward curve of the thoracic area of the spine, which leads to a hunchback or slouching position. In adults, kyphosis can be caused by degenerative joint disease, fractures, trauma, and spondylolisthesis. Symptoms stem from the location of the deformity and include mild back pain, rounded back appearance, tenderness and stiffness in the spine, and, in extreme cases, difficulty breathing,

Test-taking strategy: Analyze to determine what information the question asks for, which is location of kyphosis. Recall that the location of the deformity is located in the thoracic region, thus identifying the following regions on the illustration: cervical (neck), thoracic (upper back), lumbar (lower back), and sacral (tailbone). Review the anatomy of the musculoskeletal system and techniques for assessing the spinal column if you had difficulty answering this question.

Client needs category: Health promotion and maintenance

Client needs subcategory: None

Cognitive level: Applying

13. Upon change of shift handoff, the oncoming nurse notes that the client has rales in the bases of the lungs. Identify the area on the client's vertebrae, representing the base of the lungs, where the nurse expects the breath sounds to stop at the end of expiration.

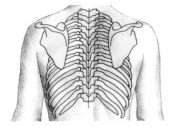

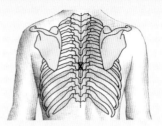

D **Rationale:** Based on posterior landmarks, the lungs extend from the cervical area to the level of the 10th thoracic vertebrae (T10) at the end of expiration.

Test-taking strategy: Analyze to determine what information the question asks for, which is the area on the posterior vertebrae where, when extending a horizontal line, the nurse anticipates to hear no further breath sounds. Recall that the lungs fill the thoracic cavity. Review the anatomy of the respiratory system and techniques for assessing the lungs if you had difficulty answering this question.

Client needs category: Health promotion and maintenance

Client needs subcategory: None

Cognitive level: Understanding

14. A nurse is performing an otoscopic examination on a client with ear pain. If the nurse suspects a potential diagnosis of otitis media, at which location would the nurse confirm the diagnosis?

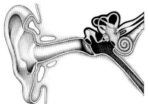

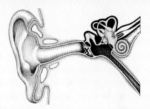

E **Rationale:** Otitis media is a middle ear infection located between the tympanic membrane and the inner ear. When an infection occurs, pressure increases, causing a bulging and red appearance of the tympanic membrane. Rupture of the tympanic membrane can occur.

Test-taking strategy: Analyze to determine what information the question asks for, which is the location of confirming evidence of otitis media. Consider the structure of the ear including the outer, middle, and inner ear. Upon otoscopic examination, a nurse can confirm symptoms associated with a middle ear infection at the location of the tympanic membrane. Review the anatomy and pathophysiology of the ear and assessment techniques if you had difficulty answering this question.

Client needs category: Physiological integrity

Client needs subcategory: Physiological adaptation

Cognitive level: Analyzing

15. A nurse is performing a cardiac assessment on a client with a suspected murmur. In which location would the nurse place the stethoscope to auscultate Erb's point?

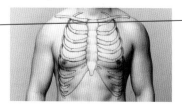

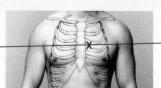

D **Rationale:** Erb's point is located at the third intercostal space, to the left of the sternum where S2 is best auscultated. Murmurs of both aortic and pulmonic origin may be heard at Erb's point.

Test-taking strategy: Analyze to determine what information the question asks for, which is the location of Erb's point. Recall that the places where valvular movement can be heard are not the actual anatomical location of the valves. Rather, the sounds represent the direction of blood flow. Review the anatomy of the cardiovascular system and techniques for assessing the heart if you had difficulty answering this question.

Client needs category: Health promotion and maintenance

Client needs subcategory: None

Cognitive level: Applying

---

16. A nurse is performing a head and neck assessment on a client who reports fatigue. When palpating the lymph nodes, in which location would the nurse palpate the occipital lymph nodes?

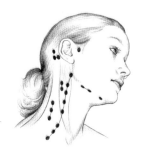

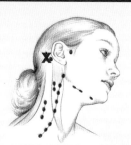

E **Rationale:** Lymph nodes are part of the lymphatic system. Lymph nodes vary in size depending upon the body status. There are clusters of head and neck lymph nodes. Using the pads of the fingers, the nurse would palpate the area behind the ears bilaterally to assess the occipital lymph nodes.

Test-taking strategy: Analyze to determine what information the question asks for, which is the location where the nurse would palpate the occipital lymph nodes. Use medical terminology (*occiput* means back of head) to identify the location of the lymph nodes. Review the anatomy of the lymphatic system and techniques for assessing lymph nodes if you had difficulty answering this question.

Client needs category: Physiological integrity

Client needs subcategory: Physiological adaptation

Cognitive level: Applying

17. The nurse is working in a public health clinic. Four clients present with various skin disorders. Which disorder requires disclosure to public health officials?

☐ **1.**

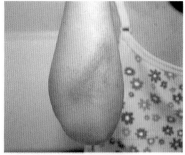

☐ **2.**

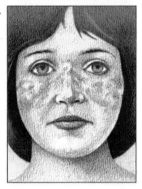

☐ **3.**

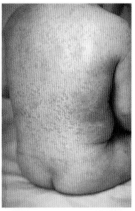

☐ **4.**

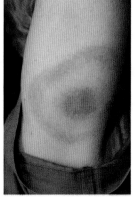

Ⓜ **Rationale**: Picture 3 is a rubella (German measles) rash. Rubella is a contagious viral infection known for its distinctive red rash. Because of vaccines, it is not seen often but is still classified as a communicable disease. Titers are drawn to document immunity. Picture 1 is poison ivy characterized by the red, raised, and sometimes fluid-filled vesicles. Picture 2 is a butterfly rash commonly seen in the autoimmune disease lupus. Picture 4 is the bull's eye rash commonly seen in Lyme's disease.

Test-taking strategy: Analyze to determine what information the question asks for, which is identification of a rash that is reportable. Recall that several communicable diseases need to be reported to the public health department because of their ability to spread from person to person. Observe each picture for defining characteristics to be able to identify the rash. Next, consider which rash is communicable in nature or in need of reporting. Review characteristics of rashes if you had difficulty answering this question.

Client needs category: Safe and effective care environment

Client needs subcategory: Safety and infection control

Cognitive level: Analyzing

18. A client has been admitted with severe abdominal pain that has lasted for the past 4 hours. Place in chronological order the correct sequence for conducting an abdominal assessment. All options must be used.

| **1.** Auscultate the client's abdomen. |
| **2.** Perform light palpation. |
| **3.** Ask the client to urinate. |
| **4.** Percuss the client's abdomen. |

G Rationale: The nurse would begin the assessment by having the client empty the bladder first. This allows the nurse to hear abdominal sounds better during auscultation. Because the client is in pain, the nurse would auscultate the abdomen before percussing it. Also, auscultation is usually performed before palpation and percussion since bowel sounds induced by percussion or palpation may mask abdominal bruits or pleural rubs. The nurse would then perform light palpation over the abdomen, leaving the painful area for last.

Test-taking strategy: Analyze to determine what information the question asks for, which is the sequence for conducting an abdominal assessment. Consider least disturbing to the abdomen first and leave painful procedures for last. Review techniques to use when assessing the abdomen if you had difficulty answering this question.

Client needs category: Physiological integrity

Client needs subcategory: Basic care and comfort

Cognitive level: Applying

19. Which is the highest **priority** performed by the nurse prior to completing this nursing action?

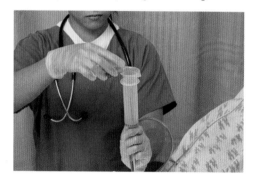

From Springhouse. *Lippincott's Visual Encyclopedia of Clinical Skills*. Philadelphia, PA: Wolters Kluwer Health, 2009.

☐ **1.** Place the client in the supine position.

☐ **2.** Assess stomach residual.

☐ **3.** Flush tube with 100 ml of water.

☐ **4.** Assess bowel sounds.

M Rationale: The picture provided is of a nurse administering a bolus tube feeding. Prior to administration, the highest priority would be to assess tube patency and stomach residual. Both can be accomplished by checking stomach residual. The client is placed in a Fowler position for feeding, not supine. It is common to flush the tube after patency and residual are assessed. Bowel sounds are assessed as part of a routine assessment.

Test-taking strategy: Analyze to determine what information the question is asking for, which is priority nursing action prior to a bolus gastrostomy tube feeding. Consider what step in the process is being completed (administering feeding) and what is a priority before this action. Always consider safety first. Determining the placement of the tube and status of the stomach is a priority. Review standard procedures for completing a gastrostomy tube feeding if you had difficulty answering this question.

Client needs category: Safe and effective care environment

Client needs subcategory: Management of care

Cognitive level: Analyzing

20. The nurse is assessing a client's deep tendon reflexes. Which graphic shows assessing the biceps reflex?

☐ **1.**

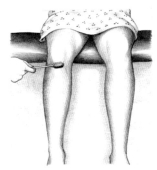

☐ **2.**

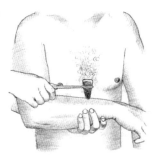

☐ **3.**

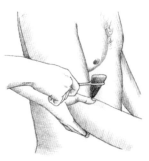

☐ **4.**

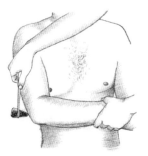

Ⓔ Rationale: To test the biceps reflex, the client's elbow is flexed at a 45° angle. The nurse places her/his thumb or index finger over the biceps tendon and strikes the digit with the pointed end of the reflex hammer, watching and feeling for the contraction of the biceps muscle and flexion of the forearm. Option 1 shows assessment of the patellar reflex. Option 2 shows assessment of the brachioradialis reflex. Option 4 shows assessment of the triceps reflex.

Test-taking strategy: Analyze to determine what information the question asks for, which is assessing the biceps reflex. Use the knowledge of anatomy to narrow the site of the reflex. Consider which illustration would elicit the bicep tendon. Review the location of bicep tendon and the proper technique for eliciting deep tendon reflexes if you had difficulty answering this question.

Client needs category: Physiological integrity
Client needs subcategory: Reduction of risk potential
Cognitive level: Analyzing

21. The nurse is assessing a client's respiratory pattern. Which graphic illustrates Kussmaul's respirations?

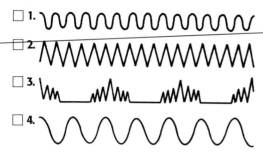

☐ 1.

☐ 2.

☐ 3.

☐ 4.

ⓜ Rationale: Kussmaul's breathing is characterized by rapid, deep breathing without pauses. Option 1 shows tachypnea (shallow breathing with an increased respiratory rate). Option 3 shows Cheyne-Stokes respirations (breaths gradually become faster and deeper than normal and then slower with intermittent periods of apnea). Option 4 shows hyperpnea (deep breathing at a normal rate).

Test-taking strategy: Analyze to determine what information the question asks for, which is characteristics of Kussmaul's breathing, and eliminate the other patterns. Recall that Kussmaul's respirations are deep and labored breathing patterns often associated with severe metabolic acidosis. Relate to the disease process and need to reduce carbon dioxide in the blood. Review Kussmaul's breathing pattern if you had difficulty answering this question.

Client needs category: Physiological integrity

Client needs subcategory: Reduction of risk potential

Cognitive level: Analyzing

---

22. A nurse is instructing a female client on the proper hygiene of wiping after toileting from front to back in order to prevent contamination of the urethra. Indicate which area of the genitourinary tract is prone to infection because of improper hygiene.

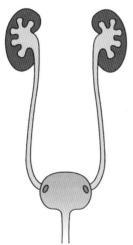

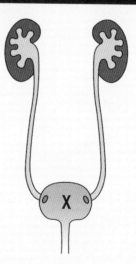

ⓜ Rationale: Because of the structure of the female genitourinary tract, bacteria causing infection can be introduced into the urethra and travel to the bladder to cause a bladder infection. One cause of a bladder infection is improper hygiene during toileting. Keeping the perineum as clean as possible diminishes the possibility of bladder infections because of contamination.

Test-taking strategy: Analyze to determine what information the question asks for, which is area of the genitourinary tract prone to infection because of improper hygiene. Consider the structure of the genitourinary tract and what structure is closest to the urethra opening. Recall that the bladder is prior to the kidney. Review the structure of the genitourinary tract if you had difficulty answering this question.

Client needs category: Physiological integrity

Client needs subcategory: Reduction of risk potential

Cognitive level: Applying

23. The nurse working in a long-term care facility notes changes in the client of confusion and change in vital signs. Upon consulting with the health care provider, lab work and a urine culture via an indwelling catheter are ordered. Place an X at the location the nurse would access the urine from the catheter.

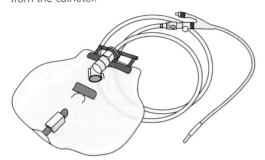

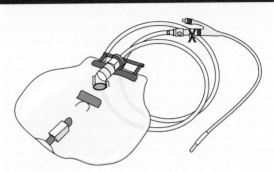

Answer:

Ⓜ Rationale: The nurse would wipe the port with an alcohol pad and then extract urine from the tubing via the port. To obtain urine via the port, clamp or kink the tubing obstructing the flow of urine through the tubing causing a "back up" of urine. This allows enough urine for the culture to be obtained.

Test-taking strategy: Analyze to determine what information the question asks for, which is procedure for accessing urine for a urine culture. First, note that the urine must be obtained via a sterile procedure since it is provided for a culture. Next, look to the catheter components that allow for urine access. Note one port is for urine samples and the other for balloon catheter inflation. Review the procedure for urine cultures via indwelling catheter if you have difficulty answering this question.

Client needs category: Physiological integrity

Client needs subcategory: Reduction of risk potential

Cognitive level: Applying

PART THREE

Medical–surgical nursing

Cardiovascular disorders

1. A client with sepsis and hypotension is being treated with dopamine hydrochloride. A nurse asks a colleague to double-check the dosage that the client is receiving. The 250-ml bag contains 400 mg of dopamine, the infusion pump is running at 23 ml/hour, and the client weighs 80 kg. How many micrograms per kilogram per minute is the client receiving? Record your answer using one decimal point.

_____ μg/kg/minute

Answer: 7.7

ⓓ Rationale: First, calculate how many milligrams per milliliter of dopamine are in the bag:

$$400 \text{ mg}/250 \text{ ml} = 1.6 \text{ mg/ml}.$$

Next, convert milligrams to micrograms:

$$1.6 \text{ mg/ml} \times 1,000 \text{ μg/mg} = 1,600 \text{ μg/ml}.$$

Lastly, calculate the dose:

$$\frac{1,600 \text{ μg}}{1 \text{ ml}} \times \frac{23 \text{ ml}}{60 \text{ minute}} \times \frac{1}{80 \text{ kg}} =$$

$$\frac{36,800 \text{ μg}}{4,800 \text{ kg/minute}} = 7.7 \text{ μg/kg/minute}$$

Test-taking strategy: Analyze to determine what information the question asks for, which is calculating the correct dosage of dopamine. Follow the steps outlined above. Logically think through the process of determining what is known and then convert to make sure that the calculation ends in the desired micrograms/kilogram/minute. Proofread your calculations. Review dosage calculations if you had difficulty answering this question.
Client needs category: Physiological integrity
Client needs subcategory: Pharmacological and parenteral therapies
Cognitive level: Analyzing

2. A client with deep vein thrombosis is receiving an intravenous infusion of heparin sodium at 1,500 units/hour. The concentration in the bag is 25,000 units/500 ml. How many milliliters would the nurse document as intake from this infusion for an 8-hour shift? Record your answer using a whole number.

_____ ml

Answer: 240

Ⓜ Rationale: First, calculate how many units are there in each milliliter of the medication:

$$25,000 \text{ units}/500 \text{ ml} = 50 \text{ units/ml}.$$

Next, calculate how many milliliters the client receives each hour:

$$1 \text{ ml}/50 \text{ units} \times 1,500 \text{ units/hour} = 30 \text{ ml/hour}.$$

Lastly, multiply by 8 hours:

$$30 \text{ ml/hour} \times 8 \text{ hours} = 240 \text{ ml}.$$

Test-taking strategy: Analyze to determine what information the question asks for, which is calculating the infusion of intravenous fluid over an 8-hour period and documenting for intake purposes. Follow the steps above to obtain the milliliters, and then multiply by the 8-hour period. Review calculation steps for giving intravenous medications based on time if you had difficulty answering this question.

Client needs category: Physiological integrity

Client needs subcategory: Pharmacological and parenteral therapies

Cognitive level: Analyzing

3. The nurse is evaluating an electrocardiogram (ECG) tracing. Which graphic shows the QT interval?

☐ **1.**

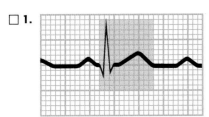

☐ **2.**

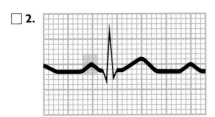

☐ **3.**

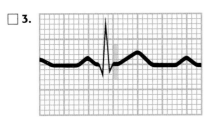

☐ **4.**

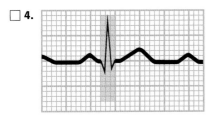

Ⓔ Rationale: The QT interval extends from the beginning of the QRS complex to the end of the T wave. It measures the time needed for ventricular depolarization and repolarization. Option 2 shows the PR interval, which is measured from the beginning of the P wave to the beginning of the QRS complex. It tracks the atrial impulse from the sinus node through the atrioventricular (AV) node. Option 3 shows the ST segment, which represents the end of ventricular depolarization. Option 4 shows the QRS duration and represents impulse conduction through the ventricles.

Test-taking strategy: Analyze to determine what information the question asks for, which is identifying the QT interval. Recall the components of the ECG waveform and what each represents in the function of the heart's conduction system. Consider which waveform is first initiated, and then follow the alphabetical sequence (P wave, then QRS complex, and lastly the T wave). Review the ECG waveform if you had difficulty answering this question.

Client needs category: Physiological integrity

Client needs subcategory: Reduction of risk potential

Cognitive level: Applying

4. A nurse is interpreting a client's ECG strip. If the PR interval measures four small blocks, how many seconds is the PR interval?

_____ seconds

Ⓜ **Rationale:** Each small block on a telemetry strip graph represents 0.04 second. So multiply as follows:

4 blocks × 0.04 second = 0.16 second.

Test-taking strategy: Analyze to determine what information the question asks for, which is the PR interval documented in seconds. An interval is a portion of the baseline and at least one wave. Intervals are measured on the horizontal axis in seconds. Recall the standard rate of each small block and multiply. Review ECG measurements and focus on second per block calculations if you had difficulty answering this question.

Client needs category: Physiological integrity

Client needs subcategory: Reduction of risk potential

Cognitive level: Applying

---

5. A nurse is caring for a client with Raynaud's phenomenon secondary to systemic lupus erythematosus (SLE). Which of the client statements demonstrates an understanding of the nurse's teaching about this disorder? Select all that apply.

☐ **1.** "My hands get pale and bluish and feel numb and painful when I'm really stressed."

☐ **2.** "I can't continue to wash dishes and do my cleaning because of this problem."

☐ **3.** "I don't need to report any other skin problems with my fingers or hands to my practitioner."

☐ **4.** "I probably got this disorder because I have lupus."

☐ **5.** "This problem is caused by a temporary lack of circulation in my hands."

☐ **6.** "Medication might help treat this problem."

Ⓜ **Rationale:** Raynaud's phenomenon causes blanching, cyanosis, coldness, numbness, and throbbing pain in the hands when the client is exposed to cold or stress. It is caused by episodic vasospasm in the small peripheral arteries and arterioles and can affect the feet as well as the hands. The phenomenon is commonly associated with connective tissue diseases such as lupus and may be alleviated by calcium channel blockers or adrenergic blockers. It does not limit the client's ability to function, although the symptoms are bothersome. Keeping the hands warm and learning to manage stressful situations effectively reduce the frequency of episodes. The disorder can progress to skin ulcerations and even gangrene in some clients, so all skin changes should be reported to the practitioner promptly.

Test-taking strategy: Analyze to determine what information the question asks for, which is correct client statements related to the Raynaud phenomenon. "Select all that apply" questions require considering each option to decide its merit. When assessing for correct statements, the true focus is correct information regarding Raynaud's phenomenon. Review the pathophysiology of Raynaud's phenomenon if you had difficulty answering this question.

Client needs category: Physiological integrity

Client needs subcategory: Physiological adaptation

Cognitive level: Analyzing

6. A nurse is evaluating the 12-lead ECG of a client experiencing an inferior wall myocardial infarction (MI). While conferring with the heath care team, which ECG changes associated with an evolving MI does the nurse correctly identify? Select all that apply.

☐ **1.** Notched T wave

☐ **2.** Presence of a U wave

☐ **3.** T-wave inversion

☐ **4.** Prolonged PR interval

☐ **5.** ST-segment elevation

Ⓒ Rationale: T-wave inversion, ST-segment elevation, and a pathological U wave (not simply a U wave that is present) are all signs of tissue hypoxia that occur during an MI. Ischemia results from inadequate blood supply to the myocardial tissue and is reflected by T-wave inversion. Injury results from prolonged ischemia and is reflected by ST-segment elevation. A notched T wave may indicate pericarditis in an adult client. A U wave may be apparent on a normal ECG; it represents repolarization of the Purkinje fibers. A prolonged PR interval is associated with first-degree AV block.

Test-taking strategy: Analyze to determine what information the question asks for, which is assessment of an MI and rhythm strip analysis. First, determine changes from a sinus rhythm and relate the changes to tissue ischemia. "Select all that apply" questions require considering each option to decide its merit. Review the clinical documentation of tissue hypoxia occurring during an MI if you had difficulty answering this question.

Client needs category: Physiological integrity

Client needs subcategory: Physiological adaptation

Cognitive level: Analyzing

7. A client with a bicuspid aortic valve has severe stenosis and is scheduled for valve replacement. The client expresses anxiety over the surgical procedure and future implications. As the nurse explains the normal blood flow through the heart, at which location would the nurse highlight the location of the faulty valve? Place an X at the valve location.

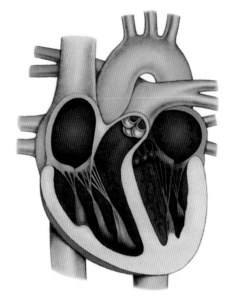

Answer:

Answer:

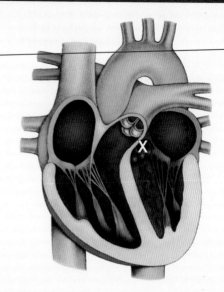

D Rationale: The aortic valve is located between the left ventricle and the aorta. It is one of the semilunar valves, which only has two leaflets instead of three. A person with a bicuspid aortic valve is at risk for aortic stenosis and aortic regurgitation. This impaired blood flow through the valve leads to increased pumping pressure of the left ventricle.

Test-taking strategy: Analyze to determine what information the question asks for, which is the location of the aortic valve. Consider the anatomy of the heart and knowledge of medical terminology to narrow the choices, if unsure. It may be helpful to visualize the path of blood flow to remind yourself of blood passing through valves. Review the placement of the aortic valve if you had difficulty answering this question.

Client needs category: Physiological integrity
Client needs subcategory: Physiological adaptation
Cognitive level: Applying

---

8. A nurse is awaiting the arrival of a client from the emergency department with a diagnosis of anterior wall myocardial infarction. In caring for this client, the nurse would be alert for which signs and symptoms of left-sided heart failure? Select all that apply.

☐ **1.** Jugular vein distention

☐ **2.** Hepatomegaly

☐ **3.** Dyspnea

☐ **4.** Crackles

☐ **5.** Tachycardia

☐ **6.** Right upper quadrant pain

Answer: 3, 4, 5

M Rationale: The right side of the heart is where the body deposits deoxygenated blood from the systematic circulation. Blood is then pumped from the right side of the heart to the lungs, where it exchanges CO_2 and picks up oxygen. Once the blood is oxygenated, it flows to the left side of the heart, which pumps to the rest of the body. Signs and symptoms of left-sided heart failure include dyspnea, orthopnea, and paroxysmal nocturnal dyspnea; fatigue; nonproductive cough and crackles; hemoptysis; point of maximal impulse displaced toward the left anterior axillary line; tachycardia; S_3 and S_4 heart sounds; and cool, pale skin. Jugular vein distention, hepatomegaly, and right upper quadrant pain are all signs of right-sided heart failure.

Test-taking strategy: Analyze to determine what information the question asks for, which is signs and symptoms of left-sided heart failure. "Select all that apply" questions require considering each option to decide its merit. Consider where the blood flows and what would happen if the left heart muscle was inefficient with pumping blood. Review the pathophysiology of heart failure, and review the differences between right- and left-sided heart failure if you had difficulty answering this question.

Client needs category: Physiological integrity

Client needs subcategory: Physiological adaptation

Cognitive level: Applying

---

9. A client is admitted to the emergency department after reporting acute chest pain radiating down the left arm. The client appears anxious, dyspneic, and diaphoretic. Which laboratory studies would the nurse anticipate? Select all that apply.

☐ **1.** Hemoglobin and hematocrit (HCT)

☐ **2.** Serum glucose

☐ **3.** Creatine kinase (CK)

☐ **4.** Troponin T and troponin I

☐ **5.** Myoglobin

☐ **6.** Blood urea nitrogen (BUN)

Answer: 3, 4, 5

Ⓒ Rationale: With myocardial ischemia or infarction, levels of CK, troponin T, and troponin I typically rise because of cellular damage. Myoglobin elevation is an early indicator of myocardial damage. Hemoglobin, HCT, serum glucose, and BUN levels do not provide information related to myocardial ischemia.

Test-taking strategy: Analyze to determine what information the question asks for, which is anticipating laboratory testing for a client with certain symptoms. First note that the client is experiencing symptoms of myocardial ischemia or infarction. Next, determine which laboratory test would provide helpful data in confirming or disproving a diagnosis. Review laboratory studies that diagnose cardiac problems or diagnostic findings for an MI if you had difficulty answering this question.

Client needs category: Physiological integrity

Client needs subcategory: Reduction of risk potential

Cognitive level: Applying

10. A client is prescribed lisinopril for the treatment of hypertension. The client asks a nurse about possible adverse effects. Which common adverse effects of angiotensin-converting enzyme (ACE) inhibitors would the nurse include in the teaching? Select all that apply.

☐ **1.** Constipation

☐ **2.** Dry cough

☐ **3.** Headache

☐ **4.** Hyperglycemia

☐ **5.** Hypotension

☐ **6.** Impotence

Ⓜ **Rationale:** ACE is a potent vasoconstrictor in the blood. By inhibiting the conversion of angiotensin I to angiotensin II, constriction of the vessel is limited. Dry cough, headache, and hypotension are all common adverse effects of lisinopril and other ACE inhibitors. Lisinopril may cause diarrhea, not constipation; it is not known to cause hyperglycemia or impotence.

Test-taking strategy: Analyze to determine what information the question asks for, which is adverse effects of ACE inhibitors. When considering adverse effects of medications, always consider an exaggerated effect of the therapeutic response. If the therapeutic response of ACE inhibitors is to lower blood pressure, the exaggerated response would be hypotension or conditions associated with hypotension. Another key to remember is what angiotensin does in the bloodstream and the response of bradykinin. Review the pharmacological class of ACE inhibitors, and focus on the common adverse effects if you had difficulty answering this question.

Client needs category: Physiological integrity

Client needs subcategory: Pharmacological and parenteral therapies

Cognitive level: Applying

11. A nurse is caring for a client who states crushing chest pressure over the sternum. The nurse places the client on oxygen and performs a 12-lead ECG. Identify the site where lead V_6 would be placed.

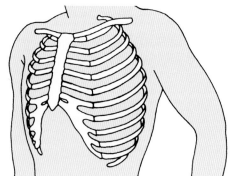

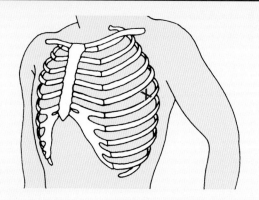

Ⓓ **Rationale:** The standard 12-lead ECG tracing is a representation of the heart's electrical activity recorded from electrodes on the body surface. The V_6 lead would be placed at the fifth intercostal space, at the midaxillary line. Correct lead placement is essential when performing a 12-lead ECG in order to accurately document the electrical potential of the heart. V_6 is one of the precordial leads and, combined with the other leads, records potential in the horizontal plane.

Test-taking strategy: Analyze to determine what information the question asks for, which is the location of an ECG lead. Review the placement of electrodes, keeping in mind that V_1 is placed medially and, as the numbers progress higher, the electrodes are placed more laterally. Visualize the placement of the leads using anatomical locations. Review ECG placement if you had difficulty answering this question.

Client needs category: Physiological integrity

Client needs subcategory: Reduction of risk potential

Cognitive level: Applying

---

12. A nurse is counseling a client about risk factors for hypertension. While reviewing the client's history, which information is consistent with the diagnosis of primary hypertension? Select all that apply.

☐ **1.** Obesity

☐ **2.** Glomerulonephritis

☐ **3.** Head injury

☐ **4.** Stress

☐ **5.** Hormonal contraceptive use

☐ **6.** High intake of sodium or saturated fat

Answer: 1, 4, 6

Ⓒ Rationale: Primary or essential hypertension has no identifiable cause and tends to develop gradually over years. Obesity, stress, high intake of sodium or saturated fat, and family history are all risk factors for primary hypertension. Diabetes mellitus, head injury, and hormonal contraceptive use are risk factors for secondary hypertension.

Test-taking strategy: Analyze to determine what information the question asks for, which is the risk factors associated with primary hypertension. Note the key word "primary" inferring original cause. Consider any cause that alone can elevate blood pressure. Review the risk factors and types of hypertension if you had difficulty answering this question.

Client needs category: Health promotion and maintenance

Client needs subcategory: None

Cognitive level: Applying

13. A client is brought to the emergency department and diagnosed with first-degree AV block. When instructing the spouse using a diagram, identify the area in the conduction cycle where this block occurs.

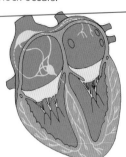

Answer:

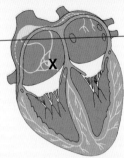

Ⓜ Rationale: An X is placed at the AV node located on the interatrial septum close to the tricuspid valve. First-degree AV block is a conduction disturbance in which electrical impulses flow normally from the sinoatrial node through the atria but are delayed at the AV node, thus prolonging the PR interval on an ECG. Although the conduction is slowed, there are no missed beats.

Test-taking strategy: Analyze to determine what information the question asks for, which is the site of specific blockage in the conduction cycle. Use the information of "AV" to narrow the location. Also, consider the electrical conduction pathway at the AV site. Review first-degree AV block and the anatomy of the heart and how it relates to cardiac electrical activity if you had difficulty answering this question.

Client needs category: Physiological integrity

Client needs subcategory: Physiological adaptation

Cognitive level: Applying

---

14. While managing a client's immediate post–cardiac catheterization period, which interventions are priorities? Select all that apply.

☐ **1.** Monitor vital signs every 15 minutes for the first hour.

☐ **2.** Assess all peripheral pulses frequently.

☐ **3.** Restrict the client to bed rest for 2 to 6 hours.

☐ **4.** Assess the catheter insertion site.

☐ **5.** Perform range-of-motion (ROM) exercises.

Answer: 1, 3, 4

Ⓒ Rationale: The key word is "immediate," indicating that care may be different throughout the recovery period. In the immediate period, the client's vital signs are typically monitored every 15 minutes for the first hour, then every 30 minutes for 2 hours or until vital signs are stable, and then every 4 hours or according to facility policy. All peripheral pulses do not require frequent assessment. (Always reflect on the word "all" in the selection.) The pulses in the affected extremity are usually assessed with every vital signs check. Clients typically remain in bed for 2 to 6 hours unless a special closure is used. The insertion site extremity is kept straight following the procedure, so ROM exercises would not be performed.

Test-taking strategy: Analyze to determine what information the question asks for, which is care of a client at a specific time. "Select all that apply" questions require considering each option to decide its merit. Focus on immediate assessment and postcatheterization care, which would include the recovery period. Consider anesthetic administered, medications, lab values, or incisions. Review post–cardiac catheterization interventions if you had difficulty answering this question.

Client needs category: Safe and effective care environment

Client needs subcategory: Management of care

Cognitive level: Applying

---

15. A nurse is caring for a client with a new prescription of digoxin. Which client statement would require further teaching about digoxin? Select all that apply.

☐ **1.** "I will take the digoxin at 9 AM daily."

☐ **2.** "I will take the digoxin with my antacids at night."

☐ **3.** "I will take my pulse before each dose of digoxin."

☐ **4.** "If I forget a dose, I will catch up by doubling the next dose."

☐ **5.** "I will notify my doctor if experiencing increased fatigue or muscle weakness."

☐ **6.** "I understand that I will need annual blood work to check therapeutic levels."

Answer: 2, 4, 6

Ⓜ **Rationale:** Digoxin is a cardiac glycoside that slows and strengthens the heart providing a more regular rhythm. Digoxin has a narrowed therapeutic window requiring every 2 weeks to monthly serum blood level monitoring initially. It is usually helpful for a client to take digoxin at a specific time each day to establish its blood level and routine for administration. The nurse would teach the client to take the pulse before each dose of digoxin and to notify the health care provider if the rate or rhythm changes, specifically if the rate drops to less than 60 beats/minute. The client would also be instructed to report increasing fatigue or muscle weakness immediately, as these are signs of digitalis (digoxin) toxicity. Antacids inhibit the absorption of digoxin, so digoxin would not be taken with these drugs. If the client forgets to take a dose of digoxin, he/she may take the missed dose only up to 12 hours later.

Test-taking strategy: Analyze to determine what information the question asks for, which is a client statement that would be incorrect or need further teaching/clarification. "Select all that apply" questions require considering each option to decide its merit. When teaching about a new medication, consider basic knowledge of therapeutic regimen, side effects, and unique considerations related to medication management. Consider factors effecting safe administration of digoxin, and review cardiac glycosides side effects if you had difficulty answering this question.

Client needs category: Health promotion and maintenance

Client needs subcategory: None

Cognitive level: Analyzing

16. A nurse is caring for a monitored client on the telemetry unit. When analyzing a cardiac monitor strip, the nurse notes an abnormality in the QRS wave on lead II. Identify the area in the conduction cycle of the heart where this abnormality occurs.

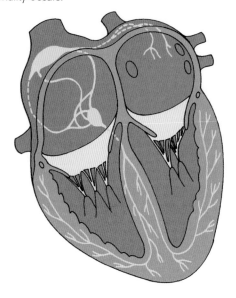

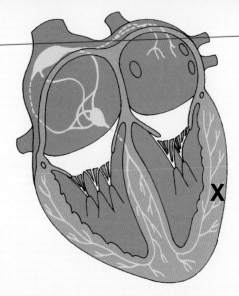

D Rationale: An X is placed on the left ventricle. The electrocardiography (ECG) shows the electrical activity of the heart over time as detected by electrodes attached to the body surface. Lead II is noted as a limb lead. The QRS complex reflects the rapid depolarization of the right and left ventricles; thus, an abnormality in the ventricular conduction will be reflected in the QRS wave.

Test-taking strategy: Analyze to determine what information the question asks for, which is the area in the conduction cycle reflected with an abnormality in the QRS wave. If unsure, remember that the QRS reflects large heart muscle activity of the ventricles and encompasses a large amount of the ECG tracing. Review the anatomy and electrical activity of the heart, and focus on the QRS wave of the cardiac cycle if you had difficulty answering this question.

Client needs category: Physiological integrity

Client needs subcategory: Physiological adaptation

Cognitive level: Analyzing

17. A nurse places electrodes on a collapsed individual who was visiting a hospitalized family member; the monitor exhibits the following. Which intervention would the nurse do **first**?

Progress notes

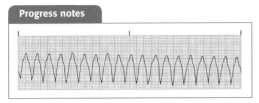

☐ **1.** Place the client on oxygen.

☐ **2.** Confirm the rhythm with a 12-lead ECG.

☐ **3.** Administer amiodarone I.V. as prescribed.

☐ **4.** Assess the client's airway, breathing, and circulation.

Answer: 4

E **Rationale:** The rhythm the client is experiencing is ventricular tachycardia (VT). Although all of the options listed are appropriate for someone with stable VT, it is not yet known whether the client's VT is stable, unstable, or pulseless. Therefore, the nurse must first assess the airway, breathing, circulation, and level of consciousness to establish the client's stability. Different actions are required if the client's VT is unstable or pulseless.

Test-taking strategy: Analyze to determine what information the question asks for, which is what intervention would be done first following rhythm/waveform analysis. Note the key word "first" indicating a priority response. Recall the unusual waveform pattern and interpret as an emergency due to the inability of the heart to perfuse. Remember to treat the client, not the rhythm strip. Review ECG waveforms and nursing action if you had difficulty answering this question.

Client needs category: Physiological integrity

Client needs subcategory: Reduction of risk potential

Cognitive level: Analyzing

---

18. A client is hospitalized following a report of dizziness, shortness of breath, and chest pain. Based on the ECG rhythm, the client is scheduled for a transesophageal echocardiogram (TEE) today. Which nursing interventions would be appropriate at this time?

Progress notes

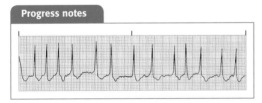

☐ **1.** Initiate a heparin drip.

☐ **2.** Encourage the client to ambulate to the bathroom.

☐ **3.** Prepare the client for immediate electrical cardioversion.

☐ **4.** Administer oxygen via nasal cannula as prescribed.

Answer: 4

M **Rationale:** After analyzing the waveform, it is noted that the client is experiencing atrial fibrillation and is symptomatic; therefore, because of the client's symptoms, the nurse would administer oxygen. Initiating a medication such as a heparin requires a health care provider order. To ensure safety, the nurse should not encourage ambulation when the client is experiencing dizziness, shortness of breath, or chest pain. A TEE is sometimes prescribed before electrical cardioversion to ensure there are no clots in the atria; if none are found, then the cardioversion can be safely performed.

Test-taking strategy: Analyze to determine what information the question asks for, which is nursing interventions prior to a TEE. First, consider the rhythm and its clinical manifestations. Once identified, relate atrial fibrillation and TEE. Review ECG waveforms, atrial fibrillation, and TEEs if you had difficulty answering this question.

Client needs category: Physiological integrity

Client needs subcategory: Reduction of risk potential

Cognitive level: Analyzing

19. A client who underwent cardiac surgery has been prescribed morphine sulfate 2 mg intravenously for pain. The morphine sulfate is packaged as 2 mg/ml. The nurse dilutes the medication in 4 ml of sterile water and prepares to administer the medication over 5 minutes. If the nurse administers 1 ml of fluid every minute, how many milligrams of morphine will be administered per minute? Record your answer using one decimal point.

_____ mg/minute

Ⓜ **Rationale:** The nurse would first determine how much fluid the medication is in.

1 ml of morphine + 4 ml of sterile water
= 5 ml of fluid

$$\frac{2\ mg}{5\ mg} = \frac{X\ ml}{1\ ml} = 2\ mg/ml = 5X$$

$$\frac{2\ mg/ml = 5X}{5} = 0.4\ mg/ml.$$

Since the nurse is administering 1 ml of fluid every minute, the nurse is administering 0.4 mg of morphine every minute.

Test-taking strategy: Analyze to determine what information the question asks for, which is amount (mg) of morphine administered. Specifically, consider how many milliliters the nurse will administer in 1 minute after diluting 1 ml of morphine with 4 ml of sterile water, and review dosage calculation formulas. Proofread your math calculations. Review drug dosage calculations when solving for X if you had difficulty answering this question.

Client needs category: Physiological integrity

Client needs subcategory: Pharmacological and parenteral therapies

Cognitive level: Analyzing

20. The nurse is preparing to interpret an ECG rhythm strip. Place the following steps for ECG rhythm analysis from first to last, in chronological order. All options must be used.

1. Measure the QRS duration.

2. Interpret the rhythm.

3. Analyze the P waves.

4. Determine the rate and rhythm.

5. Measure the PR interval.

Ⓜ Rationale: ECG rhythm strip analysis requires a systematic approach using a five-step method. First, determine the rate and rhythm of both the atria and the ventricles. Then, analyze the P waves for consistency. Next, measure the PR interval and then the QRS duration. Finally, you can interpret the rhythm with all of the information that has been collected. If the nurse has answered all five steps within normal limits, the client is in sinus rhythm. The greater the number of questions that the nurse notes inconsistent with normal limits, the greater the abnormal conduction through the heart.

Test-taking strategy: Analyze to determine what information the question asks for, which is rhythm strip analysis. Recall the above method of analysis. Note that the analysis notes deviations from normal; thus, understanding the heart's conduction is essential. Review the analysis of rhythm strips using the five-step method if you had difficulty answering this question.

Client needs category: Safe and effective care environment

Client needs subcategory: Management of care

Cognitive level: Analyzing

21. The nurse is evaluating the cardiac function of a client with history of left ventricular hypertrophy and new diltiazem administration. Which client statements indicate adequate cardiac functioning? Select all that apply.

- ☐ **1.** "I am sleeping well in the second floor bedroom."
- ☐ **2.** "I am tolerating my new low-fat diet."
- ☐ **3.** "My blood pressure has been consistently in the 130/70 range."
- ☐ **4.** "I am completing all of my activities of daily living independently."
- ☐ **5.** "In the morning, I notice 2 plus edema in my ankles."
- ☐ **6.** "My lab results reveal a serum potassium of 3.5 mEq/L (3.5 mmol/L)."

Ⓒ Rationale: When evaluating cardiac functioning, assess for client statements indicating normal client activities being completed successfully. Positive activities include sleeping well even after traveling up stairs, the blood pressure within normal limits, and completing activities of daily living independently. It is good that the client is tolerating the low-fat diet and has a normal serum potassium level, but that is not related to adequate cardiac functioning. Pitting edema in the morning is a sign of cardiac compromise.

Test-taking strategy: Analyze to determine what information the question asks for, which is statements indicating adequate cardiac function. Recall that an enlarged ventricle leads to insufficient cardiac pumping/circulation; thus, adequate functioning following medication administration allows for regular activities to be completed.

Client needs category: Physiological integrity

Client needs subcategory: Physiological adaptation

Cognitive level: Analyzing

22. A nurse is presenting health information at a community organization when one of the attendees passes out. The nurse assesses the attendee as being unresponsive. Indicate how the nurse would respond by placing the following actions in chronological order. All options must be used.

| **1.** Appoint a person to call 911. |
| **2.** Check for a pulse. |
| **3.** Deliver two rescue breaths. |
| **4.** Check for normal breathing. |
| **5.** Perform chest compressions. |
| **6.** Perform a head tilt–chin lift maneuver. |

Answer: 1, 5, 6, 4, 3, 2

Ⓓ **Rationale:** Following the 2015 American Heart Association (AHA) guidelines for cardiopulmonary resuscitation (CPR), the rescuer would attempt to awaken the victim, then activate the emergency response system, and get an automatic external defibrillator (AED) or appoint another person to do this. Past guidelines include checking for a pulse; however, current guidelines move the pulse check later in the sequence. One of the changes was removing the old "Look, Listen, and Feel" process. Lay rescuers and even experienced health care providers may have a hard time finding a pulse and spend too long looking for one before starting CPR, thus changes state to feel for a pulse for no longer than 10 seconds. The next step is to give 30 chest compressions. Next, the rescuer opens the airway with the head tilt–chin lift or jaw thrust maneuver and checks for breathing. If breathing is not detected, the rescuer gives two rescue breaths, checks for a pulse, and immediately resumes chest compressions. The rescuer would use the AED as soon as it arrives.

Test-taking strategy: Analyze to determine what information the question asks for, which is arranging the options in an order in which they would be performed during resuscitation. Note the above sequence. The 2015 AHA guidelines for CPR stress administering compressions for restoring circulation in a pulseless victim. Review current guidelines if you had difficulty answering this question.

Client needs category: Safe and effective care environment

Client needs subcategory: Management of care

Cognitive level: Applying

23. The nurse is caring for a client during the postsurgical period after having a right femoral–popliteal bypass graft. The nurse enters the room to conduct a nursing assessment and care. Order the nurse's actions according to **priority.** All options must be used.

| **1.** Offer clear fluids. |
| **2.** Assess pain using 0 to 10 scale. |
| **3.** Assess incision site. |
| **4.** Assess lung fields. |
| **5.** Assess peripheral pulses. |
| **6.** Instruct on client positioning. |

Answer: 5, 3, 2, 4, 6, 1

Ⓓ **Rationale:** Following a femoral–popliteal bypass, it is most important to assess circulation to the lower extremity by assessing the quality of the right pedal (peripheral) pulse. By assessing a strong pulse, the nurse knows that the graft is functioning. Next, the nurse assesses the incision site noting any bleeding. Lung sounds are assessed since the client had anesthesia. Lastly, the nurse assesses the client's pain level and obtains medication as appropriate. Before leaving the room, the nurse positions the client and then obtains fluids.

Test-taking strategy: Analyze to determine what information the question asks for, which is nursing priorities when a client returns from a femoral–popliteal bypass graft. Recall that assessment is completed before any intervention. Always consider the reason for the surgical procedure and potential adverse effect as an assessment priority. Review care of the postsurgical femoral–popliteal bypass graft if you had difficulty answering this question.

Client needs category: Physiological integrity

Client needs subcategory: Physiological adaptation

Cognitive level: Analyzing

Respiratory disorders

1. The nurse is caring for a client who states an increase in dyspnea. Which intervention would the nurse perform **first?**

☐ **1.**

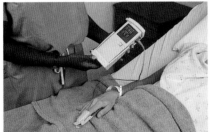

☐ **2.**

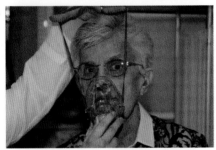

☐ **3.**

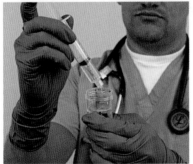

☐ **4.**

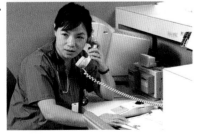

2. A nurse is caring for a client with pneumonia who was prescribed ceftriaxone oral suspension 600 mg once daily. The medication label indicates that the strength is 125 mg/5 ml. How many milliliters of medication would the nurse pour to administer the correct dose? Record your answer as a whole number.

_____ ml

Answer: 24

ⓔ **Rationale:** Use the following formula to calculate the drug dosage:

Dose on hand/quantity on hand = dose desired/X.

Plug in the values for this equation and solve for X:

$$125 \text{ mg/5 ml} = 600 \text{ mg/}X$$
$$X = 24 \text{ ml.}$$

Test-taking strategy: Analyze to determine what information the question asks for, which is the total amount of milliliters to be administered for the prescribed dose. Review dosage calculations using the ratio-and-proportion method. Recall that this method uses all known factors to determine the unknown (milliliter to be administered). Proofread your math calculations for accuracy. Review drug dosage calculations if you had difficulty answering this question.

Client needs category: Physiological integrity

Client needs subcategory: Pharmacological and parenteral therapies

Cognitive level: Applying

---

3. A nurse is caring for a client with a chest tube connected to a three-chamber drainage system without suction. On the illustration below, identify which chamber the nurse will mark to record the current drainage level.

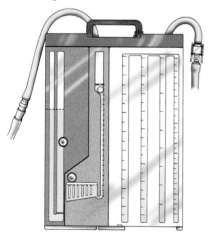

Answer:

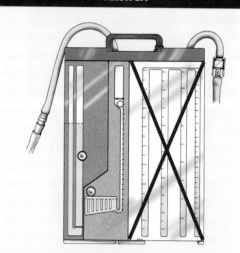

ⓔ **Rationale:** A chest tube drains blood, fluid, and air from around the lungs. The drainage system, which the nurse measures each shift, is on the right. It has three calibrated chambers that show the amount of drainage collected. When the first chamber fills, drainage empties into the second; when the second chamber fills, drainage flows into the third. The water seal chamber is located in the center. The suction control chamber is on the left.

Test-taking strategy: Analyze to determine what information the question asks for, which is where drainage is collected in a chest drainage system. Recall that at the beginning of each shift, the nurse would assess the color, consistency, and amount of drainage present. The previous nurse marks the level of drainage on the collection chamber with the date and time. Review the care and components of chest tube drainage systems if you had difficulty answering this question.

Client needs category: Physiological integrity

Client needs subcategory: Reduction of risk potential

Cognitive level: Applying

4. A client comes to the emergency department with status asthmaticus. Based on the documentation noted below, the nurse suspects that the client has what abnormality?

Progress notes	
2/1/16	Client wheezing. RR 44, BP 140/90, P 104,
1830	T 98.4°F (36.9°C). ABG results show pH 7.52,
	PaCO₂ 30 mm Hg (4.0 kPa), HCO₃⁻ 26 mEq/L
	(26 mmol/L), and PO₂ 77 mm Hg (10.2 kPa).
	——————————————— C. Wynn, RN

☐ **1.** Respiratory acidosis

☐ **2.** Respiratory alkalosis

☐ **3.** Metabolic acidosis

☐ **4.** Metabolic alkalosis

Answer: 2

Ⓔ **Rationale:** Following review of the nursing documentation, the nurse notes respiratory alkalosis related to alveolar hyperventilation. Respiratory alkalosis is marked by an increase in pH to more than 7.45 and a concurrent decrease in partial pressure of arterial carbon dioxide ($PaCO_2$) to less than 35 mm Hg (4.7 kPa). Metabolic alkalosis shows the same increase in pH but also an increased bicarbonate level and normal $PaCO_2$ (may be elevated also if compensatory mechanisms are working). Respiratory acidosis is marked by a decrease in pH and an elevated $PaCO_2$ and a normal to high bicarbonate level. Metabolic acidosis is characterized by a decreased bicarbonate level and a normal to low $PaCO_2$.

Test-taking strategy: Analyze to determine what information the question asks for, which is identification of a client's condition using data. First, consider the disease process and note abnormalities in assessment and lab data, which points to a respiratory complication. Next, evaluate lab results. Review criteria for blood gas values, acid–base disturbances, and compensation and the disease process of status asthmaticus if you had difficulty answering this question.

Client needs category: Physiological integrity

Client needs subcategory: Physiological adaptation

Cognitive level: Analyzing

5. The nurse is caring for a client following a segmental resection of the lung because of the presence of a malignant mass. The nurse explains to the family the difference between various types of lung excisions. Which picture **best** documents a segmental resection?

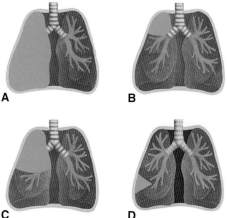

A

B

C

D

Answer: B

Ⓓ Rationale: A segmental resection is the removal of a portion of the lung smaller than an entire lobe. This procedure is often chosen when a cancerous tumor is small or the cell type in a specific area has not been determined. Picture A is a pneumonectomy, which is the removal of the entire lung. Picture C is a lobectomy, which is the removal of an entire lobe. A wedge resection removes a small piece of tissue and ensures a margin of healthy tissue surrounding.

Test-taking strategy: Analyze to determine what information the question asks for, which is identification of a segmental resection of the lung. Consider that each type removes a different amount of lung tissue. Also, use knowledge of medical terminology to identify terms such as "pneumo" meaning lung, "lobe" being a portion of the lung, and "ectomy" meaning removal. Review various lung excisions if you had difficulty answering this question.

Client needs category: Physiological integrity

Client needs subcategory: Physiological adaptation

Cognitive level: Analyzing

---

6. A nurse is preparing a staff education program on innovative devices in pulmonary circulation. Beginning with basic concepts, place the following structures in chronological order to trace the pathway of normal pulmonary circulation. All options must be used.

1. Pulmonary vein
2. Right ventricle
3. Pulmonary artery
4. Arterioles
5. Alveoli
6. Left atrium

Answer: 2, 3, 4, 5, 1, 6

Ⓜ Rationale: Pulmonary circulation is the movement of blood from the heart, to the lungs, and back to the heart again. Deoxygenated blood is ejected from the right ventricle into the pulmonary artery and then into the lungs via the arterioles and alveoli. The pulmonary vein then carries oxygenated blood back to the left atrium for circulation throughout the body.

Test-taking strategy: Analyze to determine what information the question asks for, which is the path of pulmonary circulation. Of the choices, select the right ventricle as a point of origin with deoxygenated blood. Continue through the process until oxygen-rich blood is pumped from the heart to the body systems. Review the cardiopulmonary system and pulmonary circulation if you had difficulty answering this question.

Client needs category: Physiological integrity

Client needs subcategory: Physiological adaptation

Cognitive level: Understanding

7. A client with a suspected pulmonary embolus is brought to the emergency department stating shortness of breath and chest pain. Which additional signs and symptoms are anticipated? Select all that apply.

☐ **1.** Anxiety

☐ **2.** Thick green sputum

☐ **3.** Bradycardia

☐ **4.** Frothy sputum

☐ **5.** Tachycardia

☐ **6.** Blood-tinged sputum

Ⓒ Rationale: A pulmonary embolism (PE) is a blockage to one or more arteries in the lungs. In addition to pleuritic chest pain and dyspnea, a client with a pulmonary embolus may be anxious and present with a low-grade fever, tachycardia, and blood-tinged sputum. Thick green sputum would indicate infection, and frothy sputum would indicate pulmonary edema. A client with a pulmonary embolus is tachycardic (to compensate for decreased oxygen supply), not bradycardic.

Test-taking strategy: Analyze to determine what information the question asks for, which is signs and symptoms of a PE. "Select all that apply" questions require considering each option to decide its merit. Recall that a PE is a medical emergency with symptoms of respiratory compromise. Review the pathophysiology and clinical manifestations of a PE if you had difficulty answering this question.

Client needs category: Physiological integrity

Client needs subcategory: Physiological adaptation

Cognitive level: Applying

8. A client with chronic obstructive pulmonary disease (COPD) is being evaluated for a lung transplant. Which initial assessment data would the nurse anticipate? Select all that apply.

☐ **1.** Decreased respiratory rate

☐ **2.** Dyspnea on exertion

☐ **3.** Barrel chest

☐ **4.** Shortened expiratory phase

☐ **5.** Clubbed fingers and toes

☐ **6.** Fever

Ⓒ Rationale: COPD is one of the most common lung diseases making it difficult to breathe. Severity of the illness varies. Typical findings for clients with COPD include dyspnea on exertion, a barrel chest, and clubbed fingers and toes. Clients with COPD are usually tachypneic with a prolonged expiratory phase. Fever is not associated with COPD, unless an infection is also present.

Test-taking strategy: Analyze to determine what information the question asks for, which is common symptoms of a client with severe COPD needing a lung transplant. Consider symptoms associated with severe respiratory compromise. "Select all that apply" questions require considering each option to decide its merit. Review the anatomy and physiology of the respiratory system, and focus on the pathophysiology and clinical manifestations of COPD if you had difficulty answering this question.

Client needs category: Physiological integrity

Client needs subcategory: Physiological adaptation

Cognitive level: Applying

9. A nurse is caring for a client with a wound infection who develops septic shock. The nurse notes the following arterial blood gas results: pH of 7.25, PaCO$_2$ of 43 mm Hg (43 mmol/L), partial pressure of arterial oxygen (PaO$_2$) of 70 mm Hg (9.31 kPa), and bicarbonate (HCO$_3^-$) of 18 mEq/L (18 mmol/L). According to the oxyhemoglobin dissociation curve, the nurse would be most correct to highlight which finding on shift report?

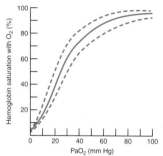

☐ **1.** The client's profile reflects alkalosis.

☐ **2.** The client's hemoglobin saturation is close to 100%.

☐ **3.** The client's oxyhemoglobin curve is shifted to the left.

☐ **4.** The client's hemoglobin saturation is close to 85%.

ⓜ The acidic condition of the blood shifts the oxyhemoglobin dissociation curve to the right. This enables oxygen molecules to unload more easily from the hemoglobin. According to the client's PaO$_2$ value of 70 mm Hg (9.31 kPa) and pH value of 7.25, his hemoglobin saturation is close to 85%.

Test-taking strategy: Analyze to determine what information the question asks for, which is using data to evaluate client status. First, note the blood pH and arterial blood gas data and relate to which statement is correct. Review concepts of arterial blood gases, oxyhemoglobin dissociation curve, and gas exchange and respiratory system physiology if you had difficulty answering this question.

Client needs category: Physiological integrity

Client needs subcategory: Physiological adaptation

Cognitive level: Evaluating

---

10. A nurse is caring for a client with a traumatic injury and developing tension pneumothorax. Which assessment data would be of concern? Select all that apply.

☐ **1.** Decreased cardiac output

☐ **2.** Flattened neck veins

☐ **3.** Tracheal deviation to the affected side

☐ **4.** Hypotension

☐ **5.** Tracheal deviation to the unaffected side

☐ **6.** Bradypnea

ⓒ **Rationale:** Tension pneumothorax results when air in the pleural space is under higher pressure than air in the adjacent lung. The site of the rupture of the pleural space acts as a one-way valve, allowing the air to enter on inspiration but not to escape on expiration. The air presses against the mediastinum, causing a tracheal shift to the unaffected side and decreased venous return (reflected by decreased cardiac output and hypotension). Neck veins bulge with tension pneumothorax. This also leads to compensatory tachycardia and tachypnea.

Test-taking strategy: Analyze to determine what information the question asks for, which is signs of a developing tension pneumothorax. "Select all that apply" questions require considering each option to decide its merit. Recall the pathophysiology of the tension pneumothorax producing tension in the thoracic cavity, and relate clinical manifestations of a high-pressure environment. Review respiratory system physiology and assessment data if you had difficulty answering this question.

Client needs category: Physiological integrity

Client needs subcategory: Physiological adaptation

Cognitive level: Applying

---

11. A nurse is caring for a client diagnosed with right middle lobe pneumonia at the last health care provider's appointment. The client has completed albuterol breathing treatments and a full dose of antibiotics. When assessing the client's lung fields, place an X at the location at which the nurse would confirm improved air movement.

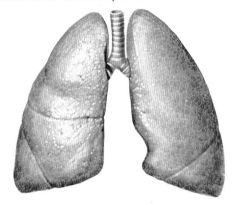

Answer:

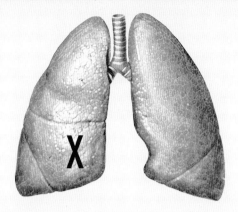

Ⓔ Rationale: Following treatment of right middle lobe pneumonia, the nurse would anticipate improved air movement throughout the right middle lobe. Note the placement of the X. The right lung is composed of three lobes: the right upper lobe, right middle lobe, and right lower lobe. The left lung is made up of only two lobes: the left upper lobe and left lower lobe. When assessing the anterior chest, the right lung is on the examiner's left.

Test-taking strategy: Analyze to determine what information the question asks for, which is identifying the area of pneumonia/area of improved air movement. The key is to recall which lung (right) has three lobes. Review the anatomy of the respiratory system and breath sound assessment techniques if you had difficulty answering this question.

Client needs category: Health promotion and maintenance

Client needs subcategory: None

Cognitive level: Applying

12. A client is prescribed continuous positive airway pressure (CPAP) therapy for sleep apnea. When troubleshooting a leak in the system, identify on the illustration below where the mechanism maintaining the positive end-expiratory pressure is located.

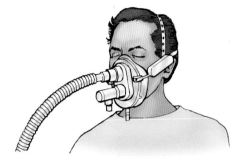

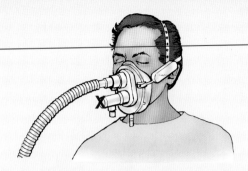

ⓓ Rationale: The X is placed on the valve below the location of the oxygen tubing connecting to the face mask. CPAP ventilation maintains positive pressure in the airways throughout the respiratory cycle. The inlet valve attaches the oxygen tubing to the face mask, and the positive end-expiratory pressure valve, located below, maintains the pressure. CPAP can be used with or without a ventilator in intubated and nonintubated clients and can be administered just nasally for a less constrictive feeling. In addition to sleep apnea, CPAP is used to treat respiratory distress syndrome, pulmonary edema, pulmonary emboli, bronchiolitis, pneumonitis, viral pneumonia, and postoperative atelectasis.

Test-taking strategy: Analyze to determine what information the question asks for, which is location of the positive pressure mechanism. If unsure, review the structure of the mask. Consider attachments for the incoming air, and look for a structure maintaining the pressure in the system and not allowing the air to escape. Review the structure and function of a CPAP machine if you had difficulty answering this question.

Client needs category: Physiological integrity

Client needs subcategory: Physiological adaptation

Cognitive level: Applying

13. A nurse is evaluating a client with primary pulmonary hypertension for a heart–lung transplant. Which medication treatment would the nurse anticipate to be included in the plan of care? Select all that apply.

☐ **1.** Oxygen therapy

☐ **2.** Aminoglycosides

☐ **3.** Diuretics

☐ **4.** Vasodilators

☐ **5.** Antihistamines

☐ **6.** Sulfonamides

Answer: 1, 3, 4

ⓜ Rationale: Pulmonary hypertension is an increase in blood pressure in the pulmonary arteries, pulmonary vein, or pulmonary capillary. This increase in pressure makes it more difficult for the blood to flow through the lungs. Oxygen, diuretics, and vasodilators are among the common medication therapies used to treat pulmonary hypertension. Other treatments include fluid restriction, digoxin, calcium channel blockers, β-adrenergic blockers, and bronchodilators. Aminoglycosides and sulfonamides are antibiotics used to treat infections. Antihistamines are indicated to treat allergies, pruritus, vertigo, nausea, and vomiting; to promote sedation; and to suppress cough.

Test-taking strategy: Analyze to determine what information the question asks for, which is medication regimens for pulmonary hypertension. "Select all that apply" questions require considering each option to decide its merit. Consider the pathophysiology of pulmonary hypertension, and focus on the benefits of each treatment. Since pulmonary hypertension decreases pulmonary blood flow, oxygen therapy is helpful. Next, focus on each medication classification and its ability to decrease hypertension. Review anticipated medical treatments for pulmonary hypertension if you had difficulty answering this question.

Client needs category: Physiological integrity

Client needs subcategory: Pharmacological and parenteral therapies

Cognitive level: Applying

14. A nurse notes crackles on a client diagnosed with right lower lobe atelectasis. In which area would the nurse place the stethoscope to assess the adventitious breath sounds?

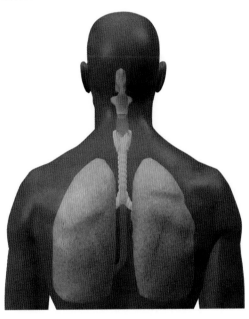

Credit: LifeART image copyright © 2016 Lippincott Williams & Wilkins. All rights reserved.

Answer:

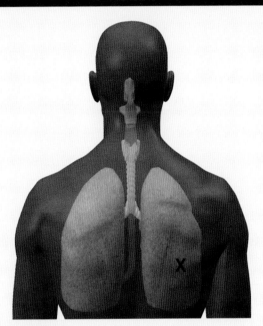

Ⓔ Rationale: Note the placement of the X. To auscultate the right lower lobe posteriorly, the nurse would place the stethoscope between T-3 and T-10 on the right side.

Test-taking strategy: Analyze to determine what information the question asks for, which is site of the right lower lobe as that is the location of the crackles. Recall the position of the lobes in the thoracic cavity. Review the thoracic cavity landmarks associated with lung/lobe positions if you had difficulty answering this question.

Client needs category: Physiological integrity

Client needs subcategory: Reduction of risk potential

Cognitive level: Applying

15. A fireman is admitted with superficial skin wounds and a sprained back following an intense fire. No respiratory concerns are verbalized. Nearly 24 hours after admission, the fireman reports dyspnea, a harsh cough, and hoarseness. Which nursing interventions would the nurse add to the plan of care? Select all that apply.

☐ **1.** Monitor for fever.

☐ **2.** Prepare the chest for chest tube insertion.

☐ **3.** Auscultate the lungs for adventitious breath sounds.

☐ **4.** Assess for increased pulse rate.

☐ **5.** Monitor for increased anxiety levels.

Answer: 3, 4, 5

Ⓜ Rationale: More than half of all clients with pulmonary involvement following inhalation injury do not immediately demonstrate pulmonary signs. Any client with possible inhalation injury must be observed for at least 24 hours for possible respiratory complications. Maintaining increased oxygen saturation levels is essential, especially following a carbon monoxide inhalation injury, to prevent the development of carboxyhemoglobin, which competes with oxygen for available hemoglobin. The client does not typically develop a fever with inhalation injury, but may progress to acute respiratory syndrome with bilateral lung infiltrates, cardiac involvement with tachycardia, and increasing anxiety because of oxygen starvation. A chest tube is not indicated.

Test-taking strategy: Analyze to determine what information the question asks for, which is nursing interventions for an inhalation injury. "Select all that apply" questions require considering each option to decide its merit. Focus on the information gathered during the nursing assessment and relate to clinical manifestations of inhalation injury. Keep in mind signs of respiratory compromise as priority nursing interventions. Review inhalation injury and respiratory interventions if you had difficulty answering this question.

Client needs category: Physiological integrity

Client needs subcategory: Physiological adaptation

Cognitive level: Analyzing

---

16. A nurse is caring for a client with history of heart failure and presenting with symptoms indicating a pulmonary embolism. The nurse documents admission findings of sudden shortness of breath, chest pain, and immobility. Which nursing diagnoses are admission priorities? Select all that apply.

☐ **1.** Activity intolerance related to inadequate oxygenation

☐ **2.** Anxiety related to breathlessness

☐ **3.** Disturbed sleep pattern related to restlessness in the night

☐ **4.** Ineffective breathing pattern related to hypoxia

☐ **5.** Risk for decreased cardiac output related to failure of the left ventricle

☐ **6.** Social isolation related to hospitalization

Answer: 1, 2, 4, 5

Ⓜ Rationale: When planning care, the nurse would select nursing diagnoses that anticipate pulmonary compromise secondary to reduction of air, blood, and gas exchange because these are ensuing complications that can develop from a pulmonary embolism, particularly in a client with a history of heart failure. The prudent nurse would analyze the client's condition and anticipate the need for safe, supportive nursing interventions related to the client's activity intolerance, anxiety, ineffective breathing, and risk for decreased oxygen output. The client history does not indicate that this client has difficulty sleeping, and although social isolation is important to consider, it is not a priority.

Test-taking strategy: Analyze to determine what information the question asks for, which is priority admission nursing diagnosis. "Select all that apply"

questions require considering each option to decide its merit. The key word is "admission," which focuses on the client's documented current symptoms. Review the pathophysiology and clinical manifestations of a pulmonary embolism as it relates to applicable nursing diagnoses if you had difficulty answering this question.

Client needs category: Safe and effective care environment

Client needs subcategory: Management of care

Cognitive level: Analyzing

---

17. The nurse is caring for a senior citizen who lives alone. When evaluating the effectiveness of adding Advair (fluticasone propionate and salmeterol) to the chronic obstructive airway disease (COPD) client's medication regimen, which client statements would support symptom improvement? Select all that apply.

☐ **1.** "I have noted an increase in sputum production."

☐ **2.** "I have begun walking up stairs to use the bathroom."

☐ **3.** "I can rely on the medication when I have an exacerbation of symptoms."

☐ **4.** "I seem to cough more in the morning hours."

☐ **5.** "I can now push my granddaughter on the swings when she visits."

☐ **6.** "The nurse aide no longer comes to the house to help me bathe."

Answer: 2, 5, 6

Ⓜ **Rationale:** Advair (fluticasone propionate and salmeterol) is a combination of steroid and bronchodilator used in the treatment of chronic asthma and chronic obstructive airway disease. The medication is intended to be used daily. It is not a rescue inhaler, and additional doses do not improve respiratory function. Evaluation of effectiveness includes improvement in respiratory status and ability to perform activities of daily living/quality-of-life activities such as walking and playing. Side effects of the medication include an increase in cough and sputum production.

Test-taking strategy: Analyze to determine what information the question asks for, which is information that would indicate improvement in respiratory status. "Select all that apply" questions require considering each option to decide its merit. Evaluate each client statement for evidence of symptom improvement or overall client activity (ADL) improvement. Review the pathophysiology and symptoms of COPD if you had difficulty answering this question.

Client needs category: Physiological integrity

Client needs subcategory: Pharmacological and parenteral therapies

Cognitive level: Evaluating

18. The nurse has been assigned to care for the following six clients. Which clients would the nurse expect to be at risk for the development of pulmonary embolism? Select all that apply.

☐ **1.** A client who is on complete bed rest following extensive spinal surgery

☐ **2.** A client who has a large venous stasis ulcer on the right ankle area

☐ **3.** A client who has recently been admitted with a broken femur and is awaiting surgery

☐ **4.** A client who has a pleural effusion secondary to infection

☐ **5.** A client who is receiving supplemental oxygen following shoulder surgery

☐ **6.** A client who has undergone a total vaginal hysterectomy and is now on estrogen replacement therapy

Answer: 1, 2, 3, 6

ⅅ **Rationale:** Bed rest, poor venous circulation, fractures, and hormone replacement therapy can cause the formation of a thromboembolus, placing these clients at risk for developing a PE. A deep vein thrombosis could break loose in the leg and travel to the lungs as a pulmonary embolus. The clot would then lodge in the pulmonary arteries or arterioles and impede blood flow. The client who is on complete bed rest is at risk for venous stasis, and the client who has a venous stasis ulcer is already demonstrating this condition. The client with a broken femur is at risk for a fat embolus, another form of PE. The client on estrogen replacement therapy is at increased risk for thromboembolic disorders. Pleural effusion and infections usually have no effect on thrombus formation, and oxygen therapy does not cause venous stasis or increase the risk of a pulmonary embolism.

Test-taking strategy: Analyze to determine what information the question asks for, which is identifying a client population who are at risk for developing a PE. "Select all that apply" questions require considering each option to decide its merit. Review the pathophysiology of thromboembolic disorders, and consider the factors that lead to blood stasis and clotting if you had difficulty answering this question.

Client needs category: Physiological integrity

Client needs subcategory: Physiological adaptation

Cognitive level: Analyzing

---

19. The nurse is caring for several clients on the respiratory unit who are receiving the β-adrenergic agonist bronchodilator albuterol in the prescribed nebulizer treatments. Which side effects would the nurse expect to assess following administration? Select all that apply.

☐ **1.** Increased tachypnea

☐ **2.** Irritability and nervousness

☐ **3.** Tachycardia

☐ **4.** Increased somnolence

☐ **5.** Insomnia

☐ **6.** Anxiety

Answer: 2, 3, 5, 6

ⅅ **Rationale:** Albuterol is prescribed to prevent and treat wheezing, difficulty breathing, and chest tightness caused by lung diseases such as asthma and chronic obstructive lung disease (COPD). Irritability, nervousness, tachycardia, insomnia, and anxiety are common side effects of β-adrenergic agonist bronchodilators that result from sympathetic nervous system stimulation. The expected therapeutic effect of a bronchodilator is decreased dyspnea and slower (not increased) breathing. Increased somnolence does not occur with sympathetic nervous system stimulation.

Test-taking strategy: Analyze to determine what information the question asks for, which is expected side effects following albuterol administration. "Select all that apply" questions require considering each option to decide its merit. Break down the classification of adrenergics (adrenaline) and agonists (mimic the action of the naturally occurring substance) and relate to sympathetic nervous system stimulation. Review the action and side effects of β-adrenergic agonists if you had difficulty answering this question.

Client needs category: Physiological integrity

Client needs subcategory: Pharmacological and parenteral therapies

Cognitive level: Applying

---

20. A nurse is caring for a client with pulmonary edema whose respiratory status is declining. Chronologically arrange the nursing interventions to prioritize care. All options must be used.

1. Administer oxygen via nasal cannula at 2 L/minute.
2. Call the physician.
3. Position the client upright at a 45° angle.
4. Prepare suctioning equipment at the bedside.
5. Administer furosemide 40 mg intravenously STAT.
6. Insert an indwelling urinary catheter.

Answer: 3, 1, 4, 2, 5, 6

Ⓓ Rationale: The order of priority moves from the simple to the complex for bedside interventions when a client is in respiratory distress. The nurse would first attempt to maximize respiratory excursion as much as possible by sitting the client up and then provide supplemental oxygen to minimize impending hypoxia. It is also important to have suction equipment readily available because the client may choke on oral secretions because of the pulmonary edema. After performing these interventions, the nurse would notify the health care provider and anticipate orders for administration of a diuretic (such as furosemide) and insertion of an indwelling urinary catheter to measure eventual output.

Test-taking strategy: Analyze to determine what information the question asks for, which is arranging nursing actions when caring for a client with a declining respiratory status. First, assess the client and determine nursing actions to improve the respiratory status and prepare for any potential emergency. Next, move from the client to notify the health care provider, and anticipate medical orders. Review priority care of individuals with pulmonary edema if you had difficulty answering this question.

Client needs category: Physiological integrity

Client needs subcategory: Reduction of risk potential

Cognitive level: Analyzing

21. A nurse is caring for a client diagnosed with pneumonia, a urinary tract infection, dehydration, and temperature of 101.4°F (38.6°C). The health care provider orders 1,000 ml of D₅W to infuse over 8 hours. The available drop factor is 20 gtt/ml. The nurse would regulate the intravenous flow rate to deliver how many drops per minute? Round your answer to the nearest whole number.

_____ gtt/min

Answer: 42

Ⓜ **Rationale:** Calculate the flow rate using the formula below:

$$\frac{\text{Total volume ordered}}{\text{Number of hours}} = \text{Flow rate}$$

$$\frac{1,000 \text{ ml}}{8 \text{ hours}} = 125 \text{ ml/hours}$$

Rounded off, this is 42 gtt/hour.

$$\frac{125 \text{ ml}}{60 \text{ minutes}} \times \frac{20 \text{ gtt}}{1 \text{ ml}} = 41.66$$

Test-taking strategy: Analyze to determine what information the question asks for, which is intravenous drops per minute. Always refer to the dosage/time or quantity that the question requires the final answer to be calculated to, which, in this case, is drops/minute. Follow the formula, setting up the equation to end with the desired dosage. Proofread your math calculations. Review the calculation of intravenous drip rates if you had difficulty answering this question.

Client needs category: Physiological integrity

Client needs subcategory: Pharmacological and parenteral therapies

Cognitive level: Applying

---

22. The registered nurse (RN) is assisting the licensed practical nurse (LPN) in performing a purified protein derivative (PPD) test on a nursing home resident. Which statements about this test are correct? Select all that apply.

☐ **1.** A PPD test is done to test for allergies.

☐ **2.** Always aspirate before injecting the PPD solution.

☐ **3.** The PPD test is an intradermal test.

☐ **4.** Hold the syringe at a 45° angle to the skin.

☐ **5.** The preferred injection site is the ventral surface of the forearm.

☐ **6.** No wheal should appear at the site following injection.

Answer: 3, 5

Ⓜ **Rationale:** The PPD test is used to determine whether a person has been exposed/infected with the _Tuberculosis_ bacillus. PPD tests should be injected intradermally in the ventral forearm, unless contraindicated, without aspiration prior to injecting. The syringe would be held at a 10° to 15° angle from the site, so the needle enters the dermis as nearly parallel to the skin as possible. A small wheal would appear; this indicates that the medication has been injected into the dermis.

Test-taking strategy: Analyze to determine what information the question asks for, which is correct statements related to the administration of a PPD. "Select all that apply" questions require considering each option to decide its merit. First, visualize the technique to place medication in the intradermal layer of the skin. Also, recall that no allergy is being tested. Review the rationale and procedure for administering a PPD test if you had difficulty answering this question.

Client needs category: Physiological integrity

Client needs subcategory: Pharmacological and parenteral therapies

Cognitive level: Applying

1. A nurse is providing discharge instructions on phenytoin to a female client with tonic–clonic seizure disorder. Which instructions would the nurse include? Select all that apply.

☐ **1.** Monitor the body for any skin rash.

☐ **2.** Maintain adequate amounts of fluid and fiber in the diet.

☐ **3.** Perform good oral hygiene, including daily brushing and flossing.

☐ **4.** Receive necessary periodic blood work.

☐ **5.** Report any problems with walking or coordination, slurred speech, or nausea.

Answer: 1, 3, 4, 5

Ⓒ Rationale: If a rash appears 10 to 14 days after starting phenytoin, the client should notify the health care provider, who may discontinue the medication. Because it may cause gingival hyperplasia, the client must practice good oral hygiene and see a dentist regularly. Periodic blood work is necessary to monitor complete blood counts, platelet count, hepatic function, and drug levels. Signs and symptoms of phenytoin toxicity include problems with walking or coordination, slurred speech, and nausea. Other signs are lethargy, diplopia, and nystagmus. These must be reported to the health care provider immediately. Although adequate amounts of fluid and fiber are part of a healthy diet, they are not required for a client taking phenytoin.

Test-taking strategy: Analyze to determine what information the question asks for, which is discharge instructions for phenytoin. "Select all that apply" questions require considering each option to decide its merit. Critically think through the distractors, consider the common side effects of phenytoin, and review the adverse and toxic effects of this classification of medications. Review the therapeutic action of phenytoin with common side effects if you had difficulty answering this question.

Client needs category: Physiological integrity

Client needs subcategory: Pharmacological and parenteral therapies

Cognitive level: Applying

2. A nurse assesses a client with suspected bacterial meningitis. Which documented findings of meningeal irritation suggest this diagnosis? Select all that apply.

☐ **1.** Generalized seizures

☐ **2.** Nuchal rigidity

☐ **3.** Positive Brudzinski's sign

☐ **4.** Positive Kernig's sign

☐ **5.** Babinski's reflex

☐ **6.** Photophobia

Answer: 2, 3, 4, 6

Ⓓ Rationale: Irritation of the meninges of the brain can be caused by a virus or bacteria. Signs of meningeal irritation include nuchal rigidity, positive Brudzinski's and Kernig's signs, and photophobia. Other signs of meningeal irritation are exaggerated and symmetrical deep tendon reflexes as well as opisthotonos (a spasm in which the back and extremities arch backward so that the body rests on the head and heels). Generalized seizures may accompany meningitis, but they are caused by irritation to the cerebral cortex, not the meninges. Babinski's reflex is a reflex action of the toes that reflects corticospinal tract disease in adults.

Test-taking strategy: Analyze to determine what information the question asks for, which is documented assessment findings that suggest bacterial meningitis. "Select all that apply" questions require considering each option to decide its merit. Review the pathophysiology and clinical manifestations of bacterial meningitis if you had difficulty answering this question.

Client needs category: Physiological integrity

Client needs subcategory: Physiological adaptation

Cognitive level: Applying

---

3. A nurse is preparing to administer phenytoin to a 99-lb (45 kg) client with a seizure disorder. The medication administration record documents phenytoin 5 mg/kg/day to be administered in three divided doses. How many milligrams of phenytoin would be administered in the first dose? Record your answer as a whole number.

_____ mg

Answer: 75

Ⓔ Rationale: First, convert the client's weight to kilograms:

$$1 \text{ kg} = 2.2 \text{ lb}$$
$$99 \text{ lb} \div 2.2 \text{ lb/kg} = 44 \text{ kg}.$$

Then, calculate the total daily dosage:

$$44 \text{ kg} \times 5 \text{ mg/kg} = 220 \text{ mg/day}.$$

Finally, divide the total daily dosage into three parts:

$$220 \text{ mg} \div 3 \text{ doses} = 75 \text{ mg/dose}.$$

Test-taking strategy: Analyze to determine what information the question asks for, which is the dose (mg) of phenytoin to be administered. First, change the weight from pounds to kilograms to fit into the equation (mg/kg). Calculate using the formula above. Note that the first dose is the same as the third dose of the day because the daily dose is divided evenly. Proofread the math calculation. Review dosage in milligrams according to body weight if you had difficulty answering this question.

Client needs category: Physiological integrity

Client needs subcategory: Pharmacological and parenteral therapies

Cognitive level: Applying

---

4. A nurse is assessing a client's extraocular eye movements as part of evaluating neurological functioning. This documents the status of which cranial nerves? Select all that apply.

☐ **1.** Optic (II)

☐ **2.** Oculomotor (III)

☐ **3.** Trochlear (IV)

☐ **4.** Trigeminal (V)

☐ **5.** Abducens (VI)

☐ **6.** Acoustic (VIII)

Answer: 2, 3, 5

🅓 **Rationale:** Assessing extraocular eye movements helps evaluate the function of cranial nerves III (oculomotor), IV (trochlear), and VI (abducens). The oculomotor nerve originates in the brain stem and controls the movement of the eyeball up, down, and inward; raises the eyelid; and constricts the pupil. The trochlear nerve rotates the eyeball downward and outward. The abducens nerve originates in the pons and rotates the eyeball laterally. Assessing the client's vision helps evaluate cranial nerve II (optic). Cranial nerve V (trigeminal) has three branches: assessing the corneal reflex helps the nurse evaluate the ophthalmic branch functions; assessing sensation to the cheek, upper jaw, teeth, lips, hard palate, maxillary sinus, and part of the nasal mucosa helps evaluate the maxillary branch functions; and assessing sensation to the lower lip, chin, ear, mucous membrane, lower teeth, and tongue helps evaluate the mandibular branch functions. Assessing hearing and balance helps evaluate the cochlear and vestibular branches of cranial nerve VIII (acoustic).

Test-taking strategy: Analyze to determine what information the question asks for, which is assessing the cranial nerves involved in extraocular movements. "Select all that apply" questions require considering each option to decide its merit. Simple recall of the 12 cranial nerves is essential in completing a neurological examination. Use of mnemonic phrases such as "On Old Olympus Towering Top, A Fin and German Viewed Some Hops" can be helpful to recall the cranial nerves and select the correct options to answer the question. Review the cranial nerves and, specifically, those involved with extraocular movements if you had difficulty answering this question.

Client needs category: Physiological integrity

Client needs subcategory: Physiological adaptation

Cognitive level: Analyzing

5. A nurse is comparing the neurological status of a client who suffered a head injury with the status on the previous shift. Using the Glasgow Coma Scale, the nurse determines that the client's score has changed from 11 to 15. Which responses did the nurse assess in this client? Select all that apply.

☐ **1.** Spontaneous eye opening

☐ **2.** Tachypnea, bradycardia, and hypotension

☐ **3.** Unequal pupil size

☐ **4.** Orientation to person, place, and time

☐ **5.** Pain localization

☐ **6.** Incomprehensible sounds

Answer: 1, 4

ⓒ Rationale: The Glasgow Coma Scale is a tool to assess a client's response to stimuli. To achieve a perfect score adding to 15 on the Glasgow Coma Scale, the client would have to open his/her eyes spontaneously (4), obey verbal commands (6), and be oriented to person, place, and time (5). Vital signs and pupil size are not assessed with the Glasgow Coma Scale. The ability to localize pain earns a motor response score of 5, not the top score of 6. Making incomprehensible sounds earns a verbal response score of 2, not a 5.

Test-taking strategy: Analyze to determine what information the question asks for, which is change or improvement in the client's neurological status. "Select all that apply" questions require considering each option to decide its merit. Recall that a perfect score of 15 would indicate normal neurological function; thus, review each option against normal functioning. Review the Glasgow Coma Scale and neurological assessment techniques if you had difficulty answering this question.

Client needs category: Physiological integrity

Client needs subcategory: Physiological adaptation

Cognitive level: Analyzing

6. The nurse is educating a client and family about macular degeneration. Which photo would be utilized to **best** illustrate what these clients typically see?

☐ **1.**

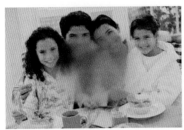

☐ **2.**

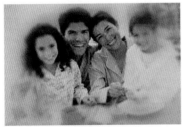

☐ **3.**

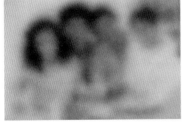

☐ **4.**

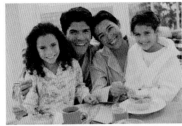

Rationale: Macular degeneration is a medical condition that typically affects the eyesight of older adults. The central vision is most affected in clients, thus revealing a blurred or distorted image in the middle of the visual field. Peripheral vision is usually maintained. The visual field is neither totally blurred, unless in an advanced case, nor completely clear.

Test-taking strategy: Analyze to determine what information the question asks for, which is the illustration that depicts a client's visual field. Recall that the macula is the center area of the retina, which provides the most detailed central vision. Degeneration in this area would compromise the center of the visual field. Review the symptoms of macular degeneration if you had difficulty answering this question.

Client needs category: Physiological integrity

Client needs subcategory: Physiological adaptation

Cognitive level: Applying

7. A nurse is caring for a client with a T5 complete spinal cord injury. Upon assessment, the nurse notes flushed skin, diaphoresis above T5, and blood pressure of 174/100 mm Hg. The client reports a severe, pounding headache. Which nursing interventions would be appropriate for this client? Select all that apply.

☐ **1.** Elevate the head of the bed to 90°.

☐ **2.** Loosen constrictive clothing.

☐ **3.** Use a fan to reduce diaphoresis.

☐ **4.** Assess for bladder distention and bowel impaction.

☐ **5.** Administer antihypertensive medication.

☐ **6.** Administer morphine as ordered.

Answer: 1, 2, 4, 5

Ⓒ Rationale: The client is exhibiting signs and symptoms of autonomic dysreflexia, a potentially life-threatening emergency caused by an uninhibited response from the sympathetic nervous system resulting from a lack of control over the autonomic nervous system. The nurse would immediately elevate the head of the bed to 90° and place the legs in a dependent position to decrease venous return to the heart and increase venous return from the brain. Because tactile stimuli can trigger autonomic dysreflexia, any constrictive clothing should be loosened. The nurse would also assess for distended bladder and bowel impaction—which may trigger autonomic dysreflexia—and correct any problems. Morphine, a narcotic, is not prescribed. Elevated blood pressure is the most life-threatening complication of autonomic dysreflexia because it can cause stroke, myocardial infarction, or seizure activity. If removing the triggering event does not reduce the client's blood pressure, intravenous antihypertensives would be administered. A fan would not be used because a cold draft may trigger autonomic dysreflexia.

Test-taking strategy: Analyze to determine what information the question asks for, which is nursing interventions for a client exhibiting signs of autonomic dysreflexia. "Select all that apply" questions require considering each option to decide its merit. Recall that this syndrome particularly occurs in individuals with spinal cord injuries at the splanchnic sympathetic outflow (T5-T6) level. Consider the hypertensive effect and the need to lower blood pressure. Review the pathophysiology of spinal cord injury and the clinical manifestations of complications such as autonomic dysreflexia if you had difficulty answering this question.

Client needs category: Physiological integrity

Client needs subcategory: Physiological adaptation

Cognitive level: Analyzing

8. A nurse is caring for a client diagnosed with a cerebral aneurysm. The health care provider orders hydralazine 15 mg intravenously every 4 hours as needed to keep the systolic blood pressure less than 140 mm Hg. To administer the correct dose, how many milliliters of medication would the nurse draw up in the syringe? Record your answer using two decimal places.

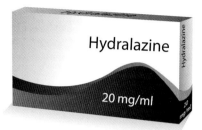

Answer: 0.75

E **Rationale:** The following formula is used to calculate drug dosages:

$$20 \text{ mg/ml} = 15 \text{ mg}/X = 0.75 \text{ ml.}$$

Test-taking strategy: Analyze to determine what information the question asks for, which is correct dosage of medication in milliliters drawn up in the syringe. Use the ratio-and-proportion strategy to align the milligram per milliliter on each side of the equation, and solve for X. Proofread the math calculation. Review medication math calculations if you had difficulty answering this question.

Client needs category: Physiological integrity

Client needs subcategory: Pharmacological and parenteral therapies

Cognitive level: Applying

---

9. A nurse is preparing to teach students in a health class about hearing pathways. Place the following steps in chronological order to match how the nurse would describe the normal pathway of sound wave transmission and hearing to the class. All options must be used.

| 1. Interpretation of sound by the cerebral cortex |
| 2. Transmission of vibrations through the hammer, anvil, and stirrup |
| 3. Stimulation of nerve impulses in the inner ear |
| 4. Transmission of vibrations to the auditory area of the cerebral cortex |
| 5. Collection of the sound waves in the pinna |

Answer: 5, 2, 3, 4, 1

M **Rationale:** Sound waves travel through the air and are collected by the pinna, which is the visible portion of the outer ear. Vibrations transmit through the canal and bones of the hammer, anvil, and stirrup. Next, there is stimulation sending nerve impulses to the inner ear. The cochlear branch of the acoustic nerve transmits these vibrations to the auditory area of the cerebral cortex. The cerebral cortex then interprets the sound.

Test-taking strategy: Analyze to determine what information the question asks for, which is pathway of sound wave transmission. Critically think through movement of the sound waves from outside the body to the inner ear and then to the brain. Review the anatomy and physiology of the ear and the physiology of the nervous system related to hearing if you had difficulty answering this question.

Client needs category: Health promotion and maintenance

Client needs subcategory: None

Cognitive level: Understanding

10. The rehabilitation nurse is caring for a client with a health history of multiple sclerosis (MS) for 10 years. Recently, the nurse has seen a significant decline in the client's function. When reevaluating the client's plan of care, the nurse considers the client's physiologic changes associated with the decline. Arrange the following degenerative changes in the order in which they occur. All options must be used.

| **1.** Degeneration of axons |
| **2.** Demyelination throughout the central nervous system |
| **3.** Periodic and unpredictable exacerbations and remissions |
| **4.** Plaque formation that interrupts nerve impulses |
| **5.** The immune system attacks myelin |

Answer: 5, 2, 1, 4, 3

Ⓓ Rationale: MS is believed to be an autoimmune disease in which the body perceives myelin to be a foreign agent and attacks it. Nursing care requires the nurse to understand the progression of degenerative changes and anticipate client needs. MS produces patches of demyelination throughout the central nervous system, resulting in myelin loss from the axis cylinders and degeneration of the axons. Plaques form in the involved area and become sclerosed, interrupting the flow of nerve impulses and resulting in a variety of symptoms. Periodic and unpredictable exacerbations and remissions occur. The prognosis varies.

Test-taking strategy: Analyze to determine what information the question asks for, which is progressive changes in clients with MS. Consider how the disease originates and then progresses causing the degenerative decline. If unsure, select the first and last in the sequence, which leaves three selections to order. Review the pathophysiology of MS progression if you had difficulty answering this question.

Client needs category: Physiological integrity

Client needs subcategory: Physiological adaptation

Cognitive level: Applying

---

11. A nurse is monitoring a client's intracranial pressure (ICP) after a traumatic head injury. The health care provider calls and asks for a report on the client's condition. Based on the documentation below, how would the nurse respond?

Flow Sheet

	0800	0805	0810	0815
ICP	20	18	18	16

☐ **1.** "The client's ICP remains elevated."

☐ **2.** "The client's ICP has decreased to lower than normal limits."

☐ **3.** "The client's ICP is within normal limits."

☐ **4.** "The client's ICP was elevated but now has returned to normal."

Answer: 1

Ⓜ Rationale: A normal ICP is between 0 and 15 mm Hg. The documentation shows pressures greater than 15 mm Hg.

Test-taking strategy: Analyze to determine what information the question asks for, which is interpretation of ICP data. Recall that ICP can normally be at 0 and then as high as 15. Memorization of the ICP parameter is essential for interpretation. Review normal values of ICP if you had difficulty answering this question.

Client needs category: Physiological integrity

Client needs subcategory: Physiological adaptation

Cognitive level: Analyzing

12. A nurse is documenting a health assessment when the client states having problems with balance as well as fine and gross motor function. When collaborating with the health team, which area on the illustration of the brain would the nurse highlight as an area of concern?

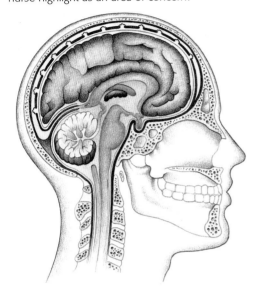

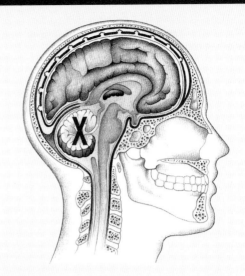

 Rationale: Note the placement of the X. The cerebellum is the portion of the brain that controls balance and fine and gross motor function. The cerebellum is located at the base of the skull and above the brain stem.

Test-taking strategy: Analyze to determine what information the question asks for, which is the area of the brain responsible for motor function. Correlate client symptoms with knowledge of anatomy and physiology of the brain. Once determined, locate the area on the illustration. Review the location and function of the lobes of the brain if you had difficulty answering this question.

Client needs category: Physiological integrity

Client needs subcategory: Physiological adaptation

Cognitive level: Analyzing

13. A nurse is performing a neurological assessment during a client's routine physical examination. To assess for a Babinski reflex, indicate the point where the nurse places the tongue blade to begin stroking the foot.

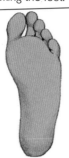

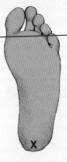

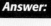 **Rationale:** To test for a Babinski reflex, use a tongue blade to slowly stroke the side of the sole (plantar aspect) of the foot. Start at the heel and move toward the great toe. The normal response in an adult is plantar flexion of the toes. Upward movement of the great toe and fanning of the little toes—Babinski's reflex—are abnormal in clients over the age of 12 to 24 months.

Test-taking strategy: Analyze to determine what information the question asks for, which is the correct procedure to assess a Babinski reflex. Recall that reflexes are predictable and uncontrolled responses to stimuli, which, in this case, are stroking the sole of the foot. Review the procedure to elicit a Babinski reflex if you had difficulty answering this question.

Client needs category: Health promotion and maintenance

Client needs subcategory: None

Cognitive level: Understanding

14. The nurse is caring for a client who is experiencing an exacerbation of gout. When providing instruction, which dietary modifications are stressed? Select all that apply.

☐ **1.** Eat a low-purine diet.

☐ **2.** Limit fluid intake to no more than 1 L/day.

☐ **3.** Eat a high-protein diet, with at least two servings of lean meat per day.

☐ **4.** Eat a high-purine diet.

☐ **5.** Limit alcohol intake.

Answer: 1, 5

Rationale: Gout is characterized by an abnormal metabolism of uric acid. Either individuals produce too much uric acid or their body is unable to metabolize and excrete it. Purines are metabolized into uric acid. The client who suffers from gout would be placed on a low-purine diet with foods such as peanut butter, cherries, rice, pasta, fruits, and vegetables. Fluids do not have to be limited. Alcohol intake would be limited as it is thought to trigger an exacerbation.

Test-taking strategy: Analyze to determine what information the question asks for, which is dietary modifications for a client with gout. "Select all that apply" questions require considering each option to decide its merit. Consider dietary modifications that relate to the production of uric acid and relate to a low-purine diet. Review dietary modifications, especially purines, if you had difficulty answering this question.

Client needs category: Physiological integrity

Client needs subcategory: Basic care and comfort

Cognitive level: Applying

15. The nurse is caring for a client who is scheduled to undergo a computed tomography (CT) scan to assess recent symptoms of muscle weakness and tingling in the extremities. Which information would the nurse include in a preprocedural teaching plan? Select all that apply.

☐ **1.** The test requires standing alone without assistance.

☐ **2.** A contrast dye may be given before the test.

☐ **3.** Throat irritation and facial flushing may occur if contrast dye is used.

☐ **4.** All medications must be withheld for 12 hours prior to the procedure.

☐ **5.** The CT scan is considered an invasive procedure, but not dangerous.

☐ **6.** It is necessary to report any known allergies to iodine or seafood prior to the procedure.

Ⓜ **Rationale:** The nurse would inform the client who is scheduled to undergo a CT scan that a contrast medium may be administered before the procedure and that the dye can cause throat irritation and facial flushing. Because the dye is iodine based, it is essential for the client to report any known allergies to iodine or seafood before testing begins. The CT scan is not invasive or dangerous. The client will need to lie still (not stand) during the procedure and will not be able to take routine medications for 24 hours beforehand.

Test-taking strategy: Analyze to determine what information the question asks for, which is teaching prior to a CT scan. "Select all that apply" questions require considering each option to decide its merit. The key word is "preprocedural," meaning preparation/teaching for the CT scan. Review procedure guidelines for a CT scan if you had difficulty answering this question.

Client needs category: Physiological integrity

Client needs subcategory: Reduction of risk potential

Cognitive level: Applying

---

16. A nurse is caring for a client, diagnosed with Alzheimer's disease, who scored a 7 (high risk) on the Hendrich II Fall Risk Model. Which nursing interventions would the nurse implement? Select all that apply.

☐ **1.** Implement a bed alarm.

☐ **2.** Request a low-dose sedative.

☐ **3.** Instruct the client to ask for help before ambulating.

☐ **4.** Maintain the bed in the lowest position.

☐ **5.** Offer toileting every 2 to 3 hours.

☐ **6.** Advise family to notify staff when leaving.

Ⓒ **Rationale:** Preventing a client from falling and causing further illness or injury is a role of the nurse. The Hendrich II Fall Risk Model is used in some acute care facilities to determine the potential for a fall. Assessment of a client's fall risk is a National Patient Safety Goal set by the Joint Commission and would be completed on admission. Nursing interventions such as implementing a bed alarm, maintaining the bed in the lowest position, offering toileting, and having the family notify staff when leaving are all appropriate nursing interventions to prevent falls. Sedating a client using chemical restraints is a last resort. Instructing a client to ask for help before ambulating is not effective in a client with Alzheimer's disease who will have difficulty remembering the instructions.

Test-taking strategy: Analyze to determine what information the question asks for, which is nursing interventions to prevent falls. "Select all that apply" questions require considering each option to decide its merit. When considering fall risk, think "safety." Always consider client-specific interventions when developing a plan of care. Because of this client's diagnosis, the ability to follow instructions will be limited. Review fall precautions if you had difficulty answering this question.

Client needs category: Physiological integrity

Client needs subcategory: Reduction of risk potential

Cognitive level: Applying

17. A client is scheduled to undergo cerebral angiography to allow for examination of the cerebral arteries. Place the following interventions in the order in which the nurse would perform them. All options must be used.

1. Administer antianxiety medication if ordered.

2. Confirm no allergies to iodine, seafood, or radiopaque dyes.

3. Make sure the client has signed an informed consent form.

4. Maintain the affected extremity in straight alignment for 6 hours as ordered.

5. Encourage the client to verbalize questions about the procedure with nurse and health care provider.

Answer: 5, 3, 2, 1, 4

D Rationale: It is important to provide the client with an opportunity to ask questions about the procedure before obtaining informed consent. The nurse would again assess and thus confirm no allergies to iodine, seafood, or radiopaque dyes because the procedure uses an iodine-based contrast medium. This would be done before administering antianxiety medication to the client. After the procedure, the affected extremity would be maintained in straight alignment for 6 hours.

Test-taking strategy: Analyze to determine what information the question asks for, which is ordered nursing actions before and after a cerebral angiography. When caring for a client prior to a procedure, think "consent and special preparation," and after the procedure think "assessment and special considerations." Consider which interventions would be completed before others. Review the nursing interventions related to cerebral angiography if you had difficulty answering this question.

Client needs category: Physiological integrity

Client needs subcategory: Reduction of risk potential

Cognitive level: Applying

18. A client presents to the emergency department with right facial droop and drooling. A diagnosis of Bell's palsy is confirmed by a neurological exam and magnetic resonance imaging (MRI). When instructing the spouse on the interventions needed to care for the client, which spouse statements need clarification by the nurse? Select all that apply.

☐ **1.** "I will buy a clothing protector for feedings."

☐ **2.** "I will obtain a walker in case symptoms progress."

☐ **3.** "I will instill eye drops to prevent symptoms of dry eyes."

☐ **4.** "I will watch for further symptoms of a stroke."

☐ **5.** "I will reinforce that symptoms are usually temporary."

☐ **6.** "I will provide sunglasses during the daytime."

Answer: 2, 4

D Rationale: Bell's palsy is a facial palsy believed to be caused by the swelling and inflammation of the nerve that controls the muscles on one side of the face. It may occur after a viral infection. Symptoms do not progress to other areas of the body and are not related to a stroke. Interventions needed are in response to the deficits from facial nerve paralysis. A clothing protector is needed while eating since the client has difficulty closing the mouth when chewing, eye drops are needed since the client has difficulty closing the eye to keep the eye moist, limiting bright lights by wearing sunglasses is protective to the inner eye, and reinforcing that the condition is temporary lessens anxiety.

Test-taking strategy: Analyze to determine what information the question asks for, which is incorrect statement regarding Bell's palsy. Consider that Bell's palsy is often incorrectly linked to a stroke because of its similar symptoms. Always focus on the impairment of cranial nerve VII and the issues involved in facial paralysis. Review the interventions and teaching related to Bell's palsy if you had difficulty answering this question.

Client needs category: Physiological integrity

Client needs subcategory: Physiological adaptation

Cognitive level: Analyzing

19. The nurse is caring for a client who sustained a head injury during a football game. The nurse is completing the following examination. Which documentation by the nurse provides normal results of this examination?

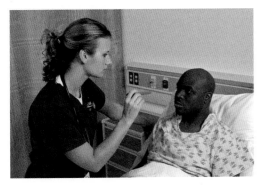

From *Lippincott's Visual Encyclopedia of Clinical Skills.* Philadelphia, PA: Wolters Kluwer Health, 2009.

☐ **1.** The client's pupils are equal and reactive to light and accommodation.

☐ **2.** The client's retina is attached, with no signs of tearing.

☐ **3.** The client's vision is 20/20 in both eyes.

☐ **4.** The client's visual field is 360°.

Answer: 1

ⓔ Rationale: The nurse in this examination is assessing the pupils and neurological function. Normal results would include that both the pupils are equal in size and reactive to light and accommodation. This examination does not assess the retina or the client's vision. The focus of the exam is the pupil reaction, not visual field assessment. The visual field does not extend to 360°.

Test-taking strategy: Analyze to determine what information the question asks for, which is documentation of normal results of a pupil light reflex test. First, identify the type of test being performed. One clue is the flashlight in the nurse's hand. Second, recall that light into the eye causes the pupil to constrict, indicating normal neurological function. Review neurological assessment tests if you had difficulty answering this question.

Client needs category: Physiological integrity

Client needs subcategory: Reduction of risk potential

Cognitive level: Applying

Gastrointestinal disorders

1. A client arrives for an annual physical examination. During the history, the client states recurrent symptoms of heartburn, a sour taste in the mouth, and hoarseness in the throat. In anticipation of client teaching, illustrate on the diagram the location of the structure that frequently enables these symptoms to occur.

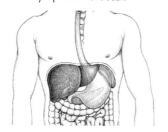

Answer:

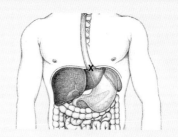

E Rationale: An X is placed on the lower esophageal sphincter, which is a ring of muscle fibers that prevents food and acid from moving backward from the stomach into the esophagus. If this sphincter does not close well, food, fluids, and stomach contents can irritate and even damage the esophagus. Symptoms include heartburn, a sour taste in the mouth, hoarseness, dysphagia, and feelings of a lump in the throat.

Test-taking strategy: Analyze to determine what information the question asks for, which is the location of the structure that prevents stomach backflow. First, correlate client symptoms to a weakening of a sphincter. Consider that this structure would need to be located at the junction between the stomach and the esophagus. Review the anatomy of the GI system and the pathophysiology of the disorder if you had difficulty answering this question.

Client needs category: Health promotion and maintenance

Client needs subcategory: None

Cognitive level: Understanding

2. As part of a routine screening for colorectal cancer, a client must undergo fecal occult blood testing. Which foods would the nurse instruct the client to avoid for 48 to 72 hours before the test and throughout the collection period? Select all that apply.

☐ **1.** High-fiber foods

☐ **2.** Red meat

☐ **3.** Turnips

☐ **4.** Cantaloupe

☐ **5.** Tomatoes

☐ **6.** Peas

Answer: 2, 3, 4

G Rationale: The client would avoid red meat, poultry, and fish as well as beets, broccoli, cauliflower, horseradish, mushrooms, and turnips. Such fruits as cantaloupe, melons, and grapefruit are also prohibited. Tomatoes and peas are acceptable. The client would be taught to maintain a high-fiber diet in order to promote colonic emptying time and fecal bulk, which aid in obtaining specimens.

Test-taking strategy: Analyze to determine what information the question asks for, which is food to avoid when having fecal occult blood testing. "Select all that apply" questions require considering each option to decide its merit. Consider that the examination tests for blood in the stool so any introduction of the blood into the GI system or irritation could cause a positive result. Also, certain food alters the test, so an understanding of the diet is essential. Review the preparation for fecal occult blood test and the role of foods in the digestive tract if you had difficulty answering the question.

Client needs category: Health promotion and maintenance

Client needs subcategory: None

Cognitive level: Applying

3. A client returns from the operating room after undergoing extensive abdominal surgery. The client is receiving 1,000 ml of lactated Ringer's solution via a central line infusion. The health care provider orders the intravenous fluid to be infused at 125 ml/hour and additional intravenous fluids based on total output of the last hour. The drip factor of the tubing is 15 gtt/ml, and the output for the previous hour was 75 ml via Foley catheter, 50 ml via nasogastric tube, and 10 ml via Jackson-Pratt tube. For how many drops (gtt) per minute would the nurse set the intravenous flow rate to deliver the correct amount of fluid? Record your answer as a whole number.

_____ gtt/minute

Answer: 65

Ⓓ **Rationale:** First, calculate the volume to be infused (in milliliters):

75 ml + 50 ml + 10 ml = 135 ml total output for the previous hour

135 ml + 125 ml ordered as a constant flow = 260 ml to be infused over the next hour.

Next, use the formula:

Volume to be infused/total minutes to be infused × drop factor = drops/minute.

In this case:

260 ml/60 minutes × 15 gtt/ml = 65 gtt/minute.

Test-taking strategy: Analyze to determine what information the question asks for, which is intravenous flow rate in drops/minute. Carefully read and calculate the volume to be infused per physician's order. Proofread your work. Next, use the standard formula calculating drip factors. Review calculation of drip rates if you had difficulty answering this question.

Client needs category: Physiological integrity

Client needs subcategory: Pharmacological and parenteral therapies

Cognitive level: Analyzing

4. A nurse is caring for a client with a retro-peritoneal abscess who is receiving gentamicin 300 mg intravenously every 8 hours. Which client data would the nurse monitor? Select all that apply.

☐ **1.** Hearing

☐ **2.** Urine output

☐ **3.** HCT

☐ **4.** BUN and serum creatinine levels

☐ **5.** Serum calcium level

☐ **6.** Muscle tone

Answer: 1, 2, 4

Ⓜ **Rationale:** Adverse effects of gentamicin include ototoxicity and nephrotoxicity; consequently, the nurse must monitor the client's hearing and instruct to report any hearing loss or tinnitus. Signs of nephrotoxicity include decreased urine output and elevated BUN and serum creatinine levels. Gentamicin does not affect the serum calcium level, HCT, or muscle tone.

Test-taking strategy: Analyze to determine what information the question asks for, which is client data that could indicate a concern. "Select all that apply" questions require considering each option to decide its merit. Recall that a peak and trough are needed to monitor therapeutic drug levels as the medication has a narrow drug index. Consider what information could be obtained from each option. Review common side effects and potential toxicity of the classification of aminoglycosides if you had difficulty answering this question.

Client needs category: Physiological integrity

Client needs subcategory: Pharmacological and parenteral therapies

Cognitive level: Analyzing

---

5. A nurse is assessing the abdomen of a client who was admitted to the emergency department with suspected appendicitis. Identify the area of the abdomen that the nurse would palpate last.

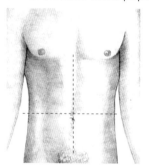

Answer:

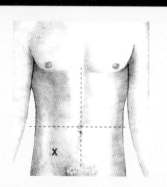

Ⓜ **Rationale:** An acute attack of appendicitis localizes as pain and tenderness in the lower right quadrant, midway between the umbilicus and the crest of the ilium. This area would be palpated last in order to determine if pain is also present in other areas of the abdomen.

Test-taking strategy: Analyze to determine what information the question asks for, which is area of the abdomen to palpate last when appendicitis is suspected. Recall that the classic sign of appendicitis is a pain when palpation and release (rebound tenderness) occurs over McBurney's point in the right lower quadrant. Since this is the classic sign, palpate last to differentiate between the other areas of the abdomen. Review the anatomy of the abdomen, and review abdominal assessment techniques, if you had difficulty answering this question.

Client needs category: Physiological integrity

Client needs subcategory: Physiological adaptation

Cognitive level: Applying

---

6. While preparing a client for an upper GI endoscopy (esophagogastroduodenoscopy), the nurse would be correct to implement which intervention? Select all that apply.

☐ **1.** Administer a preparation to cleanse the GI tract, such as GoLYTELY or Fleets Phospho-Soda.

☐ **2.** Instruct not to eat or drink for 6 to 12 hours before the procedure.

☐ **3.** Teach only to ingest a clear liquid diet for 24 hours before the procedure.

☐ **4.** Inform the client of receiving a sedative before the procedure.

☐ **5.** Encourage the client to eat and drink immediately after the procedure.

Answer: 2, 4

ⓒ **Rationale:** The client would not eat or drink for 6 to 12 hours before the procedure to ensure that the upper GI tract is clear for viewing. Before the endoscope is inserted, the client will receive a sedative that will help in relaxation, but leave conscious. GI tract cleansing and a clear liquid diet are interventions for a client having a lower GI tract procedure, such as a colonoscopy. Food and fluids must be withheld until the gag reflex returns after the procedure.

Test-taking strategy: Analyze to determine what information the question asks for, which is nursing interventions prior to an upper GI endoscopy. "Select all that apply" questions require considering each option to decide its merit. When caring for a client prior to a procedure, think "special preparation" or protocol to be followed. Review client safety and GI tract preparation, and review pre- and postendoscopy nursing interventions if you had difficulty answering this question.

Client needs category: Physiological integrity

Client needs subcategory: Reduction of risk potential

Cognitive level: Applying

---

7. A nurse is caring for a client who recently had a bowel resection. The client has a hemoglobin level of 8 g/dl and HCT of 30%. Dextrose 5% in half-normal saline solution ($D_5\frac{1}{2}NS$) is infusing through a triple-lumen central catheter at 125 ml/hour. The health care provider's orders include

■ Gentamicin 80 mg intravenous piggyback in 50 ml D_5W over 30 minutes

■ Ranitidine (Zantac) 50 mg intravenous in 50 ml D_5W piggyback over 30 minutes

■ One unit of 250 ml of packed red blood cells (RBCs) over 3 hours

■ Nasogastric tube flushes with 30 ml of normal saline solution every 2 hours

How many milliliters would the nurse document as the total intake for the 8-hour shift? Record your answer as a whole number.

_____ ml

Answer: 1,470

Ⓜ **Rationale:** Add up the total intake as follows:

I.V. of $D_5\frac{1}{2}NS$ at 125 ml × 8 hours = 1,000 ml

gentamicin piggyback = 50 ml

ranitidine piggyback = 50 ml

packed RBCs = 250 ml

+ nasogastric flushes 30 ml × 4 = 120 ml

Total = 1,470 ml.

Test-taking strategy: Analyze to determine what information the question asks for, which is total intake in milliliters for an 8-hour shift. Carefully read all information provided, and align in columns the addition equation to decrease the chance of a calculation error. Proofread your calculation.

Client needs category: Physiological integrity

Client needs subcategory: Physiological adaptation

Cognitive level: Analyzing

8. A nurse is caring for a client with history of chronic intestinal irritation. The client asks, "Is there any type of colostomy where I would not need a continuous colostomy bag?" Indicate the location where a client could have an ostomy that eventually might not require wearing an ostomy bag.

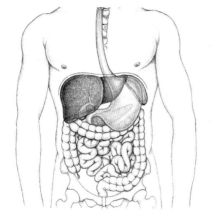

Answer:

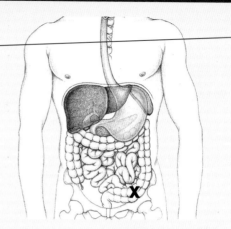

X

Ⓜ **Rationale:** With a sigmoid colostomy, the feces are solid; therefore, the client might eventually gain enough control and not need to wear a colostomy bag. With a descending colostomy, the feces are semisoft. With a transverse colostomy, the feces are soft. With an ascending colostomy, the feces are fluid. In these three latter cases, the client would be unlikely to gain control of elimination and consequently would need to continue wearing an ostomy bag.

Test-taking strategy: Analyze to determine what information the question asks for, which is site where a client may not continuously need to wear an ostomy bag. Think of how a person with a colostomy could mimic a normal bowel movement. Consider the path and contents of the colon to determine proper placement. Review the anatomy of the GI system, and review ostomy care if you had difficulty answering this question.

Client needs category: Physiological integrity

Client needs subcategory: Physiological adaptation

Cognitive level: Applying

9. A nurse is calling report to the medical–surgical floor staff regarding a client with acute diverticulitis. Which symptoms does the nurse anticipate? Select all that apply.

☐ **1.** Esophagitis.

☐ **2.** Cramping pain in the left lower abdominal quadrant

☐ **3.** Bowel irregularity

☐ **4.** Heartburn

☐ **5.** Intervals of diarrhea

☐ **6.** Hiccuping

Answer: 2, 3, 5

Ⓜ **Rationale:** Acute diverticulitis is a common digestive disease typically found in the large intestine. Signs and symptoms of acute diverticulitis include bowel irregularity, intervals of diarrhea, abrupt onset of cramping pain in the left lower abdomen, and a low-grade fever. Vomiting, heartburn, and hiccuping are not signs of the disorder.

Test-taking strategy: Analyze to determine what information the question asks for, which is signs of acute diverticulitis. "Select all that apply" questions require considering each option to decide its merit. Recall that diverticulitis occurs from an outpouching on the colon that becomes inflamed and symptoms correspond. Review the pathophysiology of diverticulitis and related signs and symptoms if you had difficulty answering this question.

Client needs category: Physiological integrity

Client needs subcategory: Physiological adaptation

Cognitive level: Applying

10. A client is admitted with inflammatory bowel syndrome (Crohn's disease). When planning care for the health care team, which would be included? Select all that apply.

☐ **1.** Lactulose therapy

☐ **2.** High-fiber diet

☐ **3.** High-protein milkshakes

☐ **4.** Corticosteroid therapy

☐ **5.** Antidiarrheal medications

Answer: 4, 5

🄓 **Rationale:** Inflammatory bowel syndrome (Crohn's disease) is an inflammatory bowel disease caused by inflammation to the lining of the digestive tract, which can lead to abdominal pain, severe diarrhea, and even malnutrition. Corticosteroids such as prednisone reduce the signs and symptoms of diarrhea, pain, and bleeding by decreasing inflammation. Antidiarrheals, such as diphenoxylate, combat diarrhea by decreasing peristalsis. Lactulose is used to treat chronic constipation and would aggravate the symptoms of Crohn's disease. A high-fiber diet and milk and milk products are contraindicated in clients with Crohn's disease because they may promote diarrhea.

Test-taking strategy: Analyze to determine what information the question asks for, which is nursing measures in the plan of care. First, consider measures to decrease inflammation in the bowel. Next, consider nursing measures to treat the symptoms. "Select all that apply" questions require considering each option to decide its merit. Review the pathophysiology and treatment of Crohn's disease, and focus on clinical manifestations and nursing interventions if you had difficulty answering this question.

Client needs category: Safe and effective care environment

Client needs subcategory: Management of care

Cognitive level: Applying

11. The nurse is caring for a client admitted with cirrhosis of the liver. Which laboratory results are consistent with the disease process? Select all that apply.

☐ **1.** Prothrombin time 22 seconds

☐ **2.** Potassium 4.0 mEq/L (4.0 mmol/L)

☐ **3.** Albumin 7.2 g/dL (72 g/L)

☐ **4.** Ammonia 96 mg/dl (68.54 mmol/L)

☐ **5.** Platelets 75,000 cells/mm³ (75 10/L)

☐ **6.** Amylase 250 units/L (4.18 μkat/L)

Answer: 1, 4, 5

ⓘ Rationale: The client with cirrhosis has liver dysfunction and impaired coagulation and rising ammonia levels. The prothrombin time is prolonged (normal is 10 to 13.0 seconds), and the platelet count is low (normal is 150,000 to 350,000 cells/mm³). A normal ammonia level is 15 to 45 mg/dl (10.71 mmol/L to 32.13 mmol/L), and this client's level is elevated, placing the client at risk for hepatic encephalopathy. A client with cirrhosis typically has hypokalemia because of the diuretic therapy used to treat the fluid retention associated with the disease. Here, the potassium level is within normal limits (3.5 to 5.0 mEq/L or 3.5 to 5.0 mmol/L). In cirrhosis, the albumin level is also typically low (normal is 3.5 to 5.0 g/dl or 35 to 50 g/L) because of alterations in protein metabolism in the liver. Levels of amylase, a pancreatic enzyme, typically increase with pancreatitis, not cirrhosis (normal level is 27 to 151 units/L or 0.45 μkat/L to 2.52 μkat/L).

Test-taking strategy: Analyze to determine what information the question asks for, which is laboratory values consistent with a diagnosis of cirrhosis of the liver. "Select all that apply" questions require considering each option to decide its merit. First, consider the functioning of the liver and laboratory values that would be elevated in the client with liver dysfunction. Next, consider the impact of other organs and the corresponding lab values. Review the pathophysiology of cirrhosis, and focus on normal and abnormal laboratory values if you had difficulty answering this question.

Client needs category: Physiological integrity

Client needs subcategory: Reduction of risk potential

Cognitive level: Analyzing

---

12. The nurse is evaluating how a client with hepatitis A understands the discharge teaching given. Which client statements indicate that further teaching is needed? Select all that apply.

☐ **1.** "I can have an occasional glass of wine with my meal as I recover."

☐ **2.** "My family and I do not need to take any special precautions as long as I take my medication."

☐ **3.** "My bath towels shouldn't be used by any other family members."

☐ **4.** "My family members should receive the hepatitis A vaccine to prevent them from getting the disease."

☐ **5.** "My spouse and I can have intercourse and kiss."

☐ **6.** "I should wear a mask when visitors come."

Answer: 1, 2, 5, 6

ⓘ Rationale: Hepatitis A is inflammation (irritation and swelling) of the liver from the hepatitis A virus. The hepatitis A virus is found mostly in the blood and stools of the infected person. Clients with hepatitis would abstain from alcohol to prevent exacerbation of the disease. Standard precautions and meticulous hand washing would be practiced by all family members. All family members would avoid close contact with the client; this includes avoiding intercourse, kissing, and the use of any personal items (such as bath towels and eating utensils) that may be contaminated with the client's feces. Because hepatitis A is transmitted by the oral–fecal route, not the respiratory route, wearing a mask is not necessary. The hepatitis A vaccine would be given prophylactically to all family members and close contacts to prevent disease transmission.

Test-taking strategy: Analyze to determine what information the question asks for, which is a client statement that indicates the need for further teaching. "Select all that apply" questions require considering each option to decide its merit. When appraising each option, look for an incorrect statement in need of further teaching. Consider the nature of the illness and mode of transmission. Review the pathophysiology and transmission route for hepatitis A if you had difficulty answering this question.

Client needs category: Health promotion and maintenance

Client needs subcategory: None

Cognitive level: Applying

13. At the beginning of the shift, the nurse is assigned a client with an ascending colostomy. Which picture identifies the correct placement where the nurse will assess the stoma?

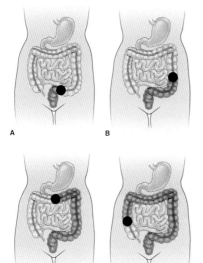

A   B

C   D

Answer: D

Ⓔ **Rationale:** A colostomy can be performed along any site of the colon. The location of an ascending colostomy is on the right side of the abdomen. An ostomy located in the ascending colon would likely produce continuous liquid output because feces in this section contain the most water and, therefore, have a liquid consistency. A sigmoid colostomy is located on the sigmoid colon and located close to the location of a descending colostomy in the left side of the abdomen. The transverse colostomy is horizontal across the middle abdomen or toward the right side of the body across the abdomen.

Test-taking strategy: Analyze to determine what information the question asks for, which is the location of an ascending colostomy. Recall that a colostomy is a surgical procedure, which brings the colon out along various locations on the abdominal wall. Note that identifying the placement uses anatomical position when reporting right and left locations. Review information on various types of colostomies if you had difficulty answering this question.

Client needs category: Physiological integrity

Client needs subcategory: Physiological adaptation

Cognitive level: Applying

14. A client has been admitted to the emergency department with severe midepigastric, upper quadrant abdominal pain. Based on the signs and symptoms and laboratory data documented in the chart below, the nurse would anticipate preparing for which diagnosis?

03/12/16	Client admitted to the emergency
0730	department with severe upper quadrant
	pain radiating to the back, nausea and
	vomiting, and fever. Laboratory results
	received via telephone as follows: glucose
	462 mg/dl (25.6 mmol/L), WBC 14,000 cells/
	mm³, lipase 214 units/L (3.6 μkat/L), and
	calcium 6.5 mg/dl (1.6 mmol/L).
	—Andrea Nichols, RN

☐ **1.** Peptic ulcer

☐ **2.** Crohn's disease

☐ **3.** Pancreatitis

☐ **4.** Irritable bowel syndrome

Answer: 3

E **Rationale:** The assessment findings combined with the laboratory results suggest pancreatitis. The pancreas is situated behind the stomach in the upper quadrant. Signs and symptoms of pancreatitis include severe midepigastric, upper quadrant abdominal pain, fever, nausea, and vomiting. Inflammation of the pancreas results in leukocytosis. Injured β-cells are unable to produce insulin, leading to hyperglycemia, which may be as high as 500 to 900 mg/dl (27.75 mmol/L to 49.95 mmol/L). Lipase and amylase levels become elevated as the pancreatic enzymes leak from injured pancreatic cells. Calcium becomes trapped as fat necrosis occurs, leading to hypocalcemia. Peptic ulcer, Crohn's disease, and irritable bowel syndrome do not cause amylase or lipase levels to increase.

Test-taking strategy: Analyze to determine what information the question asks for, which is a potential medical diagnosis obtained through assessment data. Utilize the data to provide clues to potential disorders. Begin with subjective data as reported by the client, and next consider objective data such as laboratory values. Relate to signs and symptoms of options. Review various disorders with severe midepigastric upper quadrant abdominal pain if you had difficulty answering this question.

Client needs category: Physiological integrity

Client needs subcategory: Reduction of risk potential

Cognitive level: Analyzing

---

15. The nurse is preparing to administer a 75% strength tube-feeding formula. The full-strength formula is available. To prepare 500 ml of feeding, the nurse would plan to dilute how many milliliters of the full-strength formula with water? Record your answer as a whole number.

_____ ml

Answer: 375

M **Rationale:** To determine the amount of formula to use, multiply the 500 ml of full-strength formula by 75% (0.75):

$$500 \text{ ml} \times 0.75 = 375 \text{ ml}.$$

Test-taking strategy: Analyze to determine what information the question asks for, which is the amount of formula to fluid ratio to administer a 75% concentration. Consider that a 75% concentration is less than 1; thus, multiplying by a 0.75 is correct. Review dosage calculations based on percentages if you had difficulty answering this question.

Client needs category: Physiological integrity

Client needs subcategory: Basic care and comfort

Cognitive level: Applying

---

16. The nurse is assisting a client to ambulate to the bathroom following a bowel resection for diverticulitis. Suddenly, the client reports a sharp abdominal pain. The nurse assesses the client and determines the wound has eviscerated. Prioritize the following nursing actions in chronological order to show how the nurse would respond. All options must be used.

1. Assess the client's response.

2. Call for assistance from other nursing personnel.

3. Document the incident, including the client's condition.

4. Cover the wound with sterile, nonadherent dressing moistened with sterile normal saline solution.

5. Place the client in low Fowler's position.

6. Notify the surgeon.

Ⓜ Rationale: When evisceration of an abdominal wound occurs, the nurse would remain with the client and summon help to bring necessary supplies to the client's room. The client would be placed in low Fowler's position to lessen tension on the abdomen. The nurse would not attempt to reinsert protruding organs. Instead, the nurse would moisten sterile, nonadherent dressings with warm, sterile normal saline solution and cover the wound. It is important to conduct an ongoing client assessment until the surgeon arrives because the client is at risk for shock. Documentation of the incident and the client's condition would be completed immediately after the incident.

Test-taking strategy: Analyze to determine what information the question asks for, which is nursing care when an evisceration occurs. When prioritizing, think "safety" first. Next, focus on nursing interventions related to postoperative wound dehiscence. Lastly, document as soon as possible. Review emergency care protocols related to a wound evisceration if you had difficulty answering this question.

Client needs category: Physiological integrity

Client needs subcategory: Physiological adaptation

Cognitive level: Analyzing

17. A nurse is caring for a client following gastric bypass surgery. At the six-week appointment, the client reports symptoms of nausea, abdominal pain and cramping following meals, and shakiness and sweating up to 3 hours later. Which nursing interventions would help reduce the symptoms and be included in the plan of care? Select all that apply.

☐ **1.** Eat small, frequent meals.

☐ **2.** Limit sodium intake.

☐ **3.** Reduce high concentrated sugars.

☐ **4.** Ingest fluids at the end of meals.

☐ **5.** Refer the client to a dietician.

Answer: 1, 3, 5

Ⓓ **Rationale:** Following gastric bypass surgery, many have symptoms of the dumping syndrome. Dumping syndrome occurs when food and gastric juices from the stomach move to the intestine in an uncontrollably fast manner leading to early and late symptoms. Early symptoms include the nausea and abdominal cramping. Late signs are related to the insulin surge and include symptoms of hypoglycemia. Eating small and frequent meals, reducing high concentrated sugars, and following a dietician's guidelines all are helpful in reducing symptoms. Limiting sodium intake may be a good dietary practice but is not indicated in reducing causes of dumping syndrome. There are no guidelines on when to ingest fluids other than that liquids and solids should not be taken together.

Test-taking strategy: Analyze to determine what information the question asks for, which is nursing interventions to limit symptoms of the dumping syndrome. First, relate the symptoms to food ingestion. Then, consider what would ease those symptoms. Small, frequent meals and reducing a sugar rush are notable in reducing abdominal cramping in many situations. Most individuals following gastric bypass need a dietician consultation. Review nursing interventions to decrease episodes of the dumping syndrome if you had difficulty answering this question.

Client needs category: Physiological integrity

Client needs subcategory: Physiological adaptation

Cognitive level: Applying

18. The registered nurse (RN) is assigned a client with stomach cancer, who has just returned from a subtotal gastrectomy. Which nursing interventions would be delegated to either a licensed practical/vocational nurse (LPN/VN) or a nursing assistant/unregistered health care worker (UHW)? Select all that apply.

☐ **1.** Administer carboplatin 750 mg intravenously.

☐ **2.** Document intake and output in the electronic medical record.

☐ **3.** Assess bowel sounds in all four quadrants.

☐ **4.** Place a dry dressing over an abdominal incision.

☐ **5.** Ambulate in the hall for the first time after surgery.

☐ **6.** Provide report for the oncoming shift.

Answer: 2, 4, 6

Ⓒ **Rationale:** The RN may delegate to the LPN/VN or nursing assistant the responsibilities of documentation of intake and output and dressing an abdominal wound. The LPN/VN may provide nursing report to the oncoming shift. The RN would administer carboplatin, a chemotherapeutic agent as this is out of the scope of practice of the LPN/VN. The RN would also complete any postoperative assessment such as bowel sounds and postoperative ambulation since the RN holds the responsibility of this nursing assignment. Review the management of care following a subtotal gastrectomy and delegation practices if you had difficulty answering this question.

Test-taking strategy: Analyze to determine what information the question asks for, which is delegation practice for a client returning from a subtotal gastrectomy. The key word is "surgery," meaning that the nurse assigned to the client needs to complete a thorough assessment. Also, consider the scope of practice for each level of nursing. The nurse must not complete or assign an action outside of the scope of practice. Review delegation practices if you had difficulty answering this question.

Client needs category: Safe and effective care environment

Client needs subcategory: Management of care

Cognitive level: Analyzing

Genitourinary disorders

1. A 176-lb client with minimal urine output has been prescribed dopamine at 5 µg/kg/minute. The premixed medication bag contains 800 mg of dopamine in 500 ml dextrose 5% in water. How many milliliters of solution would the nurse administer each hour? Record your answer as a whole number.

_____ ml

© **Rationale:** Factor analysis is the easiest way to solve this problem. Identify the information you have, and then use conversion factors to obtain the information you need:

$$\frac{176 \text{ lb}}{1} \times \frac{1 \text{ kg}}{2.2 \text{ lb}} \times \frac{5 \text{ µg}}{1 \text{ kg/minute}} \times \frac{1 \text{ mg}}{1{,}000 \text{ µg}}$$

$$\times \frac{500 \text{ ml}}{800 \text{ mg}} \times \frac{60 \text{ minute}}{1 \text{ hour}}$$

$$\frac{26{,}400{,}000 \text{ ml}}{1{,}760{,}000 \text{ hours}} = 15 \text{ ml / hour}$$

Test-taking strategy: Analyze to determine what information the question asks for, which is milliliters of dopamine solution to be administered each hour. Recall the steps for factor analysis and intravenous flow rate calculations. Proofread your work including the math calculations. Ask yourself, does the answer make sense? Review calculations using factor analysis if you had difficulty answering this question.

Client needs category: Physiological integrity

Client needs subcategory: Pharmacological and parenteral therapies

Cognitive level: Applying

2. A client with marked oliguria is ordered a test dose of 0.2 g/kg of 15% mannitol solution intravenously over 5 minutes. The client weighs 132 lb. How many grams would the nurse administer? Record your answer as a whole number.

_____ g

Answer: 12

Ⓔ Rationale: First, convert the client's weight from pounds to kilograms:

$$132 \text{ lb} \div 2.2 \text{ kg/lb} = 60 \text{ kg}.$$

Then, to calculate the number of grams to administer, multiply the ordered number of grams by the client's weight in kilograms:

$$0.2 \text{ g/kg} \times 60 \text{ kg} = 12 \text{ g}.$$

Test-taking strategy: Analyze to determine what information the question asks for, which is the number of grams of mannitol to administer according to the client's weight. Recall that many doses are calculated according to unit dosage (mg, g, ml, etc.) per kilogram. Be careful that the unit dosage is consistent with what the question is asking. Review intravenous calculations and weight dosing if you had difficulty answering this question.

Client needs category: Physiological integrity

Client needs subcategory: Pharmacological and parenteral therapies

Cognitive level: Analyzing

---

3. A nurse is obtaining a health history from a male senior citizen. The client states that he is having urinary hesitancy, slight dysuria, and dribbling. He denies reports of hematuria. Identify the area where the nurse anticipates the primary cause of the urinary dysfunction.

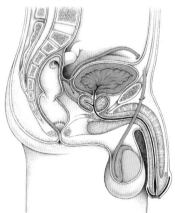

Answer:

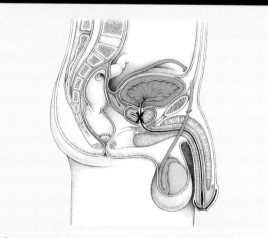

Ⓔ Rationale: Note that the X is over the prostate gland. The walnut-sized prostate gland lies beneath the bladder and surrounds the urethra. When the prostate gland becomes enlarged, which commonly occurs as a male ages, urination becomes affected as the prostate gland narrows the passage of urine through the urethra.

Test-taking strategy: Analyze to determine what information the question asks for, which is location of the cause of the urinary dysfunction. Look to the symptoms, and note the age of the client for clues of the cause of the urinary problems. Review the anatomy of the male genitourinary system and the effects of aging if you had difficulty answering this question.

Client needs category: Physiological integrity

Client needs subcategory: Physiological adaptation

Cognitive level: Applying

4. After a retropubic prostatectomy, a client needs continuous bladder irrigation. The client has an intravenous line with dextrose in 5% water infusing at 40 ml/hour and a triple-lumen urinary catheter with normal saline solution infusing at 200 ml/hour. The nurse empties the urinary catheter drainage bag three times during an 8-hour period for a total of 2,780 ml. How many milliliters would the nurse calculate as urine? Record your answer as a whole number.

_____ ml

Answer: 1,180

Ⓒ Rationale: During 8 hours, 1,600 ml of bladder irrigant has been infused (200 ml × 8 hours = 1,600 ml/8 hours). The nurse would subtract this amount from the total volume in the drainage bag to determine the urine output (2,780 ml − 1,600 ml = 1,180 ml).

Test-taking strategy: Analyze to determine what information the question asks for, which is the amount of urine production in an 8-hour shift. Focus on the output, and disregard extraneous information of the intravenous solution. Note that finding the urine amount comes from the total amount of urine minus the amount of bladder irrigation. Proofread your math calculation. Review the methods for calculating urinary elimination with bladder irrigation if you had difficulty answering this question.

Client needs category: Physiological integrity

Client needs subcategory: Basic care and comfort

Cognitive level: Applying

5. A nurse is caring for a client with chronic renal failure. The laboratory results indicate hypocalcemia and hyperphosphatemia. When assessing the client, the nurse would be alert for which occurrence? Select all that apply.

☐ **1.** Trousseau's sign

☐ **2.** Cardiac arrhythmias

☐ **3.** Constipation

☐ **4.** Decreased clotting time

☐ **5.** Drowsiness and lethargy

☐ **6.** Fractures

Answer: 1, 2, 6

Ⓒ Rationale: Chronic renal failure is the slow process of losing kidney function over time. At some point, the kidney will not be able to remove excess fluid and wastes from the body causing fluid and electrolyte complications. Hypocalcemia is a calcium deficit that causes nerve fiber irritability and repetitive muscle spasms. Signs and symptoms of hypocalcemia include Trousseau's sign, cardiac arrhythmias, diarrhea, increased clotting times, anxiety, and irritability. The calcium–phosphorus imbalance leads to brittle bones and pathologic fractures. Drowsiness and lethargy are not typically associated with hypercalcemia.

Test-taking strategy: Analyze to determine what information the question asks for, which is complications resulting from hypocalcemia and hyperphosphatemia. "Select all that apply" questions require considering each option to decide its merit. Consider the effects of calcium and phosphate in the system, and relate complications when there is an alteration of too much or too little. Review the signs and symptoms of hypocalcemia and hyperphosphatemia, and review fluids and electrolyte imbalances if you had difficulty answering this question.

Client needs category: Physiological integrity

Client needs subcategory: Reduction of risk potential

Cognitive level: Applying

6. A nurse is completing a health screening activity to identify at which point in the menstrual cycle a client's problem occurs. Place the pathophysiologic steps of the menstrual cycle listed below in the correct sequential order. All options must be used.

1. The level of estrogen in the blood peaks.

2. Peak endometrial thickening occurs.

3. The top layer of the endometrium breaks down and sloughs.

4. Increased estrogen and progesterone levels inhibit luteinizing hormone.

5. A follicle matures and ovulation occurs.

6. The endometrium begins thickening.

Answer: 4, 6, 1, 5, 2, 3

ⓘ Rationale: The nurse is performing a health screening by reviewing the steps in the menstrual cycle. The menstrual cycle begins with the first day of menstruation, when the top layer of endometrium breaks down and begins to slough off. As the endometrium thickens, the level of estrogen in the blood begins to rise and eventually peak. The follicle matures, and ovulation occurs when estrogen levels peak. After ovulation, the endometrium continues to thicken to its peak level. Increased estrogen and progesterone levels inhibit follicle-stimulating hormone, which causes a feedback loop that then decreases estrogen and progesterone production. This causes the top layer of the endometrium to break down and slough, restarting the cycle in a nonpregnant female.

Test-taking strategy: Analyze to determine what information the question asks for, which is the order of events occurring during the menstrual cycle. Carefully read each option. It can be helpful to select the first in the series and last in the series allowing a narrowing of middle options. Also, it is important to recognize that the menstrual cycle begins with the first day of menstruation. Review normal growth and development and the menstrual cycle if you had difficulty answering this question.

Client needs category: Health promotion and maintenance

Client needs subcategory: None

Cognitive level: Applying

---

7. A client requires behavioral therapies to decrease or eliminate urinary incontinence. Which procedures would the nurse expect to include in the teaching plan for this client? Select all that apply.

☐ **1.** Kegel exercises

☐ **2.** Scheduled voiding

☐ **3.** External catheters

☐ **4.** Biofeedback

☐ **5.** Self-catheterization devices

☐ **6.** Postvoid residual monitoring

Answer: 1, 2, 4

ⓘ Rationale: Clients, particularly females, have conditions relating to alterations in urinary output. Kegel exercises, scheduled voiding, and biofeedback are behavioral therapies used to decrease or eliminate urinary incontinence. Both external catheters and self-catheterization devices are used to collect urine. Postvoid residual monitoring assesses the ability to empty the bladder but does not decrease or eliminate urinary incontinence.

Test-taking strategy: Analyze to determine what information the question asks for, which is behavioral therapies to eliminate urinary incontinence. "Select all that apply" questions require considering each option to decide its merit. The key term is "behavioral therapies," providing a clue that it is teaching that provides the client control over the urinary condition. Review bladder training techniques if you had difficulty answering this question.

Client needs category: Health promotion and maintenance

Client needs subcategory: None

Cognitive level: Applying

---

8. A nurse is explaining self-catheterization to a female client who has been diagnosed with urogenic bladder. Which instructions would the nurse include in the teaching? Select all that apply.

☐ **1.** Tampons may remain in place during menstruation.

☐ **2.** The meatus would be cleaned with a towelette or soapy washcloth and then rinsed.

☐ **3.** Sterile technique is not required.

☐ **4.** A new intermittent catheterization set would be used each time.

☐ **5.** Finding the urinary meatus always requires visualization with a mirror.

Answer: 2, 3

🅓 **Rationale:** Cleaning the meatus with a towelette or soapy washcloth decreases the risk of introducing bacteria into the bladder. Sterile technique is not required during self-catheterization. Leaving a tampon in place can restrict the urethra and impede catheter insertion. It is not necessary to use a new intermittent catheter each time; washing the catheter and allowing it to air-dry after each use is usually sufficient. The urinary meatus can be found using visual or tactile techniques.

Test-taking strategy: Analyze to determine what information the question asks for, which is key points in self-catheterization. "Select all that apply" questions require considering each option to decide its merit. Focus on clean versus sterile technique during catheterization instruction. Review catheter care and self-catheterization technique if you had difficulty answering this question.

Client needs category: Health promotion and maintenance

Client needs subcategory: None

Cognitive level: Applying

---

9. The nurse is reviewing a client's urine culture and sensitivity test results. Which findings would the nurse expect to see in small amounts in normal urine? Select all that apply.

☐ **1.** Ketones

☐ **2.** Protein

☐ **3.** White blood cells

☐ **4.** Crystals

☐ **5.** Nitrates

☐ **6.** Bilirubin

Answer: 2, 3

🅓 **Rationale:** A urine culture is a test to detect and identify organisms, such as bacteria and components, within the urine. Information obtained can identify a urinary tract infection, kidney disease, or high blood glucose. Small amounts of protein and white blood cells are normal. Ketones, crystals, nitrates, and bilirubin are all abnormal findings.

Test-taking strategy: Analyze to determine what information the question asks for, which is findings in normal urine. "Select all that apply" questions require considering each option to decide its merit. Recall what information is reported in a urine culture and what information reported would be abnormal. Note that white blood cells are found in even normal cultures such as they are in normal complete blood counts. Review normal urinalysis findings and other routine urinalysis and laboratory tests if you had difficulty answering this question.

Client needs category: Physiological integrity

Client needs subcategory: Reduction of risk potential

Cognitive level: Understanding

10. A nurse is assessing a client with right flank pain, fever, and chills. A urine culture is obtained, and a diagnosis of suspected right pyelonephritis is documented. When instructing the client on the diagnosis, the nurse uses a diagram of the urinary structures. Identify with an X the area associated with the diagnosis.

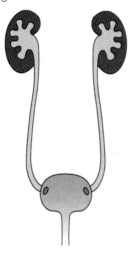

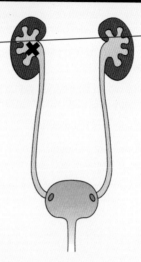

E Rationale: Pyelonephritis is a type of urinary tract infection that affects one or both kidneys. Right pyelonephritis is on the right side of the client's body but would be documented on the left in the anatomical position. Bacteria and viruses can move to the kidneys from the bladder or can be carried from other body systems through the bloodstream causing the disease process.

Test-taking strategy: Analyze to determine what information the question asks for, which is the site of right pyelonephritis. If unsure, use medical terminology to determine the site (nephro = kidney). Review the names and locations of urinary structures if you had difficulty answering this question.

Client needs category: Physiological integrity

Client needs subcategory: Physiological adaptation

Cognitive level: Understanding

11. A nurse is providing health teaching on female sexuality and provides illustration for education on the female anatomy. When discussing problems with sexual excitation, the nurse is correct to indicate which site as the area of sexual stimulation?

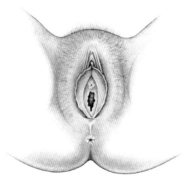

Answer:

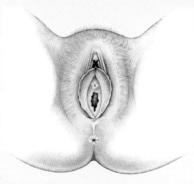

E Rationale: Sexual excitement causes various physiological changes in the female body. The area associated with sexual stimulation is located near the vaginal entrance and behind the labia minora. The clitoris is directly associated with engorgement and climax.

Test-taking strategy: Analyze to determine what information the question asks for, which is a site of female sexual stimulation. Review the anatomy of the female reproductive system and female sexuality if you had difficulty answering this question.

Client needs category: Health promotion and maintenance

Client needs subcategory: None

Cognitive level: Remembering

---

12. The nurse is caring for a client with stress incontinence who is ordered a cystometrography. The client inquires about the nature of the procedure. Place in chronological order the sequence of events for this procedure. All options must be used.

1. Client is asked to void normally.

2. Urinary catheter is inserted.

3. Fluid is instilled into the urinary catheter.

4. Any residual urine is noted.

5. Client is asked to void following instillation.

6. Urge to void is recorded.

Answer: 1, 2, 4, 6, 5, 3

D **Rationale:** A cystometrography is a urological procedure that measures the amount of pressure exerted on the bladder at various bladder volumes. First, the client is asked to void normally. Then a urinary catheter is inserted, and fluid is instilled. The first urge to void is recorded. Following the procedure, the client is instructed to void and any residual urine is noted. Finally, the catheter is removed.

Test-taking strategy: Analyze to determine what information the question asks for, which is the procedure for completing a cystometrography. Recall that the procedure measures bladder volumes and the pressure associated; thus, various volumes of fluid must be present in the bladder. Volume begins with little urine in the bladder, and then fluid volume increases. Review the physiology of the genitourinary system and the cystometrography procedure if you had difficulty answering this question.

Client needs category: Physiological integrity

Client needs subcategory: Reduction of risk potential

Cognitive level: Analyzing

13. The nurse is caring for a client with nephropathy. The health care provider orders a 24-hour urine collection. Which actions are necessary to ensure proper collection of the specimen? Select all that apply.

☐ **1.** Collect the urine in a preservative-free container and keep on ice.

☐ **2.** Inform the client to discard the last voided specimen at the conclusion of urine collection.

☐ **3.** Ask the client what his/her weight is for documentation on the container.

☐ **4.** Request an order for insertion of an indwelling urinary catheter.

☐ **5.** Encourage daily amounts of fluids.

☐ **6.** Discard the initial voiding but save all others for 24 hours.

Answer: 1, 5, 6

Ⓜ **Rationale:** All urine for a 24-hour urine collection must be saved in a container with no preservatives and refrigerated or kept on ice. Normal fluid amounts or an increase in fluids is encouraged. The first urine voided at the beginning of the collection is discarded, not the last. A self-report of weight may not be accurate, and it is typically not documented on the container. It is not necessary to have an indwelling urinary catheter inserted for urine collection.

Test-taking strategy: Analyze to determine what information the question asks for, which is proper procedure for collecting a 24-hour urine sample. Recall standard procedures for specimen collection, particularly when to begin collecting the urine and how to maintain the urine for 24 hours. As with many laboratory tests, special containers are needed for the collection. Review standard guidelines when obtaining a 24-hour urine collection if you had difficulty answering this question.

Client needs category: Physiological integrity

Client needs subcategory: Reduction of risk potential

Cognitive level: Understanding

---

14. The nurse is caring for a client who possibly may need kidney dialysis. When evaluating the client's renal function to report to the health care provider, which data will the nurse use? Select all that apply.

☐ **1.** A client's 24-hour urinary output

☐ **2.** Glomerular filtration rate

☐ **3.** Trending vital signs

☐ **4.** A client's flank pain level

☐ **5.** The blood count report

☐ **6.** Serum creatinine level

Answer: 1, 2, 6

Ⓓ **Rationale:** When evaluating renal functioning, the nurse would report to the health care provider information on the current urine output, the glomerular filtration rate, and serum creatinine levels, which identify the degree of kidney dysfunction. These objective data provide diagnostic information. Vital signs and pain level reflect the impact of the renal disease. Blood count reports do not assist in evaluating renal function.

Test-taking strategy: Analyze to determine what information the question asks for, which is data that relate information regarding the functional ability of the kidney. Consider what data provide information specifically on renal functioning. These data include actual renal output and diagnostic testing providing information on the working of the kidney. Review renal functioning indicators and symptoms associated with the disease process if you had difficulty answering this question.

Client needs category: Physiological integrity

Client needs subcategory: Physiological adaptation

Cognitive level: Evaluating

Musculoskeletal disorders

1. A nurse is caring for a client newly diagnosed with osteoporosis. Which statements would the nurse include when teaching the client about the disease? Select all that apply.

☐ **1.** Osteoporosis is common in females after menopause.

☐ **2.** Osteoporosis is a degenerative disease characterized by a decrease in bone density.

☐ **3.** The disease is inherited, caused by an inability to tolerate milk products.

☐ **4.** Osteoporosis can cause pain and injury.

☐ **5.** Passive ROM exercises can promote bone growth.

☐ **6.** Weight-bearing exercise would be avoided.

Answer: 1, 2, 4

Ⓜ **Rationale:** Osteoporosis is a degenerative metabolic bone disorder in which the rate of bone resorption accelerates and the rate of bone formation decelerates, thus decreasing bone density. Postmenopausal women are at increased risk for this disorder because of their loss of estrogen. The decrease in bone density can cause pain and injury. Osteoporosis is not an inherited disorder; however, low calcium intake because of an intolerance of milk products does contribute to it. Passive ROM exercises may be performed, but they will not promote bone growth. The client should be encouraged to participate in weight-bearing exercise because it promotes bone growth.

Test-taking strategy: Analyze to determine what information the question asks for, which is key points in osteoporosis teaching. "Select all that apply" questions require considering each option to decide its merit. Recall that the bones of the spine become less dense causing skeletal changes. Consider factors that promote bone growth. Review key points and treatments for osteoporosis if you had difficulty answering this question.

Client needs category: Physiological integrity

Client needs subcategory: Physiological adaptation

Cognitive level: Applying

2. A nurse is preparing discharge instructions for an above-the-knee amputation client. Which instructions would be a **priority** for home care? Select all that apply.

☐ **1.** Massage the residual limb in a motion away from the suture line.

☐ **2.** Avoid using heat application to ease pain.

☐ **3.** Immediately report twitching, spasms, or phantom limb pain.

☐ **4.** Avoid exposing the skin around the residual limb to excessive perspiration.

☐ **5.** Be sure to perform the prescribed exercises.

☐ **6.** Rub the residual limb with a dry washcloth for 4 minutes three times daily if the limb is sensitive to touch.

Answer: 4, 5, 6

ⓓ **Rationale:** The nurse would advise the client that perspiration on the residual limb may cause irritation. The client would exercise as instructed to minimize complications. In addition, rubbing the limb as described with a dry washcloth helps desensitize the skin. The nurse would instruct the client to massage the residual limb toward the suture line—not away from it—to mobilize the scar and prevent its adherence to the bone. Twitching, spasms, and phantom limb pain are normal reactions to an amputation and do not need to be reported. The nurse would inform the client that these symptoms might be eased by heat, massage, or gentle pressure.

Test-taking strategy: Analyze to determine what information the question asks for, which is priority discharge instructions. "Select all that apply" questions require considering each option to decide its merit. When considering instruction, think "surgical complications to watch for" and "amputation care" as priorities. Select the options that would increase the clients' ability to safely care for the new amputation. Review postoperative care to promote self-care and wound healing, and review postamputation rehabilitation if you had difficulty answering this question.

Client needs category: Physiological integrity
Client needs subcategory: Reduction of risk potential
Cognitive level: Applying

---

3. A nurse is assigned a client with an acute exacerbation of rheumatoid arthritis (RA). Which medical facts about RA are essential in developing a plan of care? Select all that apply.

☐ **1.** Onset is acute and usually occurs between ages 20 and 40.

☐ **2.** The client experiences stiff, swollen joints bilaterally.

☐ **3.** The client may not exercise once the disease is diagnosed.

☐ **4.** Erythrocyte sedimentation rate (ESR) is elevated, and x-rays show erosions and decalcification of involved joints.

☐ **5.** Inflamed cartilage triggers complement activation, which stimulates the release of additional inflammatory mediators.

☐ **6.** The first-line treatment is gold salts and methotrexate.

Answer: 2, 4, 5

ⓜ **Rationale:** RA is a chronic disorder where individuals experience stiff, swollen joints because of a severe inflammatory reaction. Elevated ESR and x-ray evidence of bony destruction are indicative of severe involvement. RA starts insidiously, with fatigue, persistent low-grade fever, anorexia, and vague skeletal symptoms, usually in middle age between the ages 35 and 50 years. Maintaining the ROM by a prescribed exercise program is essential, but clients must rest between activities. Salicylates and nonsteroidal anti-inflammatory drugs are considered the first-line treatments.

Test-taking strategy: Analyze to determine what information the question asks for, which is developing a care plan related to essential facts of RA. "Select all that apply" questions require considering each option to decide its merit. Consider that knowledge of a disease process and treatment is crucial in developing a plan of care. Understanding the severity allows for client-centered care. Review pathophysiology and treatment of RA if you had difficulty answering this question.

Client needs category: Physiological integrity
Client needs subcategory: Physiological adaptation
Cognitive level: Analyzing

---

4. A nurse is caring for a client who fell and fractured the neck of the femur. When documenting the site for the family members, place an X on the area where the fracture occurred.

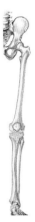

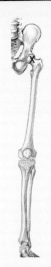

Ⓜ **Rationale:** The neck of the femur is a flattened pyramidal process of bone, connecting the femoral head with the femoral shaft just below the ball and socket. When a femoral neck fracture occurs, the ball is disconnected from the rest of the thigh bone.

Test-taking strategy: Analyze to determine what information the question asks for, which is the site of the femoral neck fracture. If unsure, use the descriptive name (femoral-femur, neck-top of the femur before ball and socket) to direct to the fractured site. Review the anatomy of the upper leg if you had difficulty answering this question.

Client needs category: Physiological integrity

Client needs subcategory: Physiological adaptation

Cognitive level: Understanding

---

5. A nurse is putting groceries in the car when an elderly client falls off of a curb. The nurse assesses the client and has a bystander call for an ambulance. Which assessment findings provide data of a suspected right hip fracture? Select all that apply.

☐ **1.** The right leg is longer than the left leg.

☐ **2.** The right leg is shorter than the left leg.

☐ **3.** The right leg is abducted.

☐ **4.** The right leg is adducted.

☐ **5.** The right leg is externally rotated.

☐ **6.** The right leg is internally rotated.

Answer: 2, 4, 5

Ⓓ **Rationale:** A hip fracture is a serious injury, particularly if you are elderly. Subjective signs of a hip fracture include the inability to move after a fall, pain, and the inability to bear weight and stiffness. Objective signs of a hip fracture include the affected leg being shorter, adducted, and externally rotated.

Test-taking strategy: Analyze to determine what information the question asks for, which is assessment data of a suspected right hip fracture. "Select all that apply" questions require considering each option to decide its merit. Note that the options are opposites; thus, there will be three correct answers. Review the clinical manifestations of fractures, specifically of the femur if you had difficulty answering this question.

Client needs category: Physiological integrity

Client needs subcategory: Physiological adaptation

Cognitive level: Applying

6. A nurse is admitting a client scheduled for a laminectomy of the L1 and L2 vertebrae. Upon returning from the surgical procedure, place an X where the nurse assesses the surgical incision.

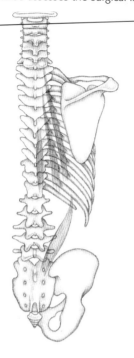

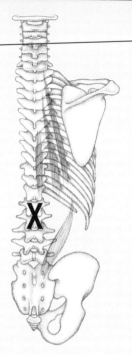

Ⓜ Rationale: Note the placement of the X in the lower back. In a laminectomy, one or more of the bony laminae that cover the vertebrae are removed. The incision for the surgery is at the site of the vertebrae. There are five lumbar vertebrae that are numbered from top to bottom. L5 is the closest to the sacrum. Count up from the sacrum to locate L1 and L2.

Test-taking strategy: Analyze to determine what information the question asks for, which is the site of the surgical procedure (L1 and L2). Recall that there are 7 cervical vertebrae, 12 thoracic vertebrae, and 5 lumbar vertebrae. Review the anatomy of the spinal column and the laminectomy surgical procedure if you had difficulty answering this question.

Client needs category: Physiological integrity

Client needs subcategory: Physiological adaptation

Cognitive level: Understanding

7. A client is being discharged to a transitional rehabilitation care facility following a hip replacement because of degenerative arthritis. When reporting to the licensed practical/vocational nurse (LPN/VN), which nursing actions would the orthopedic nurse stress as essential? Select all that apply.

☐ **1.** Place the client in high Fowler's position.

☐ **2.** Avoid any hip flexion exercises.

☐ **3.** Place two pillows between the client's knees.

☐ **4.** Place a raised toilet seat in the bathroom.

☐ **5.** Keep the client's feet elevated.

☐ **6.** Maintain the client on bed rest until the incision heals.

Answer: 2, 3, 4

Ⓜ **Rationale:** The hip is one of the body's largest joints. In a total hip replacement, the damaged bone and cartilage are removed and replaced with prosthetic components. Until healing occurs, the legs must be spread outward (abducted) away from the body by placing pillows or an abductor foam wedge between the legs. Adduction of the hip or flexion greater than 90° may dislocate the prosthesis from the joint. Raising the head of the bed 90° creates excessive hip flexion. Using a raised toilet seat is appropriate to avoid bending. The client will be out of bed for physical therapy once to twice daily. Keeping the feet elevated is not part of the hip replacement protocol.

Test-taking strategy: Analyze to determine what information the question asks for, which is nursing actions in the rehab setting for a client post hip replacement. "Select all that apply" questions require considering each option to decide its merit. Choose the options for the postoperative rehab period. Recall that positioning is very important until the hip structure heals. Review care of clients following hip replacement surgery if you had difficulty answering this question.

Client needs category: Physiological integrity

Client needs subcategory: Reduction of risk potential

Cognitive level: Applying

8. A client is suspected of having carpal tunnel syndrome. The nurse assesses for Tinel's sign. Identify the area where the nurse would percuss in an attempt to elicit Tinel's sign.

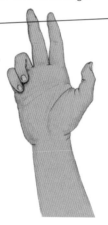

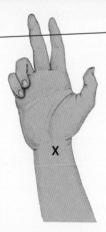

X

 Rationale: Carpal tunnel syndrome is compression of the median nerve in the wrist that supplies feeling and movement to parts of the hand. Tinel's sign may be used to help identify carpal tunnel syndrome. It is elicited by percussing lightly over the median nerve, located on the inner aspect of the wrist. If the client reports tingling, numbness, and pain, the test is considered positive.

Test-taking strategy: Analyze to determine what information the question asks for, which is site of percussion to elicit Tinel's sign. Recall that the cause of carpal tunnel syndrome is compression of the median nerve; thus, percussing over the nerve produces definitive symptoms. Review the anatomical basis for carpal tunnel syndrome and diagnostic clinical findings if you had difficulty answering this question.

Client needs category: Safe and effective care environment

Client needs subcategory: Management of care

Cognitive level: Understanding

9. A client is admitted with a possible diagnosis of osteomyelitis. Based on the documentation below, which laboratory result is the **priority** for the nurse to report to the health care provider?

Progress notes	
01/11/16 0900	Client admitted with elevated temperature, reporting bone pain and muscle spasms. Laboratory called with the following results: rheumatoid factor negative; blood culture positive for Staphylococcus aureus; alkaline phosphatase 60 IU/L; erythrocyte sedimentation rate 10 mm/hour.
	————————Susan Wright, RN

☐ **1.** Rheumatoid factor

☐ **2.** Blood culture

☐ **3.** Alkaline phosphatase

☐ **4.** ESR

Answer: 2

Ⓜ **Rationale:** Osteomyelitis is a bacterial infection of the bone and soft tissue that occurs by extension of soft tissue infection, direct bone contamination following surgery, or spreading from other infection sites in the body. A positive blood culture would be reported immediately to the physician so that specific antibiotic therapy can begin or be adjusted based on the positive culture. A negative rheumatoid factor would be expected in a possible diagnosis of osteomyelitis. An alkaline phosphatase level of 60 IU/L (1.0 μkat/L) is within the normal range, and an ESR of 10 mm/hour is also within the normal range.

Test-taking strategy: Analyze to determine what information the question asks for, which is determining priority laboratory data to be communicated to the physician. Determine laboratory data that are abnormal, and then decide the clinical implications. Always contact the health care provider with important laboratory data. Review the pathophysiology and clinical manifestations of osteomyelitis if you had difficulty answering this question.

Client needs category: Physiological integrity

Client needs subcategory: Reduction of risk potential

Cognitive level: Analyzing

---

10. The nurse is assisting the client in filling a pillbox. A client has been prescribed indomethacin for the treatment of gouty arthritis. The orders state 25 mg t.i.d. for first 5 days and then increase by 25 mg per dose at weekly intervals until the daily dose reaches a maximum of 250 mg. The client is on week 3 of treatment and has tolerated the medication without any incident thus far. By week 3, what would the daily dose of medication be? Record your answer as a whole number.

_____ mg

Answer: 225

Ⓒ **Rationale:** First, determine the first week's daily dosage: 25 mg × 3 = 75 mg. This dosage is increased by 25 mg per dose to equal the second week's daily dosage:

25 mg + 25 mg = 50 mg × 3 = 150 mg. The dosage is then increased by an additional 25 mg to equal the third week's daily dosage: 25 mg + 25 mg + 25 mg = 75 mg × 3 = 225 mg.

Test-taking strategy: Analyze to determine what information the question asks for, which is week 3's indomethacin dosage. Read carefully the health care provider order, and carefully increase each dose of medication weekly. Continue with formula until maximum dose is reached. Proofread your math calculation. Review the amount of medication per dosage, the number of daily doses, and the amount to increase the dosage weekly if you had difficulty answering this question.

Client needs category: Physiological integrity

Client needs subcategory: Pharmacological and parenteral therapies

Cognitive level: Applying

---

11. A client is scheduled for an open reduction internal fixation of the right hip. Place the following nursing interventions in chronological order to show the sequence in which the nurse would perform them. All options must be used.

1. Initiate a home care teaching plan.

2. Complete a preoperative checklist.

3. Encourage coughing, turning, and deep breathing.

4. Make sure the client has signed an informed consent form.

5. Monitor vital signs every 15 minutes × 4, every 30 minutes × 2, and every hour × 2.

6. Complete a history and physical examination.

Answer: 6, 3, 2, 5, 4, 1

Ⓜ Rationale: Initially, the nurse will complete the history and physical as part of the admission process. As part of the preoperative interventions, the nurse will witness the signing of the informed consent and complete a preoperative checklist. Postoperatively, the nurse will monitor vital signs frequently and, once the client is awake, alert, and oriented, will encourage the client to turn, cough, and deep-breathe. Finally, a home care teaching plan must be initiated before discharge.

Test-taking strategy: Analyze to determine what information the question asks for, which is nursing action for an open reduction internal fixation of the hip. Consider what actions are preoperative and those that are postoperative. Use knowledge of surgical process to chronologically order nursing actions. Review the surgical procedure and related nursing interventions, and recall that client safety is paramount if you had difficulty answering this question.

Client needs category: Physiological integrity
Client needs subcategory: Reduction of risk potential
Cognitive level: Analyzing

12. The nurse is instructing a client following right knee replacement on how to use crutches. Which instructions are included? Select all that apply.

☐ **1.** Let your armpits support your weight.

☐ **2.** Have your elbows bent when holding the crutch handles.

☐ **3.** Place crutches one foot in front of you.

☐ **4.** Step forward first on your right leg.

☐ **5.** Pivot on your left leg.

☐ **6.** Swing your left leg forward.

Answer: 2, 3, 5, 6

Ⓓ Rationale: It is very important to instruct a client to safely use crutches. Additional damage to the injured knee may result with improper crutch use. When using crutches, instruct the client to place the crutches about 1 foot (0.3 m) in front of the feet, slightly wider apart than the body. Next, lean on the handles of the crutches (not armpit) and move the body forward. Use the crutches for support. Do not step forward on the weak leg. Finish the step by swinging the left leg forward. Repeat steps to move forward. Turn by pivoting on the strong left leg, not the right leg. The armpits should not support the body weight.

Test-taking strategy: Analyze to determine what information the question asks for, which is proper crutch walking instruction. Analyze each option to ensure safety of the right knee. Consider keeping weight off of the right knee and how each option would provide for that. Review proper crutch walking with an impaired right knee if you had difficulty answering this question.

Client needs category: Safe and effective care environment
Client needs subcategory: Safety and infection control
Cognitive level: Applying

13. A client is admitted to the trauma center with a spinal cord transection at T4. Which of the physical limitations does the nurse anticipate when planning care? Select all that apply.

- ☐ **1.** The client will need ventilator support.
- ☐ **2.** The client will be unable to independently ambulate.
- ☐ **3.** The client will have no control of the bladder.
- ☐ **4.** The client will need assistance with feeding.
- ☐ **5.** The client will be unable to speak.
- ☐ **6.** The client will be cognitively impaired.

Answer: 2, 3

Ⓓ Rationale: The client with a spinal cord transection (complete tear) at the thoracic 4 location will be a paraplegic with no control of the body below midchest. The client will need assistance to ambulate (wheelchair) and assistance with urination. Clients will be able to breathe independently, speak, feed themselves, and have normal cognitive function.

Test-taking strategy: Analyze to determine what information the question asks for, which is physical limitations following a thoracic 4 spinal transection. Recall that the thoracic region is in the midregion between the cervical vertebrae and lumbar vertebrae. Also, consider that transections at the cervical vertebra are most severe resulting in quadriplegia or death. Review functional areas of the spinal cord and limitations if severed if you had difficulty answering this question.

Client needs category: Physiological integrity
Client needs subcategory: Physiological adaptation
Cognitive level: Analyzing

Immune and hematologic disorders

1. A nurse is preparing a client with systemic lupus erythematosus (SLE) for discharge. Which instructions would the nurse include in the teaching plan? Select all that apply.

- ☐ **1.** Stay out of direct sunlight.
- ☐ **2.** Do not limit activity between flare-ups.
- ☐ **3.** Monitor body temperature.
- ☐ **4.** Taper the corticosteroid dosage as prescribed when symptoms are under control.
- ☐ **5.** Apply cold packs to relieve joint pain and stiffness.

Answer: 1, 3, 4

Ⓓ Rationale: SLE is a chronic autoimmune disease that can damage any part of the body (skin, joints, and bodily organs). A client with SLE would stay out of direct sunlight and avoid other sources of ultraviolet light because they may trigger severe skin reactions and exacerbate the symptoms. The client's body temperature would be monitored and fevers reported to the primary health care provider. The corticosteroid dosage must be tapered gradually once symptoms are relieved because stopping these drugs abruptly can cause adrenal insufficiency, a potentially life-threatening condition. Fatigue can cause an SLE flare-up, so the client would pace activities and plan for rest periods. The client would apply heat, not cold, to relieve joint pain. Cold packs may aggravate Raynaud's phenomenon, which commonly occurs in clients with SLE.

Test-taking strategy: Analyze to determine what information the question asks for, which is nursing instructions for the teaching plan for a client with SLE. "Select all that apply" questions require considering each option to decide its merit. Review nursing interventions and clinical manifestations for SLE if you had difficulty answering this question.

Client needs category: Physiological integrity
Client needs subcategory: Reduction of risk potential
Cognitive level: Applying

2. A client is to receive a blood transfusion of packed RBCs for severe anemia. Place the following steps in the order a nurse would follow to administer this product. All options must be used.

1. Flush the intravenous tubing and line with normal saline solution.

2. Verify the blood bag identification, ABO group, and Rh compatibility against the client information.

3. Record baseline vital signs.

4. Remain with the client and watch for signs of a transfusion reaction.

5. Put on gloves, a gown, and a face shield.

6. Check the packed cells for abnormal color, clumping, gas bubbles, and expiration date.

Answer: 3, 6, 2, 5, 1, 4

Ⓓ Rationale: To administer a blood transfusion, the nurse would follow the steps as listed above. Begin with obtaining a baseline set of vital signs. Next, assess the blood product and verify for the client and blood accuracy. Begin the transfusion by using protective equipment, flush tubings, and administer blood products. Two client identifiers must be checked before the transfusion. Careful assessment is needed in watching for a transfusion reaction. Note that the transfusion may be withheld if the client's temperature is 100°F (37.8°C) or greater.

Test-taking strategy: Analyze to determine what information the question asks for, which is the procedure to administer a blood transfusion. When considering steps in a procedure, visualize approaching the client and ask, "What would I do first?" Early steps include obtaining a consent, teaching for the procedure, or obtaining baseline vital signs. Next, move to specific actions during the procedure and then to steps to follow/assess after a procedure. Review client safety and blood product administration if you had difficulty answering this question.

Client needs category: Physiological integrity

Client needs subcategory: Pharmacological and parenteral therapies

Cognitive level: Applying

---

3. A nurse is planning care for a client with human immunodeficiency virus (HIV). The registered nurse (RN) is delegating responsibilities to a licensed practical/vocational nurse (LPN/VN). Which statements by the LPN/VN indicate understanding of HIV transmission? Select all that apply.

☐ 1. "I will wear a gown, mask, and gloves for all client contact."

☐ 2. "I do not need to wear any personal protective equipment because nurses have a low risk of occupational exposure."

☐ 3. "I will wear a mask if the client has a cough caused by an upper respiratory infection."

☐ 4. "I will wear a mask, gown, and gloves when splashing of body fluids is likely."

☐ 5. "I will wash my hands after client care."

Answer: 4, 5

Ⓒ Rationale: When the RN delegates to the LPN/VN, it is important to make sure that the LPN/VN understands the client condition and task of delegation. In caring for a client with HIV, standard precautions include wearing gloves for any known or anticipated contact with blood, body fluids, tissue, mucous membranes, or nonintact skin. If the task may result in splashing or splattering of blood or body fluids, a mask and goggles or a face shield and a fluid-resistant gown or apron would be worn. Hands would be washed before and after client care and after removing gloves.

Test-taking strategy: Analyze to determine what information the question asks for, which is proper care and understanding of HIV transmission. "Select all that apply" questions require considering each option to decide its merit. Recall that the Centers for Disease Control and Prevention stresses standard precautions in caring for all clients in all situations where there is blood and body fluid contact. Review standard precautions at the Centers for Disease Control and Prevention isolation guidelines if you had difficulty answering this question.

Client needs category: Safe and effective care environment

Client needs subcategory: Safety and infection control

Cognitive level: Understanding

---

4. A nurse is caring for a client with moderate RA. Which nonpharmacological interventions would a nurse include in the care plan? Select all that apply.

☐ **1.** Massaging inflamed joints

☐ **2.** Avoiding ROM exercises

☐ **3.** Applying splints to inflamed joints

☐ **4.** Using assistive devices at all times

☐ **5.** Selecting clothing that has Velcro fasteners

☐ **6.** Applying moist heat to joints

Answer: 3, 5, 6

🅓 **Rationale:** RA affects more than 2 million Americans, mostly women. RA is a chronic, systematic inflammatory disorder affecting many tissues, organs, and joints. Supportive, nonpharmacological measures for the client with RA include applying splints to rest inflamed joints, using Velcro fasteners on clothing to aid in dressing, and applying moist heat to joints to relax muscles and relieve pain. Inflamed joints would never be massaged because doing so can aggravate inflammation. A physical therapy program, including ROM exercises and carefully individualized therapeutic exercises, prevents loss of joint function. Assistive devices would only be used when marked loss of ROM occurs.

Test-taking strategy: Analyze to determine what information the question asks for, which is nonpharmacological interventions for a client with moderate RA. "Select all that apply" questions require considering each option to decide its merit. Consider the main symptoms of the disease process and link with a helpful nonpharmacological intervention. Review nursing interventions and nonpharmacological pain management therapies if you had difficulty answering this question.

Client needs category: Physiological integrity

Client needs subcategory: Basic care and comfort

Cognitive level: Applying

5. A nurse is assessing a young adult with a temperature of 103°F (39.4°C), a sore throat, and swollen lymph glands. No adventitious breath sounds or cardiac disorders are noted. To complete an assessment for a potential Epstein-Barr viral infection, place an X on the quadrant of the abdomen that the nurse would be particularly careful to palpate.

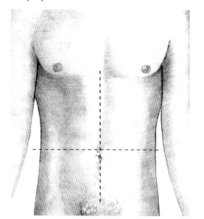

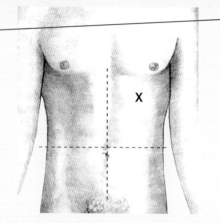

Ⓜ Rationale: An Epstein-Barr infection is a common viral infection. Symptoms include a fever, sore throat, and swollen lymph glands. Additionally, a swollen liver or spleen may develop. Assessment of the liver and spleen is essential. The spleen is located in the left upper quadrant of the abdomen. It is posterior and slightly inferior to the stomach. The nurse would stop palpating immediately if the nurse feels the spleen because compression can cause rupture.

Test-taking strategy: Analyze to determine what information the question asks for, which is area of the abdomen for palpation. The key word is area to pay "particular" attention, providing a clue that one quadrant is more important than the others. Recall the content of the abdomen in the quadrants, and relate it to the disease process. Review Epstein-Barr assessment techniques if you had difficulty answering this question.

Client needs category: Physiological integrity

Client needs subcategory: Physiological adaptation

Cognitive level: Applying

6. A client presents to the community clinic with a viral infection and swollen lymph nodes. When assessing the lymph nodes of the head and neck, the nurse notes hard and irregularly shaped nodes in the submandibular region. When documenting the site of the lymph nodes, place an X to identify the area of concern.

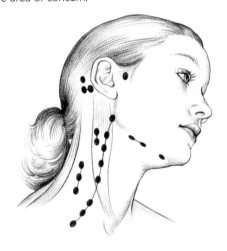

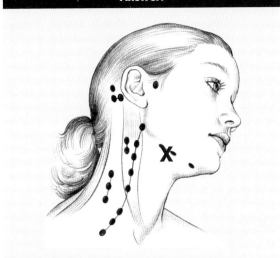

Ⓔ Rationale: The submandibular lymph nodes are found halfway between the angle and tip of the mandible. The submandibular lymph nodes account for approximately 70% of the salivary volume produced. Hard and irregularly shaped lymph nodes are a concern for more serious conditions.

Test-taking strategy: Analyze to determine what information the question asks for, which is the location of the submandibular lymph nodes. Use your knowledge of medical terminology to locate the lymph nodes. Break the word into sections such as sub–under and mandibular–mandible, and thus make a selection of the lymph node under the mandible on the illustration. Review the anatomy of the lymphatic system and the face if you had difficulty answering this question.

Client needs category: Physiological integrity

Client needs subcategory: Physiological adaptation

Cognitive level: Understanding

7. The nurse is caring for a client who is scheduled to undergo a bone marrow aspiration to assess the progression of a hematologic disorder. Which interventions would the nurse include as part of the preprocedural teaching plan? Select all that apply.

☐ **1.** Explain the procedure to the client.

☐ **2.** Maintain a pressure dressing over the aspiration site.

☐ **3.** Encourage the client to ask questions before obtaining the signed informed consent.

☐ **4.** Explain that the client will receive an analgesic prior to the procedure.

☐ **5.** Administer an anxiety-relieving medication prior to the procedure.

☐ **6.** Instruct the client to save all voided urine for 24 hours after the procedure.

Answer: 1, 3, 4, 5

Ⓓ Rationale: The preprocedure teaching extends from when the procedure is first discussed through when the procedure begins. The client would understand the procedure and the reason why it is necessary before signing an informed consent form. The client would be advised of the local analgesia or antianxiety medication to be administered before the procedure begins. Maintaining pressure over the insertion site is a nursing intervention performed after the procedure; it is not a part of the preoperative teaching. Instructing the client to save voided urine would be part of the postprocedural discharge plan.

Test-taking strategy: Analyze to determine what information the question asks for, which is the preprocedure client teaching. "Select all that apply" questions require considering each option to decide its merit. The key word is "preprocedural," indicating that which is done prior to the procedure. Analyze each option with the specific time period in mind. Review preprocedure client teaching, including guidelines on obtaining informed consent and preparation for bone marrow aspiration if you had difficulty answering this question.

Client needs category: Physiological integrity

Client needs subcategory: Basic care and comfort

Cognitive level: Applying

8. The nurse is providing discharge teaching for a client with a compromised immune system and on neutropenic precautions. When discussing types of fruits and vegetables that the client likes, which are encouraged? Select all that apply.

☐ **1.** Canned peaches

☐ **2.** Carrot sticks

☐ **3.** Broccoli florets

☐ **4.** Bananas

☐ **5.** A green salad

☐ **6.** Cooked corn

Answer: 1, 6

Ⓜ Rationale: A client with a compromised immune system and low white blood cell count (neutropenia) is at high risk for infection. Foods can introduce infections; thus, the client is encouraged to eat cooked or prepared fruits and vegetables. Canned peaches have been processed, and thoroughly cooked corn is appropriate. Raw fruits and vegetables are not allowed because they may contain microbial contamination.

Test-taking strategy: Analyze to determine what information the question asks for, which is fruits and vegetables appropriate for a neutropenic diet. Consider the impact of the immunocompromised state and the potential for each food to cause an infection. If unsure, recall that processed and cooked foods should not contain microbes because of the preparation process. Review diet considerations for the immunocompromised client if you had difficulty answering this question.

Client needs category: Health promotion and maintenance

Client needs subcategory: None

Cognitive level: Analyzing

9. The nurse is assessing a client who is suspected of having Hodgkin's disease. The client has been admitted with swollen left-sided inguinal lymph nodes. Identify the area where the nurse would be **best** able to palpate the size of these lymph nodes.

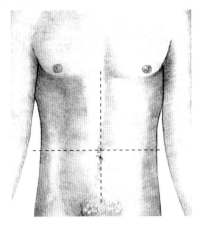

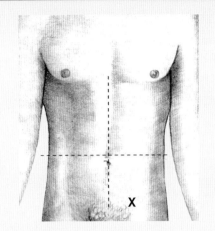

X

Ⓜ Rationale: Hodgkin's disease is a type of neoplasm involving cells of lymphoid origin. It usually begins as a painless enlargement of one or more lymph nodes. Most commonly, the lymph node enlargement involves the nodes in the neck area, but it can also involve the inguinal nodes as well. The inguinal nodes are located in the groin area.

Test-taking strategy: Analyze to determine what information the question asks for, which is a location of the left-sided inguinal lymph nodes. The key word is "inguinal" leading to the inguinal or groin region. Also, use anatomical position to distinguish between right and left sides of the body. Review the anatomy of the lymphatic system and abdomen and pathophysiology of Hodgkin's disease if you had difficulty answering this question.

Client needs category: Physiological integrity

Client needs subcategory: Physiological adaptation

Cognitive level: Applying

10. A multidisciplinary oncology team of physicians, nurses, and the social worker notes that a client who has been undergoing chemotherapy is now experiencing pancytopenia. When reviewing the laboratory data, which values support this diagnosis? Select all that apply.

☐ **1.** Decreased white blood cells

☐ **2.** Increased white blood cells

☐ **3.** Decreased platelets

☐ **4.** Increased platelets

☐ **5.** Decreased RBCs

☐ **6.** Increased RBCs

Answer: 1, 3, 5

Ⓔ **Rationale:** Pancytopenia is a deficiency of all blood cells, which includes a state of simultaneous leukopenia (decreased white blood cells), thrombocytopenia (decreased platelets), and anemia (decreased RBCs). Pancytopenia has widespread effects on the body by leading to oxygen shortage and immune function.

Test-taking strategy: Analyze to determine what information the question asks for, which is laboratory data that support a diagnosis of pancytopenia. "Select all that apply" questions require considering each option to decide its merit. Notice that there are increased and decreased options of white blood cells, platelets, and red blood cells, meaning that there should be three correct answers. Relate each option to chemotherapy side effects. Review laboratory values for the disorder, and review pertinent medical terminology (such as *pan*, meaning *universal*, and *penia*, meaning *decreased*) if you had difficulty answering this question.

Client needs category: Physiological integrity

Client needs subcategory: Physiological adaptation

Cognitive level: Applying

---

11. The nurse is completing a health history review of a client who has received long-term medical steroid therapy for lupus. Which client data does the nurse recognize as potentially linked to the steroid use? Select all that apply.

☐ **1.** A 16-lb (7.3 kg) weight loss

☐ **2.** Three infections over the course of the year

☐ **3.** Routine symptoms of nausea

☐ **4.** An increase in client blood pressure

☐ **5.** Acne noted on the forehead, cheeks, and back

Answer: 2, 5

Ⓓ **Rationale:** Suppression of the immune system occurs when a client receives long-term steroid therapy, making the client more susceptible to infections. Acne is present related to oily skin and also the overproduction of the acne bacterium, *Propionibacterium acnes*. Also, changes in metabolism occur leading to weight gain, not weight loss. Nausea and hypertension are not commonly seen with steroid use.

Test-taking strategy: Analyze to determine what information the question asks for, which is client data related to the long-term use of steroids. Consider adverse reactions of steroid use and the effect on the body. Also consider why the steroid is being administered. Review steroid use and side effects if you had difficulty answering this question.

Client needs category: Physiological integrity

Client needs subcategory: Pharmacological and parenteral therapies

Cognitive level: Analyzing

12. The nurse is caring for a client who has been newly diagnosed with systemic lupus erythematosus (SLE). Which information would be included in a teaching plan that focuses on home care? Select all that apply.

- ☐ **1.** Avoid exposure to sunlight.
- ☐ **2.** Keep exercise to a minimal level.
- ☐ **3.** Report development of a butterfly rash on the face.
- ☐ **4.** Avoid over-the-counter (OTC) medications unless approved by the physician.
- ☐ **5.** Take rest periods as needed.

© Rationale: The client who suffers from SLE has a tendency toward photosensitivity; therefore, the client would avoid exposure to sunlight. The client would also be advised to keep exercise to a minimum, to avoid OTC medications unless directed by the physician, and to rest as needed. Because the butterfly rash associated with lupus is an initial sign, the client would already have the rash and would not be reporting its development after discharge.

Test-taking strategy: Analyze to determine what information the question asks for, which is home care nursing instructions. "Select all that apply" questions require considering each option to decide its merit. The key words are "home care"; thus, instruction is specific in this situation. Review the pathophysiology of SLE, clinical manifestations, and nursing interventions if you had difficulty answering this question.

Client needs category: Physiological integrity

Client needs subcategory: Physiological adaptation

Cognitive level: Applying

---

13. The nurse is caring for a client newly diagnosed with human immunodeficiency virus (HIV) obtained from unprotected sex. The nurse is in the room when the client is explaining the disease to another person. Which statement by the client would the nurse clarify? Select all that apply.

- ☐ **1.** "My sexual practices will have to change."
- ☐ **2.** "I am afraid that I will give this disease to my nephew."
- ☐ **3.** "The disease can also be spread by body fluids."
- ☐ **4.** "I could pass this on to a baby before I give birth."
- ☐ **5.** "I will have this for the rest of my life."
- ☐ **6.** "Medications can cure the disease."

Answer: 2, 6

Ⓜ Rationale: Human immunodeficiency virus (HIV) is a sexually transmitted infection. Casual contact such as that with a family member will not spread the disease. Unfortunately, at this time, there is no cure for the disease. The client is correct in stating that sexual practices will have to change to prevent further spread of the disease and the disease can be spread by body fluids and can also be passed on to a fetus.

Test-taking strategy: Analyze to determine what information the question asks for, which is an incorrect client statement related to HIV. Look at each statement and consider if it is accurate. Recall the communicable nature of the disease and the personal nature of the spread. Review the spread of the human immunodeficiency virus (HIV) and nursing instructions if you had difficulty answering this question.

Client needs category: Health promotion and maintenance

Client needs subcategory: None

Cognitive level: Analyzing

Endocrine and metabolic disorders

1. A nurse is caring for a client who is being discharged after a thyroidectomy. Which discharge instructions would be appropriate for this client? Select all that apply.

☐ **1.** Report signs and symptoms of hypoglycemia.

☐ **2.** Take thyroid replacement medication as ordered.

☐ **3.** Watch for changes in body functioning, such as lethargy, restlessness, sensitivity to cold, and dry skin, and report these changes to the physician.

☐ **4.** Avoid all OTC medications.

☐ **5.** Carry injectable dexamethasone at all times.

Answer: 2, 3

Ⓓ Rationale: A thyroidectomy is the surgical removal of all or part of the thyroid. After removal of the thyroid gland, the client needs to take thyroid replacement medication. The client also needs to report such changes as lethargy, restlessness, cold sensitivity, and dry skin, which may indicate the need for a higher dosage of medication. The thyroid gland does not regulate blood glucose level; therefore, signs and symptoms of hypoglycemia are not relevant for this client. Injectable dexamethasone is not needed for this client. Some OTC medications (such as nonaspirin products) are allowable.

Test-taking strategy: Analyze to determine what information the question asks for, which is discharge instructions after a thyroidectomy. Use your knowledge of medical terminology to determine procedure such as "ectomy"—removal of. Recall that the thyroid gland releases hormones that affect the body's metabolism. Review the physiology of the thyroid gland and nursing interventions related to promoting rest, managing pain, and monitoring for potential complications if you had difficulty answering this question.

Client needs category: Physiological integrity

Client needs subcategory: Physiological adaptation

Cognitive level: Applying

---

2. A client is admitted with a diagnosis of diabetic ketoacidosis. An insulin drip is initiated with 50 units of insulin in 100 ml of normal saline solution administered via an infusion pump set at 10 ml/hour. The nurse determines that the client is receiving how many units of insulin each hour? Record your answer using a whole number.

_____ units/hour

Answer: 5

Ⓔ Rationale: To determine the number of insulin units the client is receiving per hour, first determine the number of units in each milliliter of fluid (50 units/100 ml = 0.5 units/ml). Next, multiply the units per milliliter by the rate of milliliters per hour (0.5 unit × 10 ml/hour = 5 units).

Test-taking strategy: Analyze to determine what information the question asks for, which is the number of units of insulin infusing per hour. First, calculate the number of units per milliliter of intravenous solution. Once determined, calculate the number of units per hour. Proofread your math calculations. Review solving for X using the ratio-and-proportion method if you had difficulty answering this question.

Client needs category: Physiological integrity

Client needs subcategory: Pharmacological and parenteral therapies

Cognitive level: Applying

---

3. A client's glucose level is 365 mg/dl (365 mmol/L). The physician orders 10 units of regular insulin to be administered. The bottle of regular insulin is labeled 100 units/ml. How many milliliters of insulin should the nurse administer? Record your answer using one decimal place.

_____ ml

4. A nurse is performing an admission assessment on a client who has been diagnosed with diabetes insipidus. Which findings does the nurse anticipate during the assessment? Select all that apply.

☐ **1.** Extreme polyuria

☐ **2.** Excessive thirst

☐ **3.** Elevated systolic blood pressure

☐ **4.** Low urine specific gravity

☐ **5.** Bradycardia

☐ **6.** Elevated serum potassium level

5. A nurse is following the progress of a client being treated for hypothyroidism. Which findings indicate that thyroid replacement therapy has been inadequate? Select all that apply.

☐ **1.** ECG changes

☐ **2.** Tachycardia

☐ **3.** Low body temperature

☐ **4.** Nervousness

☐ **5.** Bradycardia

☐ **6.** Dry mouth

Answer: 1, 3, 5

D Rationale: In hypothyroidism, the body is in a hypometabolic state. Therefore, ECG changes with bradycardia and subnormal body temperature would indicate that replacement therapy was inadequate. Tachycardia, nervousness, and dry mouth are symptoms of an excessive level of thyroid hormone; these findings would indicate that the client has received an excessive dose of thyroid hormone.

Test-taking strategy: Analyze to determine what information the question asks for, which is findings that would represent that thyroid replacement therapy is inadequate. "Select all that apply" questions require considering each option to decide its merit. The key word is "inadequate," meaning that symptoms of hypothyroidism still persist. Review the physiology of the thyroid gland and clinical manifestations of hypothyroidism if you had difficulty answering this question.

Client needs category: Physiological integrity

Client needs subcategory: Reduction of risk potential

Cognitive level: Evaluating

---

6. A client is brought to the emergency department after wandering on the street. The client is confused and verbalizes double vision, headache, and shakiness. Laboratory data reveal a serum blood glucose of 52 mg/dl (52 mmol/L). Which questions, asked by the nurse, may reveal more data related to the client's condition? Select all that apply.

☐ **1.** "What have you eaten today?"

☐ **2.** "Do you take insulin or oral antidiabetic medication?"

☐ **3.** "Have you ever felt this way before?"

☐ **4.** "Can you tell me if you are married?"

☐ **5.** "Are you having any chest pain?"

☐ **6.** "Have you been to this hospital before?"

Answer: 1, 2, 3

M Rationale: A serum blood glucose of 52 mg/dl (52 mmol/L) indicates hypoglycemia. Questions that provide information on diet, activity, medications, and daily routine can be helpful in understanding the cause of the low blood sugar. Factors that influence hypoglycemia include missed meals and strenuous activity or taking too high of a dosage of insulin/oral antidiabetic medications. Symptoms of hypoglycemia include shakiness, confusion, headache, sweating, and tingling sensations around the mouth. Questions of marital status, previous hospitalizations, and other symptoms are helpful in determining overall client status but do not provide data on hypoglycemia.

Test-taking strategy: Analyze to determine what information the question asks for, which is pertinent questions related to hypoglycemia. "Select all that apply" questions require considering each option to decide its merit. Read each option to determine how it relates to the disease process. Review the clinical manifestations of and nursing interventions for hypoglycemia if you had difficulty answering this question.

Client needs category: Physiological integrity

Client needs subcategory: Physiological adaptation

Cognitive level: Analyzing

---

7. A nurse is caring for a client with a low calcium level. Place the following options in chronological order to indicate the regulatory feedback mechanism of parathyroid hormone (PTH) release in relation to calcium levels. All options must be used.

1. High serum calcium level inhibits PTH secretion.

2. Low serum calcium level stimulates parathyroid gland.

3. Calcium is reabsorbed.

4. Parathyroid gland releases PTH.

Ⓜ **Rationale:** Simple feedback occurs when the level of one substance regulates the secretion of hormones. A low calcium level stimulates the parathyroid gland to release PTH, which promotes resorption of calcium, resulting in normalized calcium levels. When calcium levels are elevated, PTH secretion is inhibited.

Test-taking strategy: Analyze to determine what information the question asks for, which is the order when the body uses the regulatory feedback method to maintain serum calcium levels. Recall that the feedback mechanism exists when the body detects an abnormality. Once detected, the body attempts to correct the abnormality by its regulatory process. Once homeostasis reoccurs, the body returns to maintenance of body function. Review the physiology of the parathyroid gland and PTH in relation to the regulatory feedback mechanism if you had difficulty answering this question.

Client needs category: Physiological integrity

Client needs subcategory: Physiological adaptation

Cognitive level: Analyzing

8. A client with Addison's disease is scheduled for discharge after being hospitalized for an adrenal crisis. Which statements by the client would indicate that the nurse's teaching has been effective? Select all that apply.

☐ **1.** "I have to take my steroids for 10 days."

☐ **2.** "I need to weigh myself daily to be sure I don't eat too many calories."

☐ **3.** "I need to call my doctor to discuss my steroid needs before I have dental work."

☐ **4.** "I will call the doctor if I suddenly feel very weak or dizzy."

☐ **5.** "If I feel like I have the flu, I'll carry on as usual because this is an expected response."

☐ **6.** "I need to obtain and wear a Medic Alert bracelet."

Answer: 3, 4, 6

Ⓜ **Rationale:** Addison's disease is a chronic endocrine disorder that occurs when the adrenal glands do not produce enough hormones such as cortisol and aldosterone. These hormones give instruction to virtually every tissue and organ in the body. Dental work can be a cause of physical stress; therefore, the client's health care provider needs to be informed about the dental work so adjustments in the dosage of steroids can be made, if necessary. Fatigue, weakness, and dizziness are symptoms of inadequate steroid therapy; the physician should be notified if these symptoms occur. A Medic Alert bracelet allows health care providers to access the client's history of Addison's disease if the client is unable to communicate this information. A client with Addison's disease does not produce enough steroids, so routine administration of steroids is a lifetime treatment. Daily weight should be monitored to monitor changes in fluid balance, not calorie intake. Influenza is an added physical stressor that may require an increased dosage of steroids. The client should notify the physician, not "carry on as usual."

Test-taking strategy: Analyze to determine what information the question asks for, which is a correct statement by the client indicating effective teaching. "Select all that apply" questions require considering each option to decide its merit. Read each option carefully and relate to the disease process. Review the clinical manifestations and nursing interventions for Addison's disease if you had difficulty answering this question.

Client needs category: Physiological integrity

Client needs subcategory: Physiological adaptation

Cognitive level: Analyzing

---

9. A client comes to the clinic verbalizing a weight loss of 20 lb (9.1 kg) over the last month, even with a "ravenous" appetite and no change in activity level. The client is diagnosed with Graves' disease. Which other signs and symptoms of Graves' disease would the nurse assess? Select all that apply.

☐ **1.** Rapid, bounding pulse

☐ **2.** Bradycardia

☐ **3.** Heat intolerance

☐ **4.** Mild tremors

☐ **5.** Nervousness

☐ **6.** Constipation

Answer: 1, 3, 4, 5

Ⓜ **Rationale:** Graves' disease, or hyperthyroidism, is a hypermetabolic state that is associated with a rapid, bounding pulse, heat intolerance, tremors, and nervousness. Bradycardia and constipation are signs and symptoms of hypothyroidism.

Test-taking strategy: Analyze to determine what information the question asks for, which is signs and symptoms related to Graves' disease. "Select all that apply" questions require considering each option to decide its merit. Relate Graves' disease/hyperthyroidism with "speeding up" the metabolism and the related effects. Note that the correct options all relate an increased metabolism. Review the physiology of the thyroid gland and the pathophysiology of

Client needs category: Physiological integrity

Client needs subcategory: Physiological adaptation

Cognitive level: Analyzing

10. A client who suffered a brain injury after falling off a ladder has recently developed syndrome of inappropriate antidiuretic hormone (SIADH). Which findings indicate that the treatment being received for SIADH is effective? Select all that apply.

☐ **1.** Decrease in body weight

☐ **2.** Rise in blood pressure and drop in heart rate

☐ **3.** Absence of wheezing

☐ **4.** Increase in urine output

☐ **5.** Decrease in urine osmolarity

Answer: 1, 4, 5

Ⓓ Rationale: SIADH is an abnormality involving an excessive release of ADH. The predominant feature is water retention with oliguria, edema, and weight gain. Successful treatment would result in a reduction in weight, increased urine output, and a decrease in urine osmolarity (concentration). Wheezes are not typically associated with SIADH. The client's blood pressure would remain the same or decrease after treatment.

Test-taking strategy: Analyze to determine what information the question asks for, which is the reduction of symptoms from SIADH indicating effective treatment. "Select all that apply" questions require considering each option to decide its merit. First, consider which symptoms typically occur in SIADH. Next, appraise each option for normalizing of those symptoms indicating effective treatment. Review the clinical manifestations and treatment of SIADH if you had difficulty answering this question.

Client needs category: Physiological integrity

Client needs subcategory: Physiological adaptation

Cognitive level: Analyzing

11. A nurse is about to administer a client's morning dose of insulin. The client's order is for 5 units of regular insulin and 10 units of NPH (Neutral Protamine Hagedorn) insulin given as a basal dose. The client also is to receive an amount prescribed from the medium-dose sliding scale (shown below) based on morning blood glucose levels. The nurse performs a bedside blood glucose measurement, and the result is 264 mg/dl (264 mmol/L). How many total units of insulin would the nurse administer to the client?

Plasma Glucose (mg/dl)	Low Dose (Regular Insulin)	Medium Dose (Regular Insulin)	High Dose (Regular Insulin)	Very High Dose (Regular Insulin)
<70	← Call physician →			
71–140	0 units	0 units	0 units	0 units
141–180	1 unit	2 units	4 units	10 units
181–240	2 units	4 units	8 units	15 units
241–300	4 units	6 units	12 units	20 units
301–400	6 units	9 units	16 units	25 units
>400	8 units	12 units and call physician	20 units	30 units

_____ units

Answer: 21

Ⓜ **Rationale:** The basal dose for this client is 5 units of regular insulin and 10 units of NPH insulin. The medium-dose sliding scale indicates that, based on the glucose reading of 264 mg/dl (264 mmol/L), the client should receive an additional 6 units of regular insulin, totaling 21 units (5 units + 10 units + 6 units = 21 units).

Test-taking strategy: Analyze to determine what information the question asks for, which is total units of insulin. Carefully read the basal order and then add the sliding scale coverage. Proofread your math calculation. Review ordered insulin dosages if you had difficulty answering this question.

Client needs category: Physiological integrity

Client needs subcategory: Pharmacological and parenteral therapies

Cognitive level: Analyzing

---

12. A client arrives in the clinic with a possible parathyroid hormone (PTH) deficiency. When analyzing client lab data, which electrolytes would the nurse anticipate to be abnormal? Select all that apply.

☐ **1.** Sodium

☐ **2.** Potassium

☐ **3.** Calcium

☐ **4.** Chloride

☐ **5.** Glucose

☐ **6.** Phosphorus

Answer: 3, 6

Ⓜ **Rationale:** PTH deficiency is a condition of hypoparathyroidism. Primary hypoparathyroidism is a state of inadequate PTH activity. PTH is essential for maintaining the delicate balance of calcium and phosphorus levels in the blood. Sodium, chloride, potassium, and glucose are not affected by a PTH deficiency.

Test-taking strategy: Analyze to determine what information the question asks for, which is the electrolytes that are abnormal in hypoparathyroidism. "Select all that apply" questions require considering each option to decide its merit. Recall that the parathyroid glands regulate calcium, and depending on the calcium level, phosphorus levels are in balance. Review the physiology of the parathyroid gland and its effect on serum electrolytes if you had difficulty answering this question.

Client needs category: Physiological integrity

Client needs subcategory: Reduction of risk potential

Cognitive level: Applying

13. Two weeks after a partial thyroidectomy, a client is being seen for the postoperative follow-up appointment. The nurse is aware that the client is at increased risk for hypothyroidism. Which signs and symptoms would the nurse anticipate in a client with hypothyroidism? Select all that apply.

☐ **1.** Heat intolerance

☐ **2.** Hair loss

☐ **3.** Increased energy

☐ **4.** Dry skin

☐ **5.** Cold intolerance

☐ **6.** Fatigue

Answer: 2, 4, 5, 6

Ⓜ **Rationale:** Hypothyroidism refers to suboptimal levels of thyroid hormone. A client with this condition typically has hair loss, dry skin, cold intolerance, and fatigue.

Test-taking strategy: Analyze to determine what information the question asks for, which is signs and symptoms of hypothyroidism. "Select all that apply" questions require considering each option to decide its merit. Recall that in hypothyroidism, metabolism is decreased leading to a reduction in body metabolism. Review the physiology of the thyroid gland and pathophysiology of hypothyroidism if you had difficulty answering this question.

Client needs category: Physiological integrity

Client needs subcategory: Physiological adaptation

Cognitive level: Understanding

---

14. The nurse is caring for a client following a thyroidectomy assessing for a possible low calcium level related to inadvertent removal of parathyroid glands. Identify the part of the body the nurse would assess to determine a positive or negative Chvostek's sign.

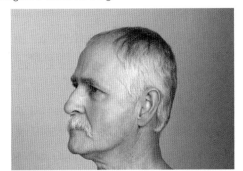

Answer:

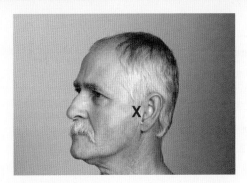

Ⓓ **Rationale:** When the facial nerve is stimulated in someone with hypocalcemia, the facial muscles contract, causing twitching of the cheek, mouth, and nose (Chvostek's sign). To elicit Chvostek's sign, tap the nerve about 2 cm anterior to the earlobe, just below the zygomatic arch.

Test-taking strategy: Analyze to determine what information the question asks for, which is the location to assess Chvostek's sign. Recall medical terminology for the definition of Chvostek's sign, which will focus you on the assessment of calcium and the facial nerve. Review postthyroidectomy care and assessment techniques if you had difficulty answering this question.

Client needs category: Physiological integrity

Client needs subcategory: Physiological adaptation

Cognitive level: Applying

---

15. The nurse is preparing the morning insulin for a diabetic client on the unit. The order is for 20 units of Humulin 70/30. The nurse knows that this dose contains a mixture of intermediate-acting insulin and fast-acting insulin. How many units of intermediate-acting insulin does this dose contain? Record your answer using a whole number.

_____ units

Answer: 14

Ⓜ Rationale: Recall that Humulin 70/30 insulin contains both intermediate-acting insulin and fast-acting insulin. The 70 and 30 represent the percentages of each kind (the first number always pertains to the percentage of intermediate-acting insulin, the second to the fast-acting insulin). Therefore, to calculate the amount of intermediate-acting insulin, the nurse must multiply the total number of units to be given by 0.7:

$$0.7 \times 20 \text{ units} = 14 \text{ units of intermediate-acting insulin.}$$

Test-taking strategy: Analyze to determine what information the question asks for, which is the calculation of the combination insulin dose. Use the formula as noted above. Proofread the math calculation. Review calculations involving percentages if you had difficulty answering this question.

Client needs category: Physiological integrity

Client needs subcategory: Pharmacological and parenteral therapies

Cognitive level: Applying

---

16. The nursing is caring for a newly admitted client with diabetes insipidus. When forming the plan of care, which nursing diagnoses are anticipated? Select all that apply.

☐ **1.** Fluid volume excess

☐ **2.** Anxiety

☐ **3.** Impaired physical mobility

☐ **4.** Self-care deficit

☐ **5.** Activity intolerance

☐ **6.** Hyperglycemia

Answer: 2, 5

Ⓓ Rationale: Diabetes insipidus is characterized by excessive output of dilute urine. Common signs and symptoms include massive diuresis, dehydration, and thirst. Additional findings include malaise, lethargy, and irritability. Nursing diagnoses that aim at providing interventions to decrease the symptoms include anxiety (irritability) and activity intolerance (because of lethargy). The client has a fluid volume deficit due to the excessive output of urine. Though the client urinates frequently, there is no reason to believe that there is an impaired physical mobility or self-care deficit. A client has symptoms of hyperglycemia with diabetes mellitus.

Test-taking strategy: Analyze to determine what information the question asks for, which is nursing diagnosis for a client with diabetes insipidus. Begin by recalling the main symptoms of the disease process, which are excessive urination and dehydration. Analyze each to see if they relate to the disease process or discard. Review nursing diagnoses related to diabetes insipidus if you had difficulty answering this question.

Client needs category: Physiological integrity

Client needs subcategory: Physiological adaptation

Cognitive level: Analyzing

17. The nurse is admitting a client with newly diagnosed diabetes mellitus and left-sided heart failure. Assessment reveals low blood pressure, increased respiratory rate and depth, drowsiness, and confusion. The client reports headache and nausea. Based on the serum laboratory results below, how would the nurse interpret the client's acid–base balance?

Lab Results	
pH	7.34
HCO_3^-	19 mEq/L (19 mmol/L)
$PaCO_2$	35 mm Hg (4.66 kPa)
PaO_2	88 mm Hg (11.70 kPa)
Potassium	5.3 mEq/L (5.3 mmol/L)
Chloride	102 mEq/L (102 mmol/L)
Calcium	10.4 mg/dl (2.6 mmol/L)
Anion gap	30 mEq/L (30 mmol/L)

☐ **1.** Metabolic alkalosis

☐ **2.** Metabolic acidosis

☐ **3.** Respiratory acidosis

☐ **4.** Respiratory alkalosis

Answer: 2

E **Rationale:** This client has metabolic acidosis, which typically manifests with a low pH, low bicarbonate level, normal to low $PaCO_2$, and normal PaO_2. The client's serum electrolyte levels also support metabolic acidosis, which include an elevated potassium level, normal to elevated chloride level, and normal calcium level. The client's anion gap of 30 mEq/L (30 mmol/L) is high, also indicative of metabolic acidosis. This kind of metabolic acidosis occurs with diabetic ketoacidosis and other disorders.

Test-taking strategy: Analyze to determine what information the question asks for, which is the interpretation of laboratory values. First, consider the diagnosis and then look to the abnormal laboratory values. Decide if there is a respiratory basis or metabolic basis to the disorder. Lastly, look to the alkalosis or acidosis findings. Review the laboratory values and physiological changes associated with diabetic ketoacidosis if you had difficulty answering this question.

Client needs category: Physiological integrity

Client needs subcategory: Reduction of risk potential

Cognitive level: Analyzing

18. When reviewing the urinalysis report of a client with newly diagnosed diabetes mellitus, the nurse would expect which urine characteristics to be abnormal? Select all that apply.

☐ **1.** Amount

☐ **2.** Odor

☐ **3.** pH

☐ **4.** Specific gravity

☐ **5.** Glucose level

☐ **6.** Ketone bodies

Answer: 1, 2, 5, 6

D **Rationale:** Diabetes mellitus is associated with increased amounts of urine, a sweet or fruity odor, and glucose and ketone bodies in the urine. It does not affect the urine's pH or specific gravity.

Test-taking strategy: Analyze to determine what information the question asks for, which is the changes in urine characteristics associated with diabetes mellitus. "Select all that apply" questions require considering each option to decide its merit. Recall that glucose is found in the urine when elevated in the serum. Also, ketones accumulate in the body when the body breaks down fat to use as energy. Ketones also spill into the urine. Review the pathophysiology and clinical manifestations of diabetes mellitus with focus on urine laboratory values if you had difficulty answering this question.

Client needs category: Physiological integrity

Client needs subcategory: Reduction of risk potential

Cognitive level: Applying

19. The nurse is caring for a client who is administering insulin for diabetes mellitus for the first time. The nurse is instructing the client on mixing Humulin N insulin and Humulin R insulin in one syringe. Arrange the instructions in order. All options must be used.

1. Withdraw Humulin N insulin.

2. Wipe with alcohol and inject air (equal to units ordered) into the Humulin N insulin.

3. Gently roll both insulins between your hands.

4. Wipe with alcohol and inject air (equal to units ordered) into the Humulin R insulin.

5. Double-check the total number of units in syringe.

6. Withdraw the Humulin R.

Answer: 3, 2, 4, 6, 1, 5

Ⓜ **Rationale:** Mixing insulin requires careful consideration. Both insulins are gently rolled to warm. Do not shake. Wipe the caps and inject air first into the Humulin N and then Humulin R. Turn the Humulin R vial upside down, and withdraw the number of units prescribed. Next, withdraw Humulin N. Double-check syringe total against order.

Test-taking strategy: Analyze to determine what information the question asks for, which is correct procedure for mixing insulin. Think of the two insulins and visualize the steps. Consider clear versus cloudy and minimizing the number of times to puncture the rubber cap. Review the standard procedure for mixing insulin if you had difficulty answering this question.

Client needs category: Health promotion and maintenance

Client needs subcategory: None

Cognitive level: Applying

---

20. The nurse is caring for a client with Cushing's disease. During change of shift report, which assessment laboratory data would the nurse anticipate communicating? Select all that apply.

☐ **1.** Serum sodium level

☐ **2.** Hemoglobin and hematocrit

☐ **3.** Serum potassium level

☐ **4.** Blood glucose level

☐ **5.** White blood cell count

☐ **6.** Creatinine clearance total

Answer: 1, 3, 4

Ⓓ **Rationale:** Cushing's disease results in an excess cortisol in the blood typically caused by a pituitary tumor secreting adrenocorticotropic hormone (ACTH). ACTH stimulates the adrenal glands to produce cortisol. Cortisol is important in controlling blood pressure and metabolism. Electrolyte disturbance is common for the nurse to report. Sodium retention is typically accompanied by potassium depletion. Clients exhibit frequent hyperglycemia. There is no impact of the blood levels or kidney function.

Test-taking strategy: Analyze to determine what information the question asks for, which is laboratory tests that need to be reported to the oncoming shift. Typically, the nurse reports those results that are abnormal or important related to the disease process. Recall the pathophysiology and the hormones excreted. Note the relation of cortisol with metabolism (hyperglycemia) and electrolyte levels. Review Cushing's disease if you had difficulty answering this question.

Client needs category: Physiological integrity

Client needs subcategory: Reduction of risk potential

Cognitive level: Analyzing

---

1. A client presents at the health care provider's office with gray-brown burrows with epidermal curved ridges and follicular papules of the skin. The health care provider diagnoses scabies. Which teaching points would a nurse review with the client? Select all that apply.

☐ **1.** The disease is only actively contagious when the lesions are open.

☐ **2.** Scabies is transmitted by close person-to-person contact or contact with infected linens and clothing.

☐ **3.** The most commonly infected areas are the hands, feet, and neck.

☐ **4.** Severe itching of the affected areas, especially at night, is a common finding.

☐ **5.** Only the infected individual needs to use the prescribed medication.

☐ **6.** All of the client's linens and clothing should be washed immediately in hot water.

Answer: 2, 4, 6

Ⓜ **Rationale:** Scabies is a contagious disorder caused by a tiny mite that burrows under the skin; it is transmitted by close person-to-person contact or contact with infected linens or clothing. It causes severe itching, especially at night, in addition to the familiar papular rash. All of the client's linens and clothing should be washed promptly in hot water to reduce the risk of reinfestation. Scabies is transmissible from the time of infection to the time the burrows and papules appear, which may occur several weeks afterward. It remains transmissible until eradicated by a prescription cream or an oral medication. Scabies is most commonly seen in the finger webs, flexor surface of the wrists, and the antecubital fossae. When a family member is diagnosed, all members of the family must be treated with medication, and their clothing and linens washed to prevent transmission and reinfestation.

Test-taking strategy: Analyze to determine what information the question asks for, which is essential teaching points of scabies. "Select all that apply" questions require considering each option to decide its merit. Typical teaching points include what scabies looks like, how to treat it, and how to prevent transfer. Review the clinical manifestations of scabies and recommended treatment if you had difficulty answering this question.

Client needs category: Physiological integrity

Client needs subcategory: Physiological adaptation

Cognitive level: Applying

---

2. At an outpatient clinic, a medical assistant interviews a client and documents the findings. The staff nurse reads the progress notes below and begins planning client care based on which nursing diagnosis?

Progress notes	
2/9/16 0900	Client very anxious because new black mole with shades of brown noted on upper outer right thigh. Asymmetrical in shape with an irregular border.————M. Rosenfeld, MA

☐ **1.** Deficient knowledge related to potential diagnosis of basal cell carcinoma

☐ **2.** Fear related to potential diagnosis of malignant melanoma

☐ **3.** Risk for impaired skin integrity related to potential squamous cell carcinoma

☐ **4.** Readiness for enhanced knowledge of skin care precautions related to benign mole

Answer: 2

Ⓔ **Rationale:** Documentation reveals that the client is anxious about the symptoms. These symptoms most closely resemble malignant melanoma. Therefore, *fear related to potential diagnosis of malignant melanoma* is the most appropriate nursing diagnosis. The nursing note does not indicate that the client presently has deficient knowledge. The characteristics of the lesion are not consistent with a basal or squamous cell carcinoma or a benign nevus (mole).

Test-taking strategy: Analyze to determine what information the question asks for, which is nursing diagnosis from the medical assistant's documentation. Look to the notation for the highest priority problem and relate to the client's symptom or statements. Review prioritizing nursing diagnosis if you had difficulty answering this question.

Client needs category: Physiological integrity

Client needs subcategory: Physiological adaptation

Cognitive level: Analyzing

3. A nurse is caring for a client who is admitted from home to a long-term care facility. During the admission assessment, the nurse documents a stage II pressure ulcer and places a referral to the enterostomal therapist (ET). When gathering supplies for a stage II ulcer, what characteristics would the ET anticipate? Select all that apply.

☐ **1.** The skin is intact.

☐ **2.** Full-thickness skin loss is evident.

☐ **3.** Undermining is present.

☐ **4.** Sinus tracts have developed.

☐ **5.** The ulcer is superficial, like a blister.

☐ **6.** Partial-thickness skin loss of the epidermis is evident.

Answer: 5, 6

Ⓜ **Rationale:** A stage II pressure ulcer involves partial-thickness skin loss of the epidermis or dermis. The ulcer is superficial and presents clinically as an abrasion, blister, or shallow crater. Intact skin is characteristic of a stage I pressure ulcer. Full-thickness skin loss, undermining, and sinus tracts are characteristic of a stage III pressure ulcer.

Test-taking strategy: Analyze to determine what information the question asks for, which is characteristics of a stage II ulcer. "Select all that apply" questions require considering each option to decide its merit. Eliminate option 1 as the skin is intact. Discriminate between the other options to select options through a partial thickness. Review the pathophysiology of pressure ulcers and ulcer staging if you had difficulty answering this question.

Client needs category: Physiological integrity

Client needs subcategory: Physiological adaptation

Cognitive level: Analyzing

---

4. The nurse is examining the back of a client and notes a rash with a discrete lesion configuration. Which graphic shows a discrete lesion configuration?

☐ **1.**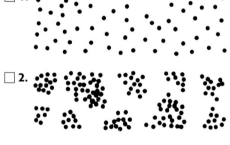

☐ **2.**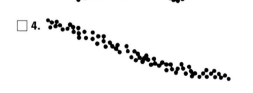

☐ **3.**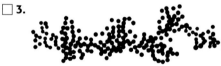

☐ **4.**

Answer: 1

Ⓜ **Rationale:** In a discrete pattern, individual lesions are separate and distinct. Option 2 shows a grouped pattern where lesions are clustered together. Option 3 is a confluent pattern. In this configuration, lesions merge so that individual lesions are not visible or palpable. Option 4 is a linear pattern in which lesions form a line.

Test-taking strategy: Analyze to determine what information the question asks for, which is identifying a discrete lesion configuration. Use knowledge of the term "discrete," meaning apart or detached from others to narrow the selection. Review skin lesion configurations and descriptions if you had difficulty answering this question.

Client needs category: Physiological integrity

Client needs subcategory: Physiological adaptation

Cognitive level: Analyzing

5. A triage nurse in the emergency department admits a client with second-degree burns on the anterior and posterior portions of both legs. Based on the rule of nines, what percentage of the body is burned?

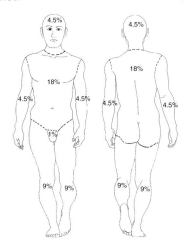

_____ %

Answer: 36

Ⓔ Rationale: The anterior and posterior portions of one leg amount to 18%. Because both legs are burned, the total is 36%.

Test-taking strategy: Analyze to determine what information the question asks for, which is percentage of body burned when the anterior and posterior portion of both legs are involved. Recall the rule of nines being a quick way of assessing the body and calculating treatment needs. Note the two areas per leg (18%), and multiply by 2. Review the areas affected and the percentage of body surface area calculation if you had difficulty answering this question.

Client needs category: Physiological integrity

Client needs subcategory: Physiological adaptation

Cognitive level: Analyzing

6. A client returns from the operating room with a partial-thickness skin graft on the left arm. The donor tissue was taken from the left hip. In planning immediate postoperative care, which interventions would the nurse include? Select all that apply.

☐ **1.** Change the dressing on the graft site every 8 hours.

☐ **2.** Elevate the left arm and provide complete rest of the grafted area.

☐ **3.** Administer pain medication every 4 hours as ordered for pain at the donor site.

☐ **4.** Perform ROM exercises to the left arm every 4 hours.

☐ **5.** Monitor the pulse in the left arm every 4 hours.

☐ **6.** Encourage the client to ambulate as desired on the first postoperative day.

Answer: 2, 3, 5

Ⓓ Rationale: Skin is the largest organ in the body representing 16% of the body weight. Skin may be harvested from one area and placed on another. In the question, the left arm should be elevated to reduce edema. Complete rest of the arm is needed to allow the graft to adhere. The donor site is usually more painful than the graft site, and the client will require pain medication to obtain relief. Because adequate circulation is needed for graft healing, it is important to monitor for the presence of a pulse. Changing the dressing every 8 hours, performing ROM exercises every 4 hours, and ambulating on the first day are inappropriate because postoperative graft sites require immobilization for 3 to 5 days.

Test-taking strategy: Analyze to determine what information the question asks for, which is the immediate postoperative care required following a skin graft. "Select all that apply" questions require considering each option to decide its merit. The key word is "immediate," and the important consideration is circulation or nourishment to the site. Review postoperative wound care and skin grafts if you had difficulty answering this question.

Client needs category: Physiological integrity

Client needs subcategory: Physiological adaptation

Cognitive level: Applying

7. During nursing rounds, a nurse checks on a client on bed rest who reports an itchy rash. The nurse assesses the client's skin for erythematous, slightly edematous areas on the client's back, posterior lower legs, and posterior elbows. The health care provider's diagnosis is an allergic contact dermatitis. Which teaching points about contact dermatitis are correct? Select all that apply.

☐ **1.** The disorder is contagious.

☐ **2.** This is an allergic reaction.

☐ **3.** Based on the location, it is likely that detergents in the bed linens caused the rash.

☐ **4.** The skin is infected wherever the rash has developed.

☐ **5.** Oatmeal (Aveeno) baths are a good treatment for a rash of this type because of the large area involved.

☐ **6.** Washing with antibacterial soap will help the rash.

Answer: 2, 3, 5

Ⓜ **Rationale:** Contact dermatitis is classified as a reaction to an allergen and can appear when skin, especially if it's moist from perspiring or other reasons, remains in contact with an irritant for an extended time. It is a hypersensitivity reaction but usually requires extended contact. This client has a presentation often seen when clients remain in bed, perspiring on detergent-cleansed bed linens or gowns. This type of sensitivity to detergents may not have produced a reaction with a shorter time contact. The rash is not contagious or infectious, although areas may become exudative and crusted. Treatment varies according to the intensity of the skin reaction and other factors, but oatmeal (Aveeno) baths are frequently prescribed.

Test-taking strategy: Analyze to determine what information the question asks for, which is teaching points of contact dermatitis. "Select all that apply" questions require considering each option to decide its merit. Consider the name "contact" to lead to answering the question correctly. Review the pathophysiology of contact dermatitis if you had difficulty answering the question.

Client needs category: Physiological integrity

Client needs subcategory: Basic care and comfort

Cognitive level: Applying

---

8. The nurse is providing an education seminar on skin care to clients and home care families. When discussing interventions, which areas have provided effective outcomes in preventing pressure ulcers? Select all that apply.

☐ **1.** Clean the skin with warm water and a mild cleaning agent, and then apply a moisturizer.

☐ **2.** When turning the client, slide and avoid lifting.

☐ **3.** Avoid raising the head of the bed more than 90°.

☐ **4.** Turn and reposition the client every 1 to 2 hours unless contraindicated.

☐ **5.** If the client uses a wheelchair, sit on a rubber or plastic doughnut.

☐ **6.** Use positioning devices to position the client and increase comfort.

Answer: 1, 4, 6

Ⓓ **Rationale:** Nursing interventions that are effective in preventing pressure ulcers include cleaning the skin with warm water and a mild cleaning agent and then applying a moisturizer; lifting—rather than sliding—the client when turning to reduce friction and shear; avoiding raising the head of the bed more than 30°, except for brief periods; repositioning and turning the client every 1 to 2 hours unless contraindicated; and using positioning devices or pillows to position the client and increase comfort. If the client uses a wheelchair, the nurse would offer a pressure-relieving cushion as appropriate. The nurse would not sit the client on a rubber or plastic doughnut because these devices can increase localized pressure at vulnerable points.

Test-taking strategy: Analyze to determine what information the question asks for, which is causes of pressure ulcer development and preventative measures. "Select all that apply" questions require considering each option to decide its merit. When thinking of pressure ulcer development, think of "skin integrity" and "pressure." Ask yourself, does this option maintain skin integrity and not create pressure on a bony prominence? Review preventative measures for pressure ulcers if you had difficulty answering this question.

Nursing process step: Implementation

Client needs category: Safe and effective care environment

Client needs subcategory: Safety and infection control

Cognitive level: Applying

---

9. A client presents to the emergency department with a foot lesion. When documenting the foot lesion in the medical record, which medical terms would a nurse use to classify the pictured lesion found below? Select all that apply.

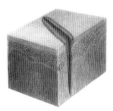

☐ **1.** Linear
☐ **2.** Flat
☐ **3.** Fissure
☐ **4.** Crack
☐ **5.** Scale
☐ **6.** Ulcer

Answer: 1, 3

ⓓ Rationale: When documenting in the medical record, it is important to use precise, descriptive terminology when documenting lesions to help aid diagnosis and track healing. The lesion depicted here is best described as a fissure, a linear crack in the skin. This type of lesion is commonly seen on clients with athlete's foot, usually between the toes.

Test-taking strategy: Analyze to determine what information the question asks for, which is accurately documenting a foot lesion. Use knowledge of medical terminology to consider each option against the pictured lesion. Review types of skin lesions, and focus on descriptors if you had difficulty answering this question.

Client needs category: Physiological integrity

Client needs subcategory: Physiological adaptation

Cognitive level: Understanding

10. The nurse is examining the back of a client who was admitted with a stage III pressure ulcer on the sacral area. Which illustration shows a stage III pressure ulcer?

☐ **1.**

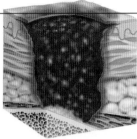

☐ **2.**

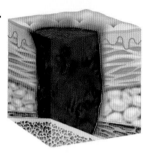

☐ **3.**

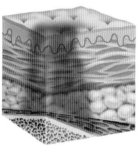

☐ **4.**

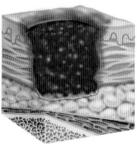

Ⓓ **Rationale:** In a stage III pressure ulcer, there is full-thickness skin loss along with damage or necrosis of the subcutaneous tissue. It may or may not extend down to (but not through) the fascia. Undermining may be present. Option 2 shows an unstageable pressure ulcer. In an unstageable pressure ulcer, the true stage of the ulcer cannot be determined until the base of the wound is exposed. Option 3 shows suspected deep tissue injury, which presents as a purple or maroon localized area of intact skin or blood-filled blister. Option 4 shows a stage IV pressure ulcer. In a stage IV ulcer, there is full-thickness skin loss with extensive tissue destruction, tissue necrosis, or damage to the muscle, bone, or support structures.

Test-taking strategy: Analyze to determine what information the question asks for, which is identification of a stage III pressure ulcer. Consider that a stage III ulcer is an advanced ulcer but not as advanced as the stage IV ulcer also depicted. Review the six pressure ulcer stages and characteristics if you had difficulty answering this question.

Client needs category: Physiological integrity

Client needs subcategory: Physiological adaptation

Cognitive level: Analyzing

11. The nurse is bathing a client and discovers a pressure ulcer on the buttocks (see photo). Which nursing intervention, following completion of the bath, is completed **first**?

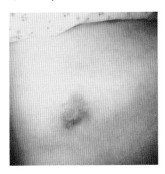

From Nettina SM. *The Lippincott Manual of Nursing Practice*, 7th ed. Philadelphia, PA: Lippincott Williams & Wilkins, 2001.

☐ **1.** Position the client off of the ulcer.

☐ **2.** Massage the ulcerated area vigorously.

☐ **3.** Place antibiotic cream over the ulcerated area.

☐ **4.** Notify the physician and await orders.

Answer: 1

Ⓔ Rationale: The first thing a nurse does after a bath would be to position the client off of the ulcer. The ulcer would not be vigorously massaged as this may increase the risk of skin breakdown. Antibiotic cream is not applied as there are signs of skin breakdown but not infection. The nurse would obtain ulcer measurements once the ulcer is discovered and notify the physician for further orders.

Test-taking strategy: Analyze to determine what information the question asks for, which is nursing intervention to be completed first after a bath. The key word is "first." Several of the actions may be completed, but when ordering the actions, what is the priority and within the scope of practice to be completed? Identify appropriate interventions, and then analyze which is to be done first. Review care of a pressure ulcer if you had difficulty answering this question.

Client needs category: Physiological integrity

Client needs subcategory: Physiological adaptation

Cognitive level: Analyzing

12. The client phones the outpatient surgery center following skin biopsy on the left shoulder. The client states that the site continues to drain pinkish drainage and is uncomfortable. Which triage questions are appropriate to evaluate the client's concern? Select all that apply.

☐ **1.** "Did you have any other skin biopsies that day?"

☐ **2.** "On which day did you have the biopsy completed?"

☐ **3.** "Can you describe the drainage that you see?"

☐ **4.** "When is your follow-up appointment?"

☐ **5.** "What is your pain level on a 0 to 10 pain scale?"

☐ **6.** "How are you cleaning the area?"

Answer: 2, 3, 5, 6

Ⓜ **Rationale:** When triaging a client's concern following a surgical biopsy, it is most important for the nurse to obtain information about the site and postoperative care. Knowing the date of the surgery allows for the nurse to determine the amount and type of drainage that is normal for that stage of healing. Understanding the characteristics of the drainage helps the nurse assess if the drainage is from a healing process or from a potential infection. Assessing the pain level provides information of the inflammatory and infectious process. The nurse compares the client's pain rating with the rating scale typically noted for this procedure. Lastly, the nurse assesses how the wound is being cleaned. The nurse wants to assess understanding regarding the cleaning process.

Test-taking strategy: Analyze to determine what information the question asks for, which is triage questions when a client with recent skin biopsy calls with concerns. When completing a triage assessment, the nurse must focus on the client problem, like the skin biopsy. Ask specific questions that would provide relevant information to answer the client's question—specifically, the when, what it looks like, and how the client is treating it. Dates of appointments and other biopsy locations are not as relevant at this time. Review triage questioning and biopsies if you had difficulty answering this question.

Client needs category: Safe and effective care environment

Client needs subcategory: Management of care

Cognitive level: Applying

Oncologic disorders

1. A nurse is caring for a terminally ill cancer client who is being transferred to hospice care. Which information regarding hospice care would the nurse include in the teaching plan? Select all that apply.

☐ **1.** The focus of care is on controlling symptoms and relieving pain.

☐ **2.** A multidisciplinary team provides care.

☐ **3.** Services are provided based on third-party insurance reimbursement.

☐ **4.** Hospice care is provided only in hospice centers.

☐ **5.** Bereavement care is provided to the family.

☐ **6.** Care is provided in the home, independent of physicians.

Answer: 1, 2, 5

Ⓜ **Rationale:** Hospice care focuses on controlling symptoms and relieving pain at the end of life. A multidisciplinary team—consisting of nurses, physicians, chaplains, aides, and volunteers—provides the care. After the client's death, hospice provides bereavement care to the grieving family. Hospice services are provided based on need, not on the ability to pay or insurance reimbursement. Hospice care may be provided in a variety of settings, such as freestanding hospice centers, the home, a hospital, or a long-term care facility. Care is provided under the direction of a physician, who is a key member of the hospice team.

Test-taking strategy: Analyze to determine what information the question asks for, which is the concepts and principles of hospice care. "Select all that apply" questions require considering each option to decide its merit. Recall the difference between acute or home health care and hospice care, which relates to the needs of a terminally ill client and extends bereavement to the family.

Client needs category: Safe and effective care environment

Client needs subcategory: Management of care

Cognitive level: Applying

---

2. An adult client with Hodgkin's disease who weighs 143 lb is to receive vincristine 25 mg/kg intravenously. What is the correct dose in micrograms that the client would receive? Record your answer as a whole number.

_____ µg

Answer: 1,625

Ⓔ **Rationale:** First, convert the client's weight from pounds to kilograms:

$$1 \text{ lb} = 2.2 \text{ kg}$$
$$143 \text{ lb} = X \text{ kg}$$
$$143 \text{ lb}/2.2 \text{ kg} = 65 \text{ kg}.$$

Next, multiply the weight in kilograms by the number of micrograms desired per kilogram:

$$65 \text{ kg} \times 25 \text{ µg} = 1,625 \text{ µg}.$$

Test-taking strategy: Analyze to determine what information the question asks for, which is micrograms of medication per client weight. Use care in reading what the question asks and follow through with a two-step problem. Proofread the math calculation. Review common conversions and drug calculations if you had difficulty answering this question.

Client needs category: Physiological integrity

Client needs subcategory: Pharmacological and parenteral therapies

Cognitive level: Applying

3. A nurse has identified the nursing diagnosis *Situational low self-esteem related to hair loss and severe fatigue* for a client with cancer. Which nursing interventions would be appropriate for this client's care? Select all that apply.

☐ **1.** Ask how the diagnosis and treatment are affecting the client's personal life and roles.

☐ **2.** Review any anticipated side effects of treatment with the client.

☐ **3.** Tell the client how to resolve specific concerns related to the effects of treatment on the personal life.

☐ **4.** As a behavioral guide, describe the experiences of friends and other clients who have had this disease and treatment.

☐ **5.** Offer information on available counseling services and support groups, if desired, explaining that these techniques are helpful to many clients.

☐ **6.** Maintain eye contact with the client and use touch during interactions, if acceptable to the client.

Answer: 1, 2, 5, 6

Ⓒ Rationale: The nursing diagnosis selected is a psychosocial diagnosis. Discussing the client's feelings about the cancer diagnosis and treatment helps identify coping-related problems. Anticipating potential adverse effects can help the client begin to adapt and prepare to cope with these events. Referral to support groups or counseling services helps provide the client with validation and assistance with problem solving. Touch and eye contact can be therapeutic in affirming individuality and acceptance and can help build self-esteem. Instructing the client in how the nurse believes problems should be resolved is not therapeutic. The nurse should help the client explore options for solving the problems in a manner consistent with the client's beliefs and values. Telling stories about others' experiences without their consent breaches confidentiality and may demonstrate a lack of listening and empathic interaction by the nurse. Validating the client's own personal story is beneficial to rebuilding self-esteem.

Test-taking strategy: Analyze to determine what information the question asks for, which is nursing interventions associated with a specific psychosocial diagnosis. "Select all that apply" questions require considering each option to decide its merit. Recall the clinical manifestations and emotional aspects of cancer, which would be a priority. Review expected outcomes for clients with cancer.

Client needs category: Psychosocial integrity

Client needs subcategory: None

Cognitive level: Applying

---

4. A client with laryngeal cancer has undergone a laryngectomy and is now receiving radiation therapy to the head and neck. The nurse would monitor the client for which adverse effects of external radiation? Select all that apply.

☐ **1.** Xerostomia

☐ **2.** Stomatitis

☐ **3.** Thrombocytopenia

☐ **4.** Cystitis

☐ **5.** Mucositis

☐ **6.** Leukopenia

Answer: 1, 2, 5

Ⓓ Rationale: Radiation of the head and neck often produces dry mouth (xerostomia), irritation of the oral mucous membranes (stomatitis, mucositis), and diminished sense of taste (dysgeusia). Thrombocytopenia (reduced platelet count) and leukopenia (reduced white blood cell count) may occur with systemic radiation; cystitis may occur with radiation of the genitourinary system.

Test-taking strategy: Analyze to determine what information the question asks for, which is the adverse effects of radiation therapy for laryngeal cancer. "Select all that apply" questions require considering each option to decide its merit. Recall the specific area being irradiated and relate localized adverse effects of radiation. Review the adverse effects of radiation therapy if you had difficulty answering this question.

Client needs category: Physiological integrity

Client needs subcategory: Reduction of risk potential

Cognitive level: Applying

5. A nurse is teaching a community program on breast self-examination (BSE). The nurse demonstrates the proper procedure for palpating each breast. In what sequence would the following actions be performed for proper self-examination? All options must be used.

1. Place the hand over the breast to be examined (use the right hand for the left breast and vice versa).

2. Lie down with one arm behind the head.

3. Palpate the breast in a perpendicular motion, going across the breast from one side to another and top to bottom.

4. Use the finger pads of the three middle fingers and touch the breast.

5. Use a circular motion to feel the breast tissue (with light, medium, and firm pressure).

Answer: 2, 1, 5, 4, 3

Ⓜ Rationale: Although the American Cancer Society (ACS) states that monthly BSEs are optional, it remains an important way to discover early breast changes. BSE is a standard procedure described by national organizations designed to ensure palpation of all breast tissue. Examination can begin when lying down, in the shower, or standing before a mirror. The examination also includes a visual inspection of the breasts while pressing the hands firmly against the hips and examining the underarms associated with each breast with the arms slightly raised.

Test-taking strategy: Analyze to determine what information the question asks for, which is the proper sequence for breast evaluation. Recall the assessment standards of palpating all areas of the breast using the pads of the fingers in a perpendicular motion. Review the method for performing BSE if you had difficulty answering this question.

Client needs category: Health promotion and maintenance

Client needs subcategory: None

Cognitive level: Applying

6. A client who is receiving chemotherapy for breast cancer develops myelosuppression. Which instructions would the nurse include in the client's discharge teaching plan? Select all that apply.

☐ **1.** Avoid people who have recently received live vaccines.

☐ **2.** Avoid activities that may cause bleeding.

☐ **3.** Wash hands frequently.

☐ **4.** Increase intake of fresh fruits and vegetables.

☐ **5.** Avoid crowded places such as shopping malls.

☐ **6.** Treat a sore throat with OTC products.

Answer: 1, 2, 3, 5

Ⓜ Rationale: Chemotherapy can cause myelosuppression, which is a decreased number of RBCs, white blood cells, and platelets. A client receiving chemotherapy needs to avoid people who have been vaccinated recently, especially by a live virus. Because platelet counts are reduced, the client also needs to avoid activities that could cause trauma and bleeding. The client would wash her hands frequently because hand washing is the best way to prevent the spread of infection. A client receiving chemotherapy would avoid crowded places as well as people with colds during flu season because she/he has a reduced ability to fight infection. Fresh fruits and vegetables would be avoided because they can harbor bacteria that cannot be removed easily by washing. Signs and symptoms of infection, such as a sore throat, fever, and a cough, are reported immediately to the health care provider.

Test-taking strategy: Analyze to determine what information the question asks for, which is the discharge teaching plan of a client with myelosuppression. First, use knowledge of medical terminology to identify that myelo = bone or bone marrow suppression. Next, consider the ramifications related to infection, which will identify several discharge teaching points. "Select all that apply" questions require considering each option to decide its merit. Review the clinical manifestations of myelosuppression, and review leukopenia, thrombocytopenia, and anemia if you had difficulty answering this question.

Client needs category: Physiological integrity

Client needs subcategory: Reduction of risk potential

Cognitive level: Applying

---

7. A client with bladder cancer undergoes surgical removal of the bladder with construction of an ileal conduit. Which assessment findings indicate that the client is developing complications? Select all that apply.

☐ **1.** Urine output greater than 30 ml/hour

☐ **2.** Dusky appearance of the stoma

☐ **3.** Stoma protrusion from the skin

☐ **4.** Mucus shreds in the urine collection bag

☐ **5.** Edema of the stoma during the first 24 hours after surgery

☐ **6.** Sharp abdominal pain with rigidity

Answer: 2, 3, 6

Ⓒ Rationale: A dusky appearance of the stoma indicates decreased blood supply to the stoma; a healthy stoma would appear beefy red. Protrusion indicates prolapse of the stoma, and sharp abdominal pain with rigidity suggests peritonitis. A urine output greater than 30 ml/hour is a sign of adequate renal perfusion and is a normal finding. Because mucous membranes are used to create the conduit, mucus in the urine is expected. Stomal edema is a normal finding during the first 24 hours after surgery.

Test-taking strategy: Analyze to determine what information the question asks for, which is abnormal findings following placement of an ileal conduit. "Select all that apply" questions require considering each option to decide its merit. Analyze the options for signs of infection or abnormal ileal conduit structure and function. Review the surgical procedure and potential complications if you had difficulty answering this question.

Client needs category: Physiological integrity

Client needs subcategory: Reduction of risk potential

Cognitive level: Analyzing

---

8. A client is ordered a dose of epoetin alfa to treat anemia related to chemotherapy. The recommended dose is 150 units/kg. The client weighs 60 kg. The vial is labeled 10,000 units/ml. How many milliliters of epoetin alfa would the nurse administer? Record your answer using one decimal place.

_____ ml

Answer: 0.9

ⓔ Rationale: First, determine the number of units of epoetin alfa the client is to receive:

$$60 \text{ kg} \times 150 \text{ units} = 9,000 \text{ units/kg.}$$

Next, determine the number of milliliters required to deliver that dose:

$$10,000 \text{ units} : 1 \text{ ml} = 9,000 \text{ units} : X$$

$$\frac{10,000 \text{ units} \times X}{10,000 \text{ units}} = \frac{9,000 \text{ units} \times 1 \text{ ml}}{10,000 \text{ units}}$$

$$X = 0.9 \text{ ml.}$$

Test-taking strategy: Analyze to determine what information the question asks for, which is correct dosage of epoetin alfa. Follow the two-step procedure noted above. Proofread your math calculation. Review drug concentration calculations if you had difficulty answering this question.

Client needs category: Physiological integrity

Client needs subcategory: Pharmacological and parenteral therapies

Cognitive level: Applying

---

9. A client who is experiencing colon cancer is scheduled to undergo a colostomy. Which interventions would be appropriate to include in a preoperative teaching plan? Select all that apply.

☐ **1.** Demonstrate turning, coughing, deep breathing, splinting, and leg ROM exercises, and provide rationales for each procedure.

☐ **2.** Instruct on dietary guidelines for healing.

☐ **3.** Arrange for an ET to speak with the client about colostomy care.

☐ **4.** Explain the need for early postoperative ambulation.

☐ **5.** Instruct the client on signs and symptoms of intestinal obstruction.

☐ **6.** Encourage the client to express feelings about changes in body image.

Answer: 1, 3, 4, 6

ⓓ Rationale: Preoperatively, the client will require instruction regarding the need for turning, coughing, deep breathing, splinting, and leg ROM exercises. The client will also need to learn about colostomy care and the reason for early postoperative ambulation. Addressing feelings about body image changes is also appropriate at this time. Learning of dietary guidelines and instructing the client about signs and symptoms of intestinal obstruction are part of the postoperative care.

Test-taking strategy: Analyze to determine what information the question asks for, which is interventions for the preoperative teaching plan. The key word is "preoperative," meaning instruction that can be given before surgery but used in the postoperative period. Review preoperative interventions and colostomy surgery if you had difficulty answering this question.

Client needs category: Physiological integrity

Client needs subcategory: Basic care and comfort

Cognitive level: Applying

10. A client has been diagnosed with lung cancer and is scheduled to undergo a left pneumonectomy. The client will have a chest tube inserted as part of the surgical procedure. Identify the area where the nurse will expect to see the chest tube inserted.

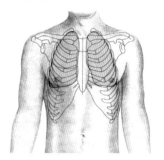

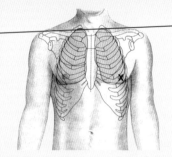

Ⓜ **Rationale:** A left pneumonectomy is the surgical removal of the left lung. Removal of one lobe of the lung is called a lobectomy. A chest tube is placed within the thoracic cavity at the site of the removed lung. Therefore, a chest tube would be placed on the left side of the chest.

Test-taking strategy: Analyze to determine what information the question asks for, which is site of chest tube insertion for a left pneumonectomy. Recall from medical terminology that pneumonectomy (pneumo—lung and ectomy—removal) means removal of the lung. Also, always use anatomical position when determining between right side and left side placement. Review the clinical manifestations of pneumonectomy and anatomical placement of a chest tube if you had difficulty answering this question.

Client needs category: Physiological integrity

Client needs subcategory: Reduction of risk potential

Cognitive level: Applying

---

11. A client has been diagnosed with breast cancer and is scheduled to begin treatment with the antineoplastic drug, doxorubicin hydrochloride. Which side effects would the nurse anticipate? Select all that apply.

☐ **1.** Hair thinning throughout the course of treatment

☐ **2.** Hepatic impairment

☐ **3.** Left ventricular failure

☐ **4.** Complete hair loss within 3 to 4 weeks

☐ **5.** Red discoloration of urine

Answer: 2, 3, 4, 5

Ⓒ **Rationale:** Doxorubicin is used in combination with other medications to treat many types of cancers. Primary side effects of this drug include cardiac changes (including left ventricular failure and arrhythmias), complete hair loss within 3 to 4 weeks of receiving the drug, hepatic impairment, and red discoloration of the urine. Methotrexate rarely causes complete hair loss but may cause thinning or no hair loss.

Test-taking strategy: Analyze to determine what information the question asks for, which is side effects of doxorubicin. Recall that a complete cardiac assessment is completed prior to the initiation of chemotherapeutic because of the cardiac changes that may occur. Also, note other common side effects of chemotherapeutic therapy. Review common side effects of chemotherapeutic agents and especially doxorubicin hydrochloride if you had difficulty answering the question.

Client needs category: Physiological integrity

Client needs subcategory: Physiological adaptation

Cognitive level: Applying

---

12. A client with pancreatic cancer has been prescribed a chemotherapeutic medication of 12 mg/kg intravenously for 4 days. If no signs of toxicity occur, the client is to receive 6 mg/kg of the medication on days 6, 8, 10, and 12. The client weighs 198 lb. At the conclusion of day 12, how many total milligrams will the client have received? Record your answer as a whole number.

_____ mg

M **Rationale:** The problem is calculated by initially converting 198 lb to kilograms:

$$1 \text{ lb} = 2.2 \text{ kg}$$
$$198 \text{ lb} = X \text{ kg}$$
$$198 \text{ lb} \div 2.2 \text{ kg} = 90 \text{ kg}.$$

Next, multiply the weight in kilograms by the number of micrograms for each of the medication days:

$$12 \text{ mg} \times 90 = 1{,}080 \text{ mg}$$
$$(1{,}080 \text{ mg} \times 4 \text{ days} = 4{,}320 \text{ mg})$$
$$6 \text{ mg} \times 90 \text{ kg} = 540 \text{ mg}$$
$$(540 \text{ mg} \times 4 \text{ days} = 2{,}160 \text{ mg})$$

Then, add these amounts together:

$$4{,}320 \text{ mg} + 2{,}160 \text{ mg} = 6{,}480 \text{ mg}.$$

Test-taking strategy: Analyze to determine what information the question asks for, which is total milligrams of chemotherapeutic medication. Note that this is a three-step problem. Begin with the conversion to kilograms. Next, obtain the titrated dosages and then add. Review all math calculations. Review conversions and calculating titrated dosages according to body weight if you had difficulty answering this question.

Client needs category: Physiological integrity

Client needs subcategory: Pharmacological and parenteral therapies

Cognitive level: Applying

13. While undergoing treatment with a caustic chemotherapeutic agent, a client experiences extravasation. Indicate how the nurse would respond to extravasation by placing the following nursing interventions in chronological order. All options must be used.

1. Notify the health care provider.

2. Follow facility policy for dealing with extravasation.

3. Implement the health care provider's orders.

4. Discontinue the intravenous infusion.

5. Document all signs and symptoms thoroughly.

6. Monitor the client throughout the shift, and give a detailed report to the oncoming shift.

Answer: 4, 2, 1, 3, 5, 6

Ⓜ **Rationale:** Extravasation is the accidental administration of intravenous fluid into the extracellular space/tissue. Immediately, the intravenous infusion would be discontinued so that the client will not continue to receive more of the medication and damage the tissue. The facility will have a policy on how to deal with extravasation (usually the application of ice) that can be implemented while the health care provider is being notified. After the health care provider is notified, the specific orders will need to be implemented. All signs and symptoms that the client is experiencing would be documented thoroughly in preparation for the report to be given to the oncoming shift.

Test-taking strategy: Analyze to determine what information the question asks for, which is nursing interventions when caring for a client with an extravasation. Safety is always a first concern, which includes discontinuing the intravenous administration. Note that options with documentation and monitoring are performed after safety and care of the client. Review the clinical manifestations of extravasation and client safety if you had difficulty answering this question.

Client needs category: Health promotion and maintenance

Client needs subcategory: None

Cognitive level: Analyzing

14. The nurse is teaching a client about breast self-examination (BSE). Which pattern of palpation would the nurse encourage based on ACS recommendations?

☐ **1.**

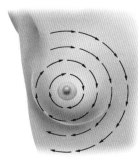

☐ **2.**

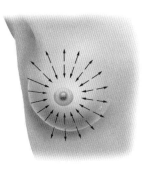

☐ **3.**

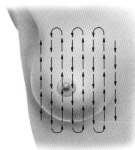

☐ **4.**

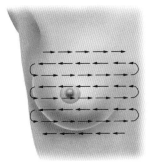

Ⓜ **Rationale:** The ACS recommends an up-and-down vertical pattern as the most effective pattern for covering the whole breast. Option 1 (circular pattern) and option 2 (wedged pattern) are alternate methods but may not be as effective. Option 4 (horizontal pattern) is not a recognized method used in BSE.

Test-taking strategy: Analyze to determine what information the question asks for, which is pattern of palpation during a BSE. Consider that the up-and-down method is a common method that covers all breast tissue. Review known patterns of palpation for BSE and the current ACS guidelines if you had difficulty answering this question.

Client needs category: Health promotion and maintenance

Client needs subcategory: None

Cognitive level: Analyzing

15. The home health nurse is caring for a client receiving chemotherapy. The client reports anorexia and has a weight loss of 15 lb (6.8 kg) over 6 weeks. Which client teaching would be helpful? Select all that apply.

☐ **1.** Eat large meals when hungry.

☐ **2.** Obtain calorie-dense foods for snack.

☐ **3.** Cook a hot meal for lunch and dinner.

☐ **4.** Have family prepare and deliver favorite meals.

☐ **5.** Eat small portions of each food group.

☐ **6.** Eat slowly and in a relaxed atmosphere.

Answer: 2, 4, 5, 6

ⓒ Rationale: The client receiving chemotherapy may experience bouts of anorexia, which leads to a weight loss. Making the most of the foods that the client ingests is important. For this reason, it is important to eat nutritious meals and snacks that are nutrient dense. The smell of food often nauseates the client; thus, having the family prepare the foods may increase the tolerance. Eating slowly and in a relaxed atmosphere may allow the client to ingest more of and enjoy the meal. Clients are often not able to eat large meals and rather have small frequent meals. Also, clients are often better able to tolerate cool or cold meals (salads, sandwiches) as opposed to hot meals for lunch and dinner.

Test-taking strategy: Analyze to determine what information the question asks for, which is helpful hints to combat anorexia and weight loss in a client receiving chemotherapy. Recall that chemotherapeutic agents often affect the digestive system causing anorexia and nausea. Think "nutrient dense" and "small frequent" when considering how to maximize nutrients and meal times. "Select all that apply" questions require considering each option to decide its merit in improving nutrition and increasing client weight. Review client nutrition during chemotherapy if you had difficulty answering this question.

Client needs category: Physiological integrity

Client needs subcategory: Physiological adaptation

Cognitive level: Applying

16. The nurse is caring for a client, newly diagnosed with cancer, who speaks limited English. The client's family speaks limited English also, and a friend drives him to his doctor's appointments. The nurse selects *Deficient knowledge* as a priority. Which nursing interventions are appropriate? Select all that apply.

☐ **1.** Ask the client's driver to interpret the conversation.

☐ **2.** Provide a brochure on the cancer and treatment options.

☐ **3.** Work with an interpreter to discuss the situation.

☐ **4.** Assess any community resources for support groups and communication.

☐ **5.** Obtain a "type to speak" computerized translation dictionary to express information.

☐ **6.** Obtain common pictures to provide a common ground for understanding.

Answer: 3, 4, 5, 6

Ⓒ Rationale: It is very difficult to discuss specific cancer treatments and options when there is a language barrier. Clients have a difficult time with medical terminology associated with diagnosis and treatment. To improve the knowledge base, it is best to have an interpreter, with medical background if possible, become part of the health care team. Most agencies ask all health care workers if they speak another language and then will pull on this group as needed. It is not appropriate to have the client's driver interpret unless this is approved by the client. Also, the health care providers are unsure if the driver understands the information to translate. Community resources can be helpful as well as a pictorial guide or "type to speak" dictionary. Brochures are not helpful unless the client understands the information provided.

Test-taking strategy: Analyze to determine what information the question asks for, which is nursing interventions that are helpful to a client with limited English knowledge. Look to each option for assistance with communication. Review communication with a client with limited English skills if you had difficulty answering this question.

Client needs category: Psychosocial integrity

Client needs subcategory: None

Cognitive level: Applying

PART FOUR

Maternal–neonatal nursing

Antepartum period

1. During her first prenatal visit, a client asks a nurse what physiological changes she can expect during pregnancy. The nurse begins the discussion with the presumptive changes of pregnancy. Put the following presumptive changes in ascending chronological order according to when they occur. All options must be used.

| **1.** Frequent urination |
| **2.** Breast changes |
| **3.** Quickening |
| **4.** Appearance of linea nigra, melasma, and striae gravidarum |
| **5.** Uterine enlargement in which the uterus can be palpated over the symphysis pubis |

Answer: 2, 1, 5, 3, 4

Ⓓ Rationale: Presumptive changes are subjective and can be caused by other medical conditions. Breast changes occur approximately 2 weeks after implantation of the embryo; frequent urination, at 3 weeks; fatigue and uterine enlargement over the symphysis pubis, at 18 weeks; quickening, between 18 and 20 weeks; and the appearance of linea nigra, melasma, and striae gravidarum, at 24 weeks.

Test-taking strategy: Analyze to determine what information the question asks for, which is the progression of the presumptive changes of pregnancy. The key word is "progression" as the question states that all five options are presumptive changes. The earliest signs can lead from hormonal changes; thus, breast changes are first. Next, look to the end and critically think what would be last. The appearance of the linea nigra group of changes refers to a stretched abdomen making it the last choice. Discriminate through the remaining three options to fill in the middle. Review the physiologic changes of pregnancy with presumptive signs if you had difficulty answering this question.

Client needs category: Health promotion and maintenance
Client needs subcategory: None
Cognitive level: Applying

2. A 30-year-old client comes to the office for a routine prenatal visit. After reading the chart entry below, the nurse would prepare the client for which test?

Progress notes

| 6/8/15 1320 | Client is 11 weeks pregnant; urine sample shows glycosuria. Client has a family history of diabetes. ———— Chrissy Franks, RN |

☐ **1.** Triple screen
☐ **2.** Indirect Coombs' test
☐ **3.** 1-Hour glucose tolerance test
☐ **4.** Amniocentesis

Answer: 3

Ⓔ Rationale: A 1-hour glucose tolerance test is recommended to screen for gestational diabetes if the client is obese, has glycosuria or a family history of diabetes, or lost a fetus for unexplained reasons or gave birth to a large-for-gestational-age neonate. A triple screen tests for chromosomal abnormalities. The indirect Coombs' test screens maternal blood for red blood cell antibodies. Amniocentesis is used to detect fetal abnormalities.

Test-taking strategy: Analyze to determine what information the question asks for, which is identifying an abnormal finding, requiring further testing, in the documentation provided. Note that all abnormal findings such as "glycosuria" and "diabetes" lead to a test for gestational diabetes. Review laboratory studies during pregnancy, especially related to gestational diabetes, if you had difficulty answering this question.

Client needs category: Physiological integrity
Client needs subcategory: Reduction of risk potential
Cognitive level: Applying

3. A nurse is preparing to teach a client about fetal growth and development during the first 3 months of pregnancy. The nurse is assembling teaching aids by milestones. In ascending order (month 1, month 2, month 3, and months 4 to 9), how would the nurse arrange the aids? All options must be used.

1. Teeth and bones begin to appear, the kidneys start to function, and, at the end of the month, gender is distinguishable.

2. The embryo has a definite form; the head, trunk, and tiny buds for arms and legs develop; and the cardiovascular system begins to function.

3. Internal and external fetal growth continues at a rapid rate, and the fetus stores the fats and minerals it needs to live outside the womb.

4. The eyes, ears, nose, lips, tongue, and tooth buds develop; the umbilical cord has a definite form; and the external genitalia are present.

Ⓜ Rationale: Significant growth and development take place during the first 3 months. By the first month, the embryo has a definite form; the head, trunk, and tiny buds for arms and legs develop; and the cardiovascular system begins to function. By the second month, the eyes, ears, nose, lips, tongue, and tooth buds develop; the umbilical cord has a definite form; and the external genitalia are present. By the third month, teeth and bones begin to appear, the kidneys start to function, and, at the end of the month, gender is distinguishable. By the fourth month, internal and external fetal growth begins accelerating at a more rapid rate; the fetus stores the fats and minerals it needs to live outside the womb, and growth continues until the fetus is full-term.

Test-taking strategy: Analyze to determine what information the question asks for, which is order of prenatal development milestones. Read each grouping carefully to identify the sequence. Recall that large structures appear first such as head and trunk. Also note the last option, fetal stores for outside the womb. Fill in the middle two options, but note umbilical cord development as first. Review fetal development by milestones if you had difficulty answering this question.

Client needs category: Health promotion and maintenance

Client needs subcategory: None

Cognitive level: Applying

4. A woman at 15 weeks of gestation comes to the clinic for an amniocentesis. If an abnormal result is found, which characteristics or problems could be identified? Select all that apply.

☐ **1.** Fetal lung maturity

☐ **2.** Gestational diabetes

☐ **3.** Chromosomal defects

☐ **4.** Neural tube defects

☐ **5.** Polyhydramnios

☐ **6.** Sex of the fetus

Answer: 3, 4, 6

Ⓒ Rationale: In early pregnancy, amniocentesis can be used to identify chromosomal and neural tube defects and to determine the sex of the fetus. It can also be used to evaluate fetal lung maturity during the last trimester of pregnancy. According to the U.S. Preventive Health Task Force, a blood test performed after 24 weeks of gestation is used to screen for gestational diabetes. Ultrasound is used to identify polyhydramnios; amniocentesis can be used to treat polyhydramnios by removing excess fluid.

Test-taking strategy: Analyze to determine what information the question asks for, which is the characteristics/problems that can be identified with an amniocentesis. "Select all that apply" questions require considering each option to decide its merit. Understanding basic facts, such as fetal development at 15 weeks (approximately 4 months) of gestation and the benefits of amniocentesis, is a must. When considering each option, ask if the option would be able to be identified at that gestation and if amniocentesis would identify it. Both must fit to be chosen for the answer. Review gestational development and amniocentesis if you had difficulty answering this question.

Client needs category: Physiological integrity
Client needs subcategory: Reduction of risk potential
Cognitive level: Applying

---

5. A nurse is caring for a postterm client at 41 weeks of gestation who is about to undergo a biophysical profile (BPP) to evaluate her fetus's well-being. The client asks, "What will be able to be determined from this test?" The nurse is correct to answer which? Select all that apply.

☐ **1.** Fetal tone

☐ **2.** Fetal breathing

☐ **3.** Femur length

☐ **4.** Amniotic fluid volume

☐ **5.** Biparietal diameter

☐ **6.** Crown–rump length

Answer: 1, 2, 4

Ⓜ Rationale: A BPP is an ultrasound assessment of fetal well-being that includes the following components: nonstress test, fetal tone, fetal breathing, fetal motion, and volume of amniotic fluid. It is used to confirm the health of the fetus or identify abnormalities. Crown–rump length is used to assess gestational age during the first trimester. Biparietal diameter and femur length are also used to assess gestational age and are done in the second and third trimesters.

Test-taking strategy: Analyze to determine what information the question asks for, which is components of a BPP. "Select all that apply" questions require considering each option to decide its merit. First, identify the options that provide information about "well-being." Next, add that information to the five parameters of a BPP. Determine those options that differentiate growth from well-being. Review BPP information if you had difficulty answering this question.

Client needs category: Physiological integrity
Client needs subcategory: Reduction of risk potential
Cognitive level: Applying

---

6. A nurse is caring for a client who is at 32 weeks of gestation and performs Leopold's maneuvers to confirm that the fetus is in the cephalic position. To identify fetal heart tones, place an X where the nurse would place the Doppler transducer.

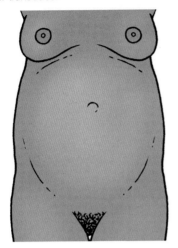

Answer:

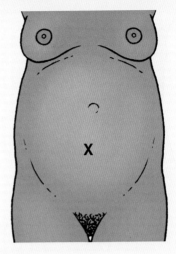

Ⓜ Rationale: When the fetus is in the cephalic position (head down), fetal heart tones are best auscultated midway between the symphysis pubis and the umbilicus. When the fetus is in the breech position, fetal heart tones are best heard at or above the level of the umbilicus.

Test-taking strategy: Analyze to determine what information the question asks for, which is placement of transducer to hear fetal heart sound when the fetus is in the cephalic position. Use the clues from medical terminology (cephalo—head). Cephalic position means head first in the birth canal. With that knowledge, visualize where the heart sounds would best be heard. Review fetal positions related to the fetal head placement if you had difficulty answering this question.

Client needs category: Health promotion and maintenance

Client needs subcategory: None

Cognitive level: Analyzing

7. A nurse is caring for a primigravida client. At 20 weeks of gestation, identify the location where the nurse anticipates the uterine fundus.

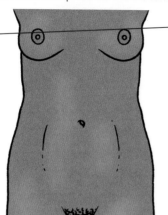

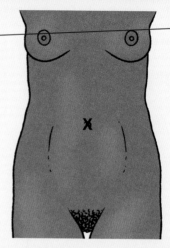

Ⓜ **Rationale:** At 20 weeks, the uterine fundus would be palpated approximately at the umbilicus. Fundal height would be measured from the symphysis pubis to the top of the uterus (McDonald's method). Serial measurements assess fetal growth over the course of the pregnancy. Between weeks 22 and 34, the number of centimeters measured correlates approximately with the week of gestation. However, if the client is very tall or short, fundal height will differ.

Test-taking strategy: Analyze to determine what information the question asks for, which is the location of the uterine fundus at a specific time (20 weeks of gestation). Recall that the uterine fundus is the top portion of the uterus, opposite the cervix. At 20 weeks, the fundal height is at the level of the umbilicus and increases 1 cm per week thereafter; thus, as pregnancy progresses, the fundal height increases. Review changes in fundal height throughout pregnancy if you had difficulty answering this question.

Client needs category: Health promotion and maintenance

Client needs subcategory: None

Cognitive level: Applying

8. A nurse is caring for a client who is 32 weeks pregnant and being monitored in the antepartum unit for pregnancy-induced hypertension. The client suddenly reports continuous abdominal pain and vaginal bleeding. Which nursing interventions are priorities? Select all that apply.

☐ **1.** Evaluate maternal vital signs.

☐ **2.** Prepare for vaginal birth.

☐ **3.** Reassure the client that she will be able to continue the pregnancy.

☐ **4.** Auscultate fetal heart tones.

☐ **5.** Monitor the amount of vaginal bleeding.

☐ **6.** Monitor intake and output.

Ⓒ Rationale: The client's symptoms indicate that she is experiencing abruptio placentae. The nurse must immediately evaluate the mother's vital signs, auscultate fetal heart tones, monitor the amount of blood loss, and evaluate volume status by monitoring intake and output. After the severity of the abruption has been determined and blood and fluid have been replaced, a prompt cesarean (not vaginal) birth is indicated if the fetus is in distress.

Test-taking strategy: Analyze to determine what information the question asks for, which is priority nursing interventions of a client experiencing abdominal pain and vaginal bleeding. "Select all that apply" questions require considering each option to decide its merit. Recall that vaginal bleeding and abdominal pain can be ominous signs related to life-threatening disorders for the mother and baby. Consider the assessment data needed to relate important data to the health care provider. Review disorders of pregnancy related to abdominal pain and vaginal bleeding if you had difficulty answering this question.

Client needs category: Physiological integrity

Client needs subcategory: Physiological adaptation

Cognitive level: Analyzing

9. A nurse is obtaining a pregnancy history at the first antepartal visit. The client states common symptoms of a nagging abdominal pain and a pulling sensation. Place an X where the nurse anticipates these normal symptoms in early pregnancy.

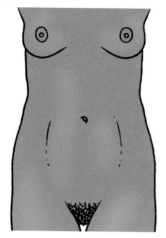

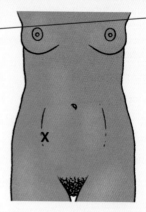

D **Rationale:** The nurse must be aware of common symptoms encountered in the antepartum period. New mothers especially can express concerns regarding the nature and significance of the discomfort. As the uterus grows in early pregnancy, it deviates physically to the right. This shift, or dextrorotation, is because of the presence of the rectosigmoid colon in the left lower quadrant. As a result, many women report pain in the right lower quadrant.

Test-taking strategy: Analyze to determine what information the question asks for, which is the abdominal site of discomfort in early pregnancy. Consider the effects of a growing fetus in the abdominal cavity, and relate these to the impact on other abdominal muscles and organs. Review maternal anatomy especially with the enlarging uterus if you had difficulty answering this question.

Client needs category: Health promotion and maintenance

Client needs subcategory: None

Cognitive level: Analyzing

---

10. During a prenatal visit, a health care provider decides to admit a client to the hospital. Based on the nurse's admission note below, which complication of pregnancy would the health care provider suspect?

Progress notes	
2/2/16	30-year-old female admitted with nausea and
1100	vomiting. Client is 16 weeks pregnant and
	reports of thirst and vertigo. BP 120/70 mm
	Hg, RR 20, P 104, Temp 100° F (37.8°C). Client
	has had nothing to eat or drink for 24 hours.
	—S. Thomas, RN

☐ **1.** Iron deficiency anemia

☐ **2.** Placenta previa

☐ **3.** Pregnancy-induced hypertension

☐ **4.** Hyperemesis gravidarum

E **Rationale:** Hyperemesis gravidarum is severe nausea and vomiting that persists after the first trimester. If untreated, it can lead to weight loss, starvation, dehydration, fluid and electrolyte imbalances, and acid–base disturbances. The client may report thirst, hiccups, oliguria, vertigo, and headache. A rapid pulse and elevated or subnormal temperature can also occur. Signs and symptoms of iron deficiency anemia include fatigue, pallor, and exercise intolerance. Placenta previa causes painless, bright red, vaginal bleeding after 20 weeks of pregnancy. Pregnancy-induced hypertension usually develops after 20 weeks of pregnancy; the client reports sudden weight gain and presents with hypertension.

Test-taking strategy: Analyze to determine what information the question asks for, which is a complication as documented in the nurse's admission note. Begin by focusing on abnormal findings in the note (nausea/vomiting, thirst, vertigo, and nothing by mouth for 24 hours). Next, relate those symptoms to the options. If unsure, note that hyperemesis contains the word emesis, which is an abnormal symptom in the admission note. Review the assessment findings and relate to complications of pregnancy if you had difficulty answering this question.

Client needs category: Physiological integrity

Client needs subcategory: Physiological adaptation

Cognitive level: Applying

---

11. A client at 32 weeks of gestation has mild preeclampsia. She is discharged home with instructions to remain in bed rest. She would also be instructed to call her health care provider if she experiences which of the following symptoms? Select all that apply.

☐ **1.** Headache

☐ **2.** Increased urine output

☐ **3.** Blurred vision

☐ **4.** Difficulty sleeping

☐ **5.** Epigastric pain

☐ **6.** Severe nausea and vomiting

Answer: 1, 3, 5, 6

Ⓜ **Rationale:** The care of a client with mild preeclampsia can be managed at home with proper instructions. Headache, blurred vision, epigastric pain, and severe nausea and vomiting can indicate worsening preeclampsia. Decreased, not increased, urine output is a concern because preeclampsia is associated with decreased renal perfusion, leading to a reduction in the glomerular filtration rate and decreased urine output. Difficulty sleeping, a common concern during the third trimester, is only a concern if it is caused by any of the other symptoms.

Test-taking strategy: Analyze to determine what information the question asks for, which is discharge instructions for mild preeclampsia. "Select all that apply" questions require considering each option to decide its merit. Even though the client's preeclampsia is mild, it is still considered dangerous. Select the options that relate to decreased perfusion and increased blood pressure. Review the management of client symptoms of preeclampsia in the home if you had difficulty answering this question.

Client needs category: Physiological integrity

Client needs subcategory: Reduction of risk potential

Cognitive level: Applying

12. The nurse is caring for a client approaching a term pregnancy. When assessing fetal presentation using Leopold's maneuvers, the nurse alerts the health care provider to the need of an external version. Place an X where the nurse assesses the fetal head.

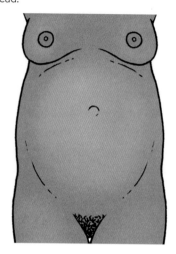

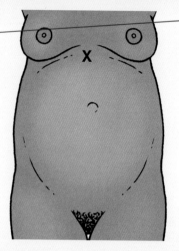

Rationale: An external version is a procedure that externally rotates the fetus from a breech presentation to a vertex presentation. If the fetal head is palpated at the top of the uterus, the fetus is in the breech position. That is, the head is not the presenting part and the health care provider may consider external version to convert the fetus to the head-down position. This is accomplished by applying pressure on the maternal abdomen to turn the infant over, as in a somersault.

Test-taking strategy: Analyze to determine what information the question asks for, which is the location of the fetal head if external version is needed. Recall that the correct position for the fetus approaching a term pregnancy is in the pelvis preparing for birth. The client would note lightening at this time marking the descent of the fetus. External version, if successful, will place the head in the correct position for birth. Review the gestational age of the fetus and the expected fetal position if you had difficulty answering this question.

Client needs category: Physiological integrity
Client needs subcategory: Reduction of risk potential
Cognitive level: Analyzing

13. A nurse is counseling a couple with history of infertility. The nurse instructs on the female reproductive tract and area for fertilization. Place an X over the area that the nurse instructs where fertilization **most** often occurs.

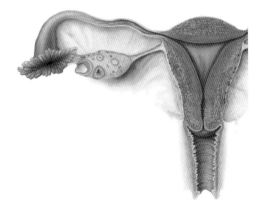

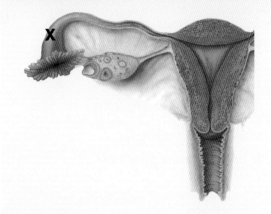

D **Rationale:** After ejaculation, the sperm travel by flagellar movement through the cervical mucus into the fallopian tube to meet the descending ovum in the ampulla. Fertilization occurs in the ampulla (outer third) of the fallopian tube.

Test-taking strategy: Analyze to determine what information the question asks for, which is the location of ovum fertilization. Follow the path of the illustration for sperm movement, and note the egg erupting from the follicle. Recall that the location of fertilization is different from the area of implantation. Review female anatomy and physiology as related to fertilization if you had difficulty answering this question.

Client needs category: Health promotion and maintenance

Client needs subcategory: None

Cognitive level: Understanding

14. The nurse is giving prenatal instructions to a 32-year-old primigravida. Which nutritional instructions would the nurse review? Select all that apply.

☐ **1.** Caloric intake would be increased by 300 cal/day.

☐ **2.** Protein intake would be increased to more than 30 g/day.

☐ **3.** Vitamin intake would not increase from prepregnancy requirements.

☐ **4.** Folic acid intake would be increased to 800 mg/day.

☐ **5.** Intake of all minerals, especially iron, would be increased.

☐ **6.** Water intake would be doubled.

Answer: 1, 2, 4, 5

C **Rationale:** A pregnant woman would increase her caloric intake by 300 cal/day. The protein requirements (76 g/day) of a pregnant woman exceed those of a nonpregnant woman by 30 g/day. All mineral requirements, especially iron, are increased in a pregnant woman. The woman would also increase her intake of all vitamins; a prenatal vitamin is usually recommended. Folic acid intake is particularly important to help prevent fetal anomalies such as neural tube defect. Intake would be increased from 400 to 800 mg/day. Nonpregnant females are encouraged to drink six 8 oz glasses of water daily. Pregnant females increase that amount to eight.

Test-taking strategy: Analyze to determine what information the question asks for, which is nutritional requirements in pregnancy. "Select all that apply" questions require considering each option to decide its merit. Consider increases needed as the maternal body uses its resources to develop a fetus. Most nutritional building blocks will be increased for this reason. Review nutritional requirements of pregnancy, including calorie, protein, vitamin, and mineral needs if you had difficulty answering this question.

Client needs category: Health promotion and maintenance

Client needs subcategory: None

Cognitive level: Applying

15. A nurse is palpating the fundal height of a pregnant woman at 40 weeks of gestation. Identify the area on the abdomen where the nurse would expect to feel the uterine fundus.

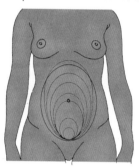

Answer:

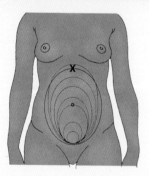

M **Rationale:** Uterine height is measured from the top of the maternal symphysis pubis to the top of the uterine fundus. By the 36th week, the uterine fundus would touch the xiphoid process. About 2 weeks before term (the 38th week), the fetal head settles into the pelvis to prepare for birth and the uterus returns to the height it was at 36 weeks.

Test-taking strategy: Analyze to determine what information the question asks for, which is fundal height at 40 weeks of gestation, prior to childbirth.

Recall that the uterus has expanded to largest position and now will decrease because of lightening. Review the fundal height as related to the gestational age and fetal position if you had difficulty answering this question.

Client needs category: Health promotion and maintenance

Client needs subcategory: None

Cognitive level: Applying

---

16. A 35-year-old client who is 28 weeks pregnant is admitted for testing. After reading the nursing notes below, which rationale **best** explains why a pregnant client would lie on her left side when resting or sleeping in the later stages of pregnancy?

Progress notes	
5/12/15 1430	Client admitted to short-term procedure unit for testing. States "I'm feeling a little faint." Skin slightly diaphoretic to touch. Client assisted to left side. VS stable. States "I'm feeling better now." ———— S. Brown, RN

☐ **1.** To facilitate digestion

☐ **2.** To facilitate bladder emptying

☐ **3.** To prevent compression of the vena cava

☐ **4.** To prevent development of fetal anomalies

Answer: 3

Ⓔ Rationale: The weight of the pregnant uterus is sufficiently heavy to compress the vena cava, which could impair blood flow to the uterus, possibly decreasing oxygen to the fetus. The client may experience supine hypotension syndrome (faintness, diaphoresis, and hypotension) from the pressure on the inferior vena cava. The side-lying position puts the weight of the fetus on the bed, not on the woman. The side-lying position has not been shown to prevent fetal anomalies, nor does it facilitate bladder emptying or digestion.

Test-taking strategy: Analyze to determine what information the question asks for, which is rationale for left side lying in later stages of pregnancy. Note the documented client symptoms. Analyze the options to relate position change to improvement of condition. Review fetal positioning as related to maternal anatomy, particularly with respect to supine and side-lying positions if you had difficulty answering this question.

Client needs category: Physiological integrity

Client needs subcategory: Reduction of risk potential

Cognitive level: Analyzing

17. A client is at risk for seizures because of pregnancy-induced hypertension. The health care provider orders 4-g magnesium sulfate in 250-ml D_5W to be infused at 1 g/hour following a loading dose. What is the flow rate in milliliters per hour? Round your answer to the nearest whole number.

_____ ml/hour

Answer: 63

Ⓜ **Rationale:** To solve this, first set up a proportion and then solve for X:

$$4 \text{ g}/250 \text{ ml} = 1 \text{ g}/X \text{ ml}$$
$$4 \times X = 250$$
$$X = \frac{250 \text{ ml}}{4}$$
$$X = 62.5 \text{ ml.}$$

Rounded off to a whole number, this is 63 ml/hour.

Test-taking strategy: Analyze to determine what information the question asks for, which is flow rate in milliliters per hour of a magnesium sulfate infusion. Read the question thoroughly eliminating any extraneous information (loading dose). Solve for X using the ratio–proportion method and aligning both sides of the equation consistently using known data. Proofread the math calculation.

Client needs category: Physiological integrity

Client needs subcategory: Pharmacological and parenteral therapies

Cognitive level: Applying

---

18. When teaching an antepartum client about the passage of the fetus through the birth canal during labor, the nurse describes the cardinal mechanisms of labor. Using a teaching pelvis and fetus, the nurse demonstrates which sequence during childbirth? Place these events in the proper sequence. All options must be used.

1. Flexion
2. External rotation
3. Descent
4. Expulsion
5. Internal rotation
6. Extension

Answer: 3, 1, 5, 6, 2, 4

Ⓓ **Rationale:** As the fetus moves through the bony and narrow birth canal, it goes through position changes to ensure that the smallest diameter of fetal head presents to the smallest diameter of the birth canal. Termed the cardinal mechanisms of labor, these position changes occur in the following sequence: descent, flexion, internal rotation, extension, external rotation, and expulsion.

Test-taking strategy: Analyze to determine what information the question asks for, which is position changes during the birth process. If unsure, identify the first (descent) and last (expulsion) to narrow the options. Also, consider the birth canal and fetal adjustment to fit through the canal. Review the relationship of the fetal head diameter, diameter of the birth canal, and cardinal movements to aid in birth if you had difficulty answering this question.

Client needs category: Health promotion and maintenance

Client needs subcategory: None

Cognitive level: Applying

---

19. A nurse is caring for a client who is anxious to know her baby's due date. The nurse instructs the client on how to determine the baby's due date according to Nägele's rule. The client is correct to state which of the following when discussing the use of the rule? Select all that apply.

☐ **1.** "I need to know the date of intercourse."

☐ **2.** "I will calculate 9 months from my last menstrual period."

☐ **3.** "Nägele's rule provides a good approximation of the due date."

☐ **4.** "I will add 7 days to the first day of my last menstrual period and count back 3 months."

☐ **5.** "Nägele's rule may be used in conjunction with other assessment findings."

Answer: 3, 4, 5

Ⓜ Rationale: Nägele's rule is one method of determining the estimated due date. When using Nägele's rule, add 7 days to the first day of the last menstrual period, and count back 3 months. Nägele's rule may be used with other assessment findings, especially in situations when the last menstrual period is in question. Nägele's rule does not use dates of intercourse or adding 9 months to the last menstrual period to determine the due date.

Test-taking strategy: Analyze to determine what information the question asks for, which is correct responses indicating an understanding of Nägele's rule. Recall that Nägele's rule uses a calculation based upon the last menstrual period. Consider that it is used frequently along with other assessment data to determine the gestational age of a fetus. Review Nägele's rule if you had difficulty answering this question.

Client needs category: Health promotion and maintenance

Client needs subcategory: None

Cognitive level: Applying

---

20. The obstetric nurse is performing a non-stress test on a 30-week primigravida client sent from a health care provider's office. The client reports a decrease in fetal movement over the past 24 hours. The nurse documents the following nursing note.

Progress notes	
7/27/15 1100	Client placed on fetal monitor. No fetal movement or reactivity noted over 20 minutes on monitor. No fetal heart rate heard. Client repositioned with no change. Health care provider notified.——— ———————————S. Brown, RN

Which nursing statement is appropriate at this time?

☐ **1.** "Let's have you change your position and lie on your left side."

☐ **2.** "I will check with the health care provider to see if further tests are needed."

☐ **3.** "I bet you are excited about the baby."

☐ **4.** "Have you done anything different today?"

Answer: 2

Ⓔ Rationale: At this time, fetal demise is anticipated because of a lack of fetal heart rate and movement. An ultrasound may be ordered to confirm status. Having the client lie on her side is not necessary if a fetal demise is suspected. Talking about the baby is inappropriate at this time. Asking if the client did something differently today may be interpreted as blaming the client for the fetal demise.

Test-taking strategy: Analyze to determine what information the question asks for, which is appropriate communication when fetal demise is anticipated. The nurse, though concerned of the fetal status, would notify the health care provider and await further orders. It is the health care provider who will make the final determination of fetal status and speak with the client. Consider the impact of the fetal demise on the client. Review communication and nurse action when fetal demise is suspected if you had difficulty answering this question.

Client needs category: Psychosocial integrity

Client needs subcategory: None

Cognitive level: Applying

21. The nurse is admitting a client with suspected diagnosis of abruptio placentae. When assessing client symptoms, which symptoms require health care provider notification of this medical emergency? Select all that apply.

☐ **1.** Overt vaginal bleeding

☐ **2.** Pain rated 2 out of 10 on the pain scale

☐ **3.** A rigid abdomen

☐ **4.** Gastrointestinal upset

☐ **5.** Increased blood pressure

☐ **6.** Rapid uterine contractions

Answer: 1, 3, 5, 6

Ⓜ **Rationale:** Abruptio placentae occurs when the there is a partial or complete detachment of the placenta from the uterus. One third of infants die from this complication of pregnancy. Symptoms include dark red vaginal bleeding; a rigid, boardlike abdomen; rapid uterine contractions with little relief in between; and severe pain. An elevated heart rate and blood pressure are commonly noted early from the pain and anxiety. Gastrointestinal upset is not a common symptom.

Test-taking strategy: Analyze to determine what information the question asks for, which is symptoms indicating an abruptio placentae. Relate an abruption to bleeding. Consider all of the effects of internal bleeding in the uterus. Select all choices related to bleeding in the reproductive tract and the accompanying pain. Review abruption placentae if you had difficulty answering this question.

Client needs category: Physiological integrity

Client needs subcategory: Physiological adaptation

Cognitive level: Applying

Intrapartum period

1. A nurse is evaluating a client who is 34 weeks pregnant for preterm rupture of the membranes (PROM). Which findings indicate that PROM has occurred? Select all that apply.

☐ **1.** Fernlike pattern when vaginal fluid is placed on a glass slide and allowed to dry

☐ **2.** Acidic pH of fluid when tested with nitrazine paper

☐ **3.** Presence of amniotic fluid in the vagina

☐ **4.** Cervical dilation of 6 cm

☐ **5.** Alkaline pH of fluid when tested with nitrazine paper

☐ **6.** Contractions occurring every 5 minutes

Answer: 1, 3, 5

Ⓓ **Rationale:** The fernlike pattern that occurs when vaginal fluid is placed on a glass slide and allowed to dry, the presence of amniotic fluid in the vagina, and an alkaline pH of fluid are all signs of ruptured membranes. The fernlike pattern is a result of the high sodium and protein content of the amniotic fluid. The presence of amniotic fluid in the vagina results from the expulsion of the fluid from the amniotic sac. Amniotic fluid tests as an alkaline, not acidic, fluid. Cervical dilation and regular contractions are signs of progressing labor, but they do not indicate PROM.

Test-taking strategy: Analyze to determine what information the question asks for, which is definitive data of a premature rupture of membranes. "Select all that apply" questions require considering each option to decide its merit. Consider the definitive presence of amniotic fluid as being the pattern displayed on the slide, actual presence of amniotic fluid, and alkaline pH on Nitrazine paper. Review the clinical manifestations of PROM if you had difficulty answering this question.

Client needs category: Physiological integrity

Client needs subcategory: Physiological adaptation

Cognitive level: Analyzing

2. A client in the first stage of labor is being monitored using an external fetal monitor. After the nurse reviews the monitoring strip from the client's chart (shown below), into which of the following positions would the nurse assist the client?

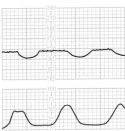

☐ **1.** Left lateral

☐ **2.** Right lateral

☐ **3.** Supine

☐ **4.** Prone

ℰ **Rationale:** The fetal heart rate monitoring strip shows late decelerations, which indicate uteroplacental circulatory insufficiency and can lead to fetal hypoxia and acidosis if the underlying cause is not corrected. The client would be turned onto her left side to increase placental perfusion and decrease contraction frequency. In addition, the intravenous fluid rate may be increased and oxygen administered. The right lateral, supine, and prone positions do not increase placental perfusion.

Test-taking strategy: Analyze to determine what information the question asks for, which is client position following monitor strip analysis. Interpret the data from the monitor strip by aligning the fetal heart rate (top line) with contraction sequence (bottom line). Compare reaction of fetal heart rate against contractions, and conclude late decelerations. Recall that throughout pregnancy, having the client lie on the left side aids in placental perfusion. Review fetal heart rate patterns and uterine contractions if you had difficulty answering this question.

Client needs category: Physiological integrity

Client needs subcategory: Reduction of risk potential

Cognitive level: Analyzing

3. The nurse is caring for a client in active labor. As the nurse is evaluating the waveform below, identify the area of concern that suggests umbilical cord compression.

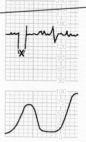

ⓔ Rationale: The X is placed at the site where the fetal heart rate decreases. Variable decelerations are decreases in fetal heart rate that are not related to the timing of contractions. They are characteristic of umbilical cord compression, which reduces blood flow between the placenta and fetus. These decelerations generally occur as drops of 10 to 60 beats/minute below the baseline.

Test-taking strategy: Analyze to determine what information the question asks for, which is waveform location suggesting umbilical cord compression. The key term is "compression," indicating an interruption in circulation and heart rate leading to the placement of the X. Review fetal oxygen depletion causing a decrease in fetal heart rate if you had difficulty answering this question.

Client needs category: Physiological integrity

Client needs subcategory: Reduction of risk potential

Cognitive level: Analyzing

4. A client who is 29 weeks pregnant comes to the labor and birth unit. She states that she is having contractions every 8 minutes. The client is also 3 cm dilated. Which of the following can the nurse expect to administer? Select all that apply.

☐ **1.** Folic acid

☐ **2.** A β-2 agonist

☐ **3.** Betamethasone

☐ **4.** Rh₀(D) immune globulin (RhoGAM)

☐ **5.** Intravenous fluids

☐ **6.** Nalbuphine

ⓔ Rationale: The nurse can expect that a β-2 agonist that relaxes smooth muscle will be administered to halt contractions; that betamethasone, a corticosteroid, will be administered to decrease the risk of respiratory distress to the neonate if preterm birth occurs; and that intravenous fluids will be given to expand the intravascular volume and decrease contractions if dehydration is the cause. Folic acid is a mineral recommended throughout pregnancy (especially in the first trimester) to decrease the risk of neural tube defects. RhoGAM is given to Rh-negative clients who have been, or may have been, exposed to Rh-positive fetal blood. Nalbuphine is an opioid analgesic used during labor and childbirth.

Test-taking strategy: Analyze to determine what information the question asks for, which is medications given to a client who is 29 weeks pregnant and in labor. "Select all that apply" questions require considering each option to decide its merit. First, determine that the client is in preterm labor (29 weeks). Next, consider the options that would help stop the progression of labor or be beneficial to the fetus if the birth occurs early. Review interventions to suppress preterm labor and medications used if you had difficulty answering this question.

Client needs category: Physiological integrity

Client needs subcategory: Pharmacological and parenteral therapies

Cognitive level: Analyzing

---

5. A registered nurse is delegating the monitoring of a client who is receiving oxytocin to induce labor to a new graduate nurse. When discussing adverse side effects of oxytocin, which conditions would the graduate nurse notify the registered nurse of immediately? Select all that apply.

☐ **1.** A blood pressure of 170/92 mm Hg

☐ **2.** Jaundice in the sclera

☐ **3.** Lab work suggesting dehydration

☐ **4.** Fluid overload with crackles in the lung fields

☐ **5.** Palpable uterine tetany

☐ **6.** A heart rate of 60 beats/minute

Answer: 1, 4, 5

Ⓓ Rationale: Adverse effects of oxytocin in the mother include hypertension, fluid overload, uterine tetany, and tachycardia, not bradycardia. The antidiuretic effect of oxytocin increases renal reabsorption of water, leading to fluid overload, not dehydration. Jaundice and bradycardia are adverse reactions that may occur in the neonate.

Test-taking strategy: Analyze to determine what information the question asks for, which is maternal adverse effects of oxytocin. "Select all that apply" questions require considering each option to decide its merit. Recall that the therapeutic action of oxytocin is to induce contractions. When considering adverse reactions, consider effects that suggest an exaggerated effect of the medication. Review the therapeutic action and adverse effects of oxytocin if you had difficulty answering this question.

Client needs category: Physiological integrity

Client needs subcategory: Pharmacological and parenteral therapies

Cognitive level: Analyzing

6. A nurse is evaluating the external fetal monitoring strip (shown below) of a client who is in labor. Which nursing intervention would the nurse implement?

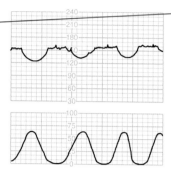

☐ **1.** Increase the intravenous fluid rate to boost intravascular volume.

☐ **2.** Reassure the client and continue to monitor the fetal heart rate.

☐ **3.** Elevate the client's legs.

☐ **4.** Administer supplemental oxygen.

☐ **5.** Require the client to lie on her left side.

---

7. A client in labor is 8 cm dilated. The fetus, which is in vertex presentation, is 75% effaced and at 0 station. In the illustration below, identify the level of the fetus's head.

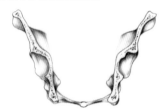

Answer: 2

Ⓒ Rationale: The monitoring strip from this client's chart shows early decelerations. These can result from head compression during normal labor and do not indicate fetal distress. The nurse would reassure the client and continue to monitor the fetal heart rate. The other nursing interventions are not appropriate.

Test-taking strategy: Analyze to determine what information the question asks for, which is nursing intervention determined following monitor strip analysis. First, analyze the monitor strip noting timing and sequence of heart rate and contractions. Consider that the heart rate decreases with contraction onset peak and then returns to baseline. Recall that this occurs in the normal labor process. Review the relationship between fetal heart rate patterns and uterine contraction patterns if you had difficulty answering this question.

Client needs category: Physiological integrity

Client needs subcategory: Physiological adaptation

Cognitive level: Analyzing

Answer:

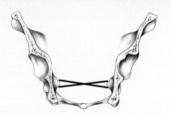

Ⓓ Rationale: Station refers to the level of the presenting part in relation to the pelvic inlet and the ischial spines. A 0 station indicates that the presenting part lies at the level of the ischial spines. Other stations are defined by their distance in centimeters above or below the ischial spines.

Test-taking strategy: Analyze to determine what information the question asks for, which is level of the infant's head in the specific circumstance. The key words are "0 station" and the only information needed to answer the question when in the vertex position. Recall that the 0 station is the level of the ischial spines that present inward in the pelvis. Review maternal anatomy as it relates to fetal presentation and position if you had difficulty answering this question.

Client needs category: Health promotion and maintenance

Client needs subcategory: None

Cognitive level: Applying

---

8. A nurse is evaluating a fetal monitoring strip to time the contractions of a client in labor. Identify the beginning of the contraction in the illustration below.

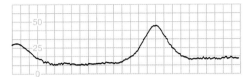

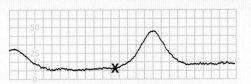

Ⓜ **Rationale:** An X is placed at the beginning of a contraction, identified by a rise in pressure in the uterus, and indicated on the monitoring strip by movement of the waveform away from the baseline.

Test-taking strategy: Analyze to determine what information the question asks for, which is beginning of a contraction of the monitoring strip. First, identify the baseline on the illustration. Next, recall that any change in the baseline, such as contraction, moves the waveform from baseline. Review uterine contraction waveforms if you had difficulty answering this question.

Client needs category: Health promotion and maintenance

Client needs subcategory: None

Cognitive level: Applying

---

9. A nurse is caring for a client who is in the third stage of labor. Which characteristic behaviors does the nurse anticipate at this stage? Select all that apply.

☐ **1.** The client is excited about the process.

☐ **2.** The client is focused on the neonate's condition.

☐ **3.** The client is exhausted from the labor process.

☐ **4.** The client states she has discomfort from uterine contractions.

☐ **5.** The client is apprehensive about the process.

☐ **6.** The client is feeling embarrassed as she has an urge to defecate.

Answer: 2, 4

Ⓒ **Rationale:** In the third stage of labor, the client focuses on the neonate's condition. Before the placenta is expelled, she may also state that she is experiencing discomfort from uterine contractions. Excitement and apprehension are characteristic of the first stage of labor. Exhaustion is common in the second stage of labor. The urge to defecate is noted prior to birth at the end of the second stage of labor when the fetus is pushing on the rectum.

Test-taking strategy: Analyze to determine what information the question asks for, which is the behavior of the mother in the third stage of labor. "Select all that apply" questions require considering each option to decide its merit. Recall that during this stage of labor, the focus is on the delivery of the placenta. Consider the process physiologically within the mother and emotionally as the neonate is born. Review maternal behaviors in the stages of labor if you had difficulty answering this question.

Client needs category: Psychosocial integrity

Client needs subcategory: None

Cognitive level: Applying

10. The nurse is caring for a client in labor. Which assessment findings would prompt the nurse to notify the health care provider? Select all that apply.

☐ **1.** The client is moaning in pain during contractions.

☐ **2.** The fetal heart rate baseline is between 140 and 150 beats/minute.

☐ **3.** The client is anxious and requests that someone help her.

☐ **4.** The client's membranes rupture, and the amniotic fluid is green.

☐ **5.** Late decelerations are noted on the external fetal monitor strip.

☐ **6.** Blood-tinged mucus is noted upon internal examination.

Answer: 4, 5

Ⓜ **Rationale:** The presence of green amniotic fluid indicates that the fetus has passed a meconium stool in utero and is a strong possibility of fetal distress. Late decelerations are caused by uteroplacental insufficiency resulting from decreased blood flow and oxygen transfer to the fetus through the intervillous spaces during uterine contractions. Both assessment findings would be related to the health care provider. Experiencing pain and maternal anxiety are common, especially during the transition period of labor. A fetal heart rate between 140 and 150 beats/minute is normal. Blood-tinged mucus indicates the progression of labor. As the pregnancy becomes postterm, it is important to note that the incidence of meconium in the amniotic fluid steadily increases because of the maturity of the fetus.

Test-taking strategy: Analyze to determine what information the question asks for, which is assessment data prompting health care provider notification. "Select all that apply" questions require considering each option to decide its merit. Consider any option indicating fetal complications. Recall that amniotic fluid is colorless; thus, green fluid is abnormal and late decelerations could indicate fetal compromise. Review signs and symptoms of fetal distress if you had difficulty answering this question.

Client needs category: Physiological integrity

Client needs subcategory: Physiological adaptation

Cognitive level: Analyzing

---

11. A client is being admitted to the labor and birth unit. Her GTPAL classification is 5-2-1-1-2. When providing shift handoff, which information would the nurse include? Select all that apply.

☐ **1.** The client has had four previous pregnancies.

☐ **2.** The client has had five previous pregnancies.

☐ **3.** The client has had one full-term child, one abortion, and one premature child.

☐ **4.** The client has had two full-term children, one premature child, and one abortion.

☐ **5.** The client has three living children and is pregnant again.

☐ **6.** The client has two living children and is pregnant again.

Answer: 1, 4, 6

Ⓜ **Rationale:** Detailed information about a client's obstetric history is described using the GTPAL classification system. G represents gravida, or the number of times the client has been pregnant, including the current pregnancy. T is the number of full-term infants born (after 37 weeks); P is the number of preterm infants born (before 37 weeks); A is the number of induced or spontaneous abortions; and L is the number of living children.

Test-taking strategy: Analyze to determine what information the question asks for, which is correct obstetric history as identified by the GTPAL. "Select all that apply" questions require considering each option to decide its merit. Recall what each letter of the GTPAL pregnancy status classification system represents and relate to each option. Realize that each correct option would be included in shift report. Review the GTPAL classification system if you had difficulty answering this question.

Client needs category: Health promotion and maintenance

Client needs subcategory: None

Cognitive level: Applying

---

12. A nurse is assisting in the birthing room. The health care provider prepares to perform a midline episiotomy. On the illustration below, identify the area where the health care provider makes the incision.

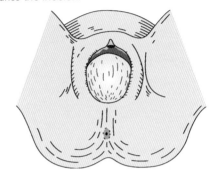

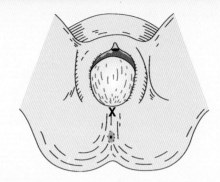

Rationale: An X is placed in the center of the perineum for a midline episiotomy. An episiotomy is a surgical enlargement of the vaginal opening that allows easier birth of the fetus and prevents tearing of the perineum. The incision is made in the perineum and can be midline or right or left mediolateral.

Test-taking strategy: Analyze to determine what information the question asks for, which is location for a midline episiotomy. Use the anatomical terms to determine the location (midline = in the middle) of the perineal incision. Review maternal anatomy and the purpose of an episiotomy if you had difficulty answering this question.

Client needs category: Physiological integrity

Client needs subcategory: Reduction of risk potential

Cognitive level: Applying

13. The nurse is performing Leopold's maneuvers to determine fetal presentation and position. Which illustration shows the third maneuver?

☐ **1.**

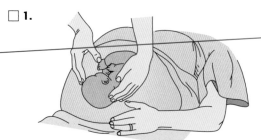

☐ **2.**

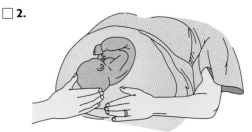

☐ **3.**

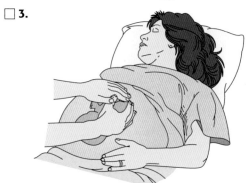

☐ **4.**

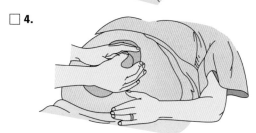

Ⓜ **Rationale:** To perform the third maneuver, the nurse gently grasps the lower portion of the abdomen just above the symphysis pubis between the thumb and index finger and presses them together to determine any movement and whether the part is firm or soft. This maneuver determines the part of the fetus at the inlet and its mobility. Option 1 shows the fourth maneuver of locating the fetal brow; option 3 shows the first maneuver of palpating the upper abdomen to determine the size, shape, and mobility of the fetus; and option 4 shows the second maneuver of determining the location of the fetal back.

Test-taking strategy: Analyze to determine what information the question asks for, which is identifying the third maneuver within Leopold's maneuvers. Visualize the sequence of observing and palpating the client's abdomen to determine fetal presentation and position. Recall that the maneuvers begin with general information with the first and second maneuvers being the fundal grip and then umbilical grip. The third and fourth maneuvers provide data on engagement for the birthing process. Review Leopold's maneuvers if you had difficulty answering this question.

Client needs category: Physiological integrity

Client needs subcategory: Reduction of risk potential

Cognitive level: Applying

14. The nurse is assisting with the birth of a fetus in a frank breech presentation. Which graphic illustrates that position?

☐ **1.**

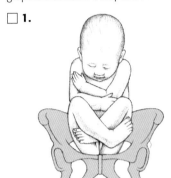

☐ **2.**

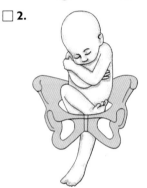

☐ **3.**

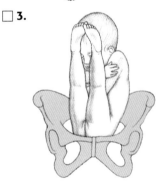

☐ **4.**

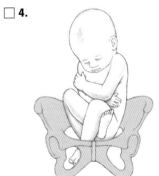

Ⓜ Rationale: In a frank breech presentation, the buttocks are the presenting part, with the hips flexed and the knees remaining straight. In a complete breech (option 1), the knees and hips are flexed. In a footling breech (option 2), neither the hips nor lower legs are flexed, and one or both feet may present. In an incomplete breech (option 4), one or both hips remain extended, and one or both feet or knees lie below the breech.

Test-taking strategy: Analyze to determine what information the question asks for, which is identifying the characteristics of a frank breech presentation. Recall that breech = buttocks. The defining characteristic of the frank breech is the straight legs with feet by head. Review the various breech presentations if you had difficulty answering this question.

Client needs category: Physiological integrity

Client needs subcategory: Reduction of risk potential

Cognitive level: Analyzing

15. A primigravida client arrives at the labor and birth unit at 39 weeks' gestation. After completing the initial assessment, the nurse documents the following:

Progress notes	
7/27/15	The client presents to the labor and child-
0700	birth unit stating pain radiating from the
	back to abdomen. Contractions are noted on
	the fetal monitor varying between every 8 to
	10 minutes. Accelerations with movement and
	moderate variability noted. The fetal heart
	rate is 120 beats/minute. Client verbalizes a
	6 on the 0-10 pain scale during contractions.
	Membranes intact. Cervical dilation 4 cm.
	Health care provider notified.
	———— S. Brown, RN

Which nursing action is initiated?

- ☐ **1.** Providing discharge home with instruction to ambulate
- ☐ **2.** Admitting the client to the labor and birth unit
- ☐ **3.** Instructing the client to rest and turn on the left side
- ☐ **4.** Preparing the client for a cesarean section

Answer: 1

Ⓒ Rationale: The nurse identifies the client as being in early labor by symptoms of back pain, varying contractions, moderate pain, and cervical dilation of 4 cm. The nurse identifies the normal progress of labor thus far and conveys to the health care provider. Until the health care provider admits the client, it is appropriate to have the client discharged with instruction to ambulate. Typically, the client is instructed to return to the birthing center/hospital when contractions are 4 to 5 minutes apart. Ambulation may progress the labor process. The client does not need to turn on her left side as there is no sign of fetal compromise. The client is considered a full-term pregnancy. There is no indication of a need for a cesarean section.

Test-taking strategy: Analyze to determine what information the question asks for, which is nursing action following analysis of client symptoms. Note key pieces of information from the nurse's note such as primigravida. Ask yourself, "How is this helpful in determining what a nurse would do?" Recall that women delivering first babies typically are in labor longer. Next, look at the physical symptoms, and ask how that information fits into the clinical picture. Relate to the options provided. Review characteristics of the labor process if you had difficulty answering this question.

Client needs category: Health promotion and maintenance

Client needs subcategory: None

Cognitive level: Analyzing

16. The nurse is performing an assessment of a client progressing through labor. Place the following findings in the order in which they occur. All options must be used.

1. Uncontrollable urge to push

2. Cervical dilation of 7 cm

3. 100% cervical effacement

4. Strong Braxton Hicks contractions

5. Mild contractions lasting 20 to 40 seconds

Answer: 4, 5, 2, 3, 1

Ⓜ Rationale: Strong Braxton Hicks contractions typically occur prior to the onset of true labor and are considered a preliminary sign. During the latent phase of the first stage of labor, contractions are mild, lasting about 20 to 40 seconds. As the client progresses through labor, contractions increase in intensity and duration, and cervical dilation occurs. Cervical dilation of 7 cm indicates that the client has entered the active phase of the first stage of labor. Cervical effacement also occurs, and effacement of 100% characterizes the transition phase of the first stage of labor. Progression into the second stage of labor is noted by the client's uncontrollable urge to push.

Test-taking strategy: Analyze to determine what information the question asks for, which is characteristics of the stages of labor. Sequence the progression through the stages of labor beginning with Braxton Hicks contractions and ending with the uncontrollable urge to push the neonate out. Arrange the middle sections from mild contractions through dilation and effacement. Review the stages of labor if you had difficulty answering this question.

Client needs category: Health promotion and maintenance

Client needs subcategory: None

Cognitive level: Applying

---

17. A nurse is monitoring the contractions of a client in the first stage of labor. Order the phases of a uterine contraction from the beginning of contraction to its conclusion. All options must be used.

1. Acme

2. Relaxation

3. Decrement

4. Increment

Answer: 4, 1, 3, 2

Ⓜ Rationale: A contraction consists of three phases: the increment (when the intensity of the contraction increases), the acme (when the contraction is at its strongest), and the decrement (when the intensity decreases). Between contractions, the uterus relaxes. As labor progresses, the relaxation intervals decrease from 10 minutes early in labor to only 2 to 3 minutes later. The duration of contractions also changes, increasing from 20 to 30 seconds to a range of 60 to 90 seconds.

Test-taking strategy: Analyze to determine what information the question asks for, which is order of the phases of the contractions. If unsure, focus on the definition of terms to help determine the sequence. Review the phases as a contraction progresses if you had difficulty answering this question.

Client needs category: Physiological integrity

Client needs subcategory: Physiological adaptation

Cognitive level: Understanding

1. The nurse is caring for a client on her second postpartum day. Before providing discharge instructions, at what area of the abdomen does the nurse anticipate the level of the fundus?

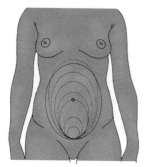

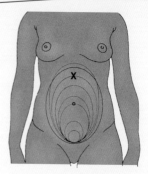

D **Rationale:** The nurse anticipates the fundus being at or slightly above the umbilicus following birth. During involution, the fundus descends one fingerbreadth each day. Since this is the client's second postpartum day, the fundus would be anticipated at 2 fingerbreadths below the umbilicus.

Test-taking strategy: Analyze to determine what information the question asks for, which is anticipated location of the uterine fundus on the second postpartum day. Recall the role of the umbilicus in determining descent and the use of fingerbreadths (one day = 1 fingerbreadth). Review uterine involution if you had difficulty answering this question.

Client needs category: Physiological integrity

Client needs subcategory: Reduction of risk potential

Cognitive level: Applying

2. A nurse is caring for a client with history of a warm, reddened, painful area in the breast diagnosed as mastitis as well as cracked and fissured nipples. The client expresses the desire to continue breast-feeding throughout treatment. Which instructions would the nurse include to prevent a recurrence of this condition? Select all that apply.

☐ **1.** Wash the nipples with soap and water.

☐ **2.** Change the breast pads frequently.

☐ **3.** Expose the nipples to air for part of each day.

☐ **4.** Wash hands before handling the breast and breast-feeding.

☐ **5.** Make sure that the baby grasps the nipple only.

☐ **6.** Release the baby's grasp on the nipple before removing the baby from the breast.

Answer: 2, 3, 4, 6

C **Rationale:** Mastitis is an infection of the breast tissue usually caused by *Staphylococcus aureus*. This infection typically occurs in the second or third postpartum week and is more frequent in primigravidas. To help prevent mastitis, the nurse would suggest measures to prevent cracked and fissured nipples. Changing breast pads frequently and exposing the nipples to air for part of the day help keep the nipples dry and prevent irritation. Washing hands before handling the breast reduces the chance of accidentally introducing organisms into the breast. Releasing the baby's grasp on the nipple before removing the baby from the breast also reduces the chance of irritation. Nipples would be washed with water only; soap tends to remove the natural oils and increases the chance of cracking. The baby would grasp both the nipple and areola.

Test-taking strategy: Analyze to determine what information the question asks for, which is instruction to prevent a reoccurrence of symptoms related to mastitis. "Select all that apply" questions require considering each option to decide its merit. Note that correct options, including hand hygiene, reduce the chances of reopening the fissures and causing infection. Review the principles of infection control and methods to prevent the reoccurrence of mastitis if you had difficulty answering this question.

Client needs category: Health promotion and maintenance

Client needs subcategory: None

Cognitive level: Applying

---

3. A nurse is caring for a 1-day postpartum client. The progress note below informs the nurse that the client is in which phase of the postpartum period?

Progress notes	
5/24/15	Mother verbalizing labor and delivery
1715	experience. Doesn't appear confident about
	holding baby or changing diapers. Asking
	appropriate questions.———— J. Conners, RN

☐ **1.** Letting go

☐ **2.** Taking in

☐ **3.** Holding out

☐ **4.** Taking hold

Answer: 2

M **Rationale:** The taking-in phase is normally the first postpartum phase. During this phase, the mother feels overwhelmed by the responsibilities of newborn care and is still fatigued from childbirth. Taking hold is the next phase, when the client has rested and can learn mothering skills with confidence. Letting go is the final stage, when the client adapts to parenthood, her new role as a caregiver, and her new baby as a separate entity. Holding out is not a valid phase.

Test-taking strategy: Analyze to determine what information the question asks for, which is the phase of the postpartum period as documented in a nursing note. Analyze the nurse's note for clues such as verbalizing labor and birth, not confident and asking questions. Relate to early stages in the postpartum period. Review the mother's behavior and postpartum phases if you had difficulty answering this question.

Client needs category: Psychosocial integrity

Client needs subcategory: None

Cognitive level: Analyzing

4. A nurse observes several interactions between a client and her neonate son. Which behaviors by the mother would the nurse identify as evidence of mother–infant attachment? Select all that apply.

☐ **1.** Talks to and coos at her son

☐ **2.** Cuddles her son close to her

☐ **3.** Does not make eye contact with her son

☐ **4.** Requests that the nurse take the baby to the nursery for feedings

☐ **5.** Encourages the father to hold the baby

☐ **6.** Takes a nap when the baby is sleeping

Answer: 1, 2

C **Rationale:** Talking to, cooing at, and cuddling with her son are positive signs that the client is adapting to her new role as a mother. Eye contact, touching, and speaking help establish attachment with a neonate. Avoiding eye contact is a nonbonding behavior. Feeding a neonate is an important role of a new mother and facilitates attachment. Encouraging the father to hold the neonate will facilitate attachment between the neonate and his father. Resting while the neonate is sleeping will conserve needed energy and allow the mother to be alert and awake when her infant is awake; however, it is not evidence of bonding.

Test-taking strategy: Analyze to determine what information the question asks for, which is evidence of mother–infant attachment. "Select all that apply" questions require considering each option to decide its merit. Consider that evidence means factual actions related to demonstrating bonding. Review behaviors that relate to maternal–infant bonding if you had difficulty answering this question.

Client needs category: Psychosocial integrity
Client needs subcategory: None
Cognitive level: Analyzing

---

5. A nurse is caring for a postpartum client suspected of developing postpartum psychosis. Which statements accurately characterize this disorder? Select all that apply.

☐ **1.** Symptoms appear at the 6-month screening.

☐ **2.** The disorder is common in postpartum women.

☐ **3.** Symptoms include delusions and hallucinations.

☐ **4.** Suicide and infanticide are uncommon in this disorder.

☐ **5.** The disorder rarely occurs without a psychiatric history.

Answer: 3, 5

D **Rationale:** A postpartum client would be suspected of psychosis if she exhibits delusions or hallucinations, generally starting within 4 weeks of postpartum. Typically, the woman has a past history of a psychiatric disorder and treatment. A history of bipolar disorder is an important risk factor. The disorder occurs in less than 1% of postpartum mothers. It is considered a medical emergency. Suicide and infanticide are common.

Test-taking strategy: Analyze to determine what information the question asks for, which is correct characterization of postpartum psychosis. "Select all that apply" questions require considering each option to decide its merit. The key word is "psychosis." Use your knowledge of medical terminology to identify options related to delusions. Review the onset, symptoms, and etiology of postpartum psychosis and the differences with postpartal blues and depression if you had difficulty answering this question.

Client needs category: Psychosocial integrity
Client needs subcategory: None
Cognitive level: Analyzing

---

6. A mother with a history of varicose veins has just delivered her first baby. The nurse suspects that the mother has developed a pulmonary embolus. Which data below would lead to this nursing judgment? Select all that apply.

☐ **1.** Sudden dyspnea

☐ **2.** Chills, fever

☐ **3.** Diaphoresis

☐ **4.** Cough

☐ **5.** Confusion

☐ **6.** Chest pain

Answer: 1, 3, 4, 5, 6

D Rationale: Sudden dyspnea with diaphoresis, chest pain, and confusion are classic signs and symptoms of a pulmonary embolus. The client could also have a cough with blood-tinged sputum. In this disorder, a thrombus (stationary blood clot) dislodges from a varicose vein and becomes lodged in the pulmonary circulation. Chills and fever would indicate an infection.

Test-taking strategy: Analyze to determine what information the question asks for, which is data supporting the possibility of a pulmonary embolism. "Select all that apply" questions require considering each option to decide its merit. Use knowledge of medical terminology to determine that pulmonary = lung and embolism = clot. Consider symptoms that would occur with an interruption of blood flow. Review the pathophysiology and clinical manifestations of a pulmonary embolism if you had difficulty answering this question.

Client needs category: Physiological integrity

Client needs subcategory: Physiological adaptation

Cognitive level: Analyzing

---

7. A nurse is palpating the uterine fundus of a client who delivered her neonate 8 hours ago. Identify the area where the nurse would expect to feel the fundus.

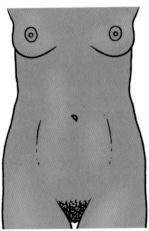

Answer:

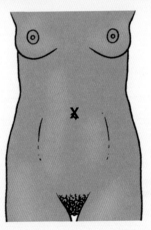

E Rationale: Note the X at the level of the umbilicus. The uterus would be felt at the level of the umbilicus from about 1 to 24 hours after birth.

Test-taking strategy: Analyze to determine what information the question asks for, which is fundal height at 8 hours postpartum. Consider the time frame of 8 hours as key data. Recall the involution process and that fundal height decreases one fingerbreadth (1 cm) per day. Review the involution process if you had difficulty answering this question.

Client needs category: Physiological integrity

Client needs subcategory: Reduction of risk potential

Cognitive level: Applying

8. A nurse is caring for a client in the fourth stage of labor. Based on the nurse's note below, which postpartum complication has the client developed?

Progress notes

6/7/15	Client's 24-hour blood loss is 600 ml. Uterus
1745	is soft and relaxed on palpation and client
	has a full bladder. Assisted client in emptying
	bladder and notified Dr. G. McMann of
	findings. Vital signs stable at present. See
	graphic sheet for ongoing assessments and
	perineal pad weights.————— S. Jones, RN

- ☐ **1.** Postpartum hemorrhage
- ☐ **2.** Puerperal infection
- ☐ **3.** Deep vein thrombosis (DVT)
- ☐ **4.** Mastitis
- ☐ **5.** Uterine rupture

Answer: 1

Ⓔ Rationale: Blood loss from the uterus that exceeds 500 ml in a 24-hour period is considered postpartum hemorrhage. If uterine atony is the cause, the uterus feels soft and relaxed. A full bladder can prevent the uterus from contracting completely, increasing the risk of hemorrhage. Puerperal infection is an infection of the uterus and structures above; its characteristic sign is fever. Two major types of DVT occur in the postpartum period: pelvic and femoral. Each has different signs and symptoms, but both occur later in the postpartum period (femoral, after 10 days postpartum; pelvic, after 14 days). Mastitis is an inflammation of the mammary glands that disrupts normal lactation and usually develops 1 to 4 weeks postpartum. Uterine rupture is a potentially catastrophic event during childbirth where the wall of the uterus ruptures. A uterine rupture is a life-threatening event for the mother and fetus.

Test-taking strategy: Analyze to determine what information the question asks for, which is a complication during the fourth stage of labor as identified in the nurse's note. Analyze the nurse's note to determine clues (blood loss of 600 ml, uterus soft and relaxed) and relate to the options. Review complications during the fourth stage of labor if you had difficulty answering this question.

Client needs category: Physiological integrity

Client needs subcategory: Reduction of risk potential

Cognitive level: Analyzing

---

9. A nurse assesses a client's vaginal discharge on the first postpartum day and describes it in the progress note (shown below). Which term **best** identifies the discharge?

Progress notes

3/30/15	Perineal pad changed two times this
1645	shift for moderate amount of red
	discharge.————————J. Jones, RN

- ☐ **1.** Lochia alba
- ☐ **2.** Lochia
- ☐ **3.** Lochia serosa
- ☐ **4.** Lochia rubra

Answer: 4

Ⓔ Rationale: For the first 3 days after birth, the discharge is called lochia rubra. It consists almost entirely of blood, with only small particles of decidua and mucus. Lochia alba is a creamy white or colorless discharge that occurs 10 to 14 days postpartum. Lochia serosa is a pink or brownish discharge that occurs 4 to 14 days postpartum. The term *lochia* alone is not a correct description of the discharge.

Test-taking strategy: Analyze to determine what information the question asks for, which is the best description of postpartum vaginal discharge. First note that option 2 has no descriptor, eliminating that choice. Recall knowledge of medical terminology that rubra = red. Review vaginal discharge from birth to 14 days postpartum if you had difficulty answering this question.

Client needs category: Physiological integrity

Client needs subcategory: Physiological adaptation

Cognitive level: Applying

10. A home care lactation nurse has asked a client to keep a record of her intake, including calories, and output for 1 day. After reviewing the flow sheet that the client used to document the results (shown below), the nurse would make which assessments?

Intake and output

Time period	Fluids (ml)	Calories	Output (ml)
0700 to 1100	Milk 240	Breakfast 510	60
	Orange juice 60		
1100 to 1500	Coffee 240	Lunch 350	250
	Orange juice 120	Snack 80	200
	Water 240		200
1500 to 2300	Water 240	Dinner 500	100
	Water 240	Snack 350	230
	Water 240		200
2300 to 0700	Water 240		300

☐ **1.** The client consumed an adequate amount of calories and fluids for breast-feeding.

☐ **2.** The client consumed an adequate amount of calories but not enough fluids for breast-feeding.

☐ **3.** The client consumed an adequate amount of fluids but not enough calories for breast-feeding.

☐ **4.** The client consumed an inadequate amount of fluids and calories for breast-feeding.

Answer: 4

Ⓓ Rationale: In general, new mothers who are breast-feeding should consume 2 to 3 L of fluids and 2,300 to 2,700 cal daily. Consuming less than 1,500 to 1,800 cal/day may put the mother's milk supply at risk.

Test-taking strategy: Analyze to determine what information the question asks for, which is analysis of 24-hour intake and output for a lactating mother. First, calculate intake, calories, and output, and compare with standard needs. Recall that an increased fluid intake is important to maintain milk production. Also, an increase in calories and nutrients is needed to meet the nutritional requirements of the mother and baby. Calculate the total calories and fluid intake and relate them to the nutritional needs of the lactating client if you had difficulty answering this question.

Client needs category: Health promotion and maintenance

Client needs subcategory: None

Cognitive level: Analyzing

11. During physical assessment of a client who gave birth 3 hours ago, a nurse finds that the client has completely saturated a perineal pad within 15 minutes. Which nursing actions would be appropriate? Select all that apply.

- ☐ **1.** Begin an intravenous infusion of lactated Ringer's solution.
- ☐ **2.** Assess the client's vital signs.
- ☐ **3.** Palpate the client's fundus.
- ☐ **4.** Place the client in high Fowler's position.
- ☐ **5.** Administer a pain medication.

Answer: 2, 3

Ⓒ Rationale: Saturating a perineal pad within 15 minutes indicated excessive bleeding. Checking vital signs provides information about the client's circulatory status and identifies significant changes that may need to be reported to the health care provider. By palpating the client's fundus, the nurse also gains valuable data. A boggy uterus may lead to excessive bleeding. Starting an intravenous infusion requires a health care provider's order. Placing the client in high Fowler's position may lower the blood pressure and be harmful to the client. Administration of a pain medication does not address the current problem.

Test-taking strategy: Analyze to determine what information the question asks for, which is nursing actions when assessment findings reveal a saturated perineal pad indicating excessive bleeding. "Select all that apply" questions require considering each option to decide its merit. Choose the options that directly relate to interventions for bleeding. Review nursing actions related to excessive bleeding if you had difficulty answering this question.

Client needs category: Physiological integrity

Client needs subcategory: Reduction of risk potential

Cognitive level: Applying

---

12. The nurse is caring for a postpartum client with symptoms of swelling and tenderness in the left leg. The nurse suspects a developing deep vein thrombosis (DVT). When assessing for a DVT, identify the area on the body below, where the nurse would perform a focused assessment.

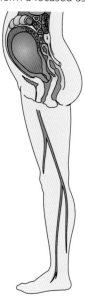

Answer:

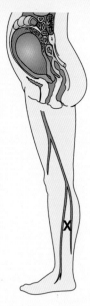

Ⓔ Rationale: Note that an X is placed on the calf. To assess for the presence of a DVT, the nurse performs a Homans' sign. To elicit Homans' sign, the client dorsiflexes her ankle and then the nurse assesses for pain in the calf during that motion. If a positive Homans' sign is noted, the health care provider may order an ultrasound or venography for a definitive diagnosis.

Test-taking strategy: Analyze to determine what information the question asks for, which is site of a focused assessment when a DVT is suspected. Recall the area where thrombosis usually develops, and consider how to assess if a thrombosis blocking blood flow is present. Review Homans' sign for assessing a DVT if you had difficulty answering this question.

Client needs category: Physiological integrity

Client needs subcategory: Physiological adaptation

Cognitive level: Applying

---

13. The nurse is assessing a client who is 4 hours postpartum. Based on the findings documented by the nurse below, which action is **most** appropriate at this time?

Progress notes	
06/11/15 1830	Client's vital signs stable at present. Perineal pad changed for moderate amount of red drainage. Uterus palpated at the level of the umbilicus and to the left side of the abdomen.————————N. Green, RN

☐ **1.** Ask the client to empty her bladder.

☐ **2.** Raise the head of the bed.

☐ **3.** Straight catheterize the client immediately.

☐ **4.** Call the client's primary health care provider for direction.

☐ **5.** Straight catheterize the client for half of her urine volume.

☐ **6.** Notify the charge nurse of the assessment findings.

Answer: 1

🅔 **Rationale:** A full bladder may displace the uterine fundus to the left or right of the abdomen. A straight catheterization is unnecessarily invasive if the client can urinate on her own. Nursing interventions would be completed before notifying the primary health care provider or charge nurse in a nonemergency situation. Raising the head of the bed is not helpful to change the position of the uterus.

Test-taking strategy: Analyze to determine what information the question asks for, which is nursing action needed following focused assessment and documentation. Analyze the nurse's note to determine any abnormal data. Note the position of the uterus and consider causes. Recall that a filled bladder sits adjacent to the uterus and can dislocate the uterus. Review assessment findings as they relate to the postpartal uterus if you had difficulty answering this question.

Client needs category: Physiological integrity

Client needs subcategory: Reduction of risk potential

Cognitive level: Applying

14. A postpartum client has been ordered 500 mg of ampicillin oral suspension. The label reads *ampicillin 125 mg/5 ml*. How many milliliters would the client receive? Record your answer using a whole number.

_____ ml

E **Rationale:** To solve this problem, set up proportions as follows:

$$5 \text{ ml}/125 \text{ mg} = X \text{ ml}/500 \text{ mg}$$
$$X \times 125 \text{ mg} = 5 \text{ ml} \times 500 \text{ mg.}$$

Solve for *X* by dividing both sides of the equation by 125 mg: $X \times 125 \text{ mg} = 5 \text{ ml} \times 500 \text{ mg}$

$$\frac{X \times 125 \text{ mg}}{125 \text{ mg}} = \frac{5 \text{ ml} \times 500 \text{ mg}}{125 \text{ mg}}$$

$$X = \frac{2,500 \text{ ml}}{125}$$

$$X = 20 \text{ ml.}$$

Test-taking strategy: Analyze to determine what information the question asks for, which is dosage of ampicillin oral suspension. Use the proportion method aligning both sides of the equation consistently using known data. Proofread the math calculation. Review calculations using proportions and solving for *X* if you had difficulty answering this question.

Client needs category: Physiological integrity

Client needs subcategory: Pharmacological and parenteral therapies

Cognitive level: Applying

---

15. Five days postpartum following an uneventful vaginal birth, a client phones the obstetrician's office stating various symptoms and requesting an appointment. As the nurse is documenting symptoms, which indicate a potential puerperal infection? Select all that apply.

☐ **1.** Temperature of 100.8°F (38.2°C)

☐ **2.** Pink drainage from vagina

☐ **3.** Frequent abdominal pain requiring medication

☐ **4.** Reddened area increasing around episiotomy

☐ **5.** Slight edema to perineum

☐ **6.** Ecchymosis in the perineal area

M **Rationale:** The nurse must analyze normal symptoms following childbirth (5 days postpartum) and abnormal symptoms, which may indicate a puerperal infection. Abnormal symptoms include a temperature over 100.8°F or 38.2°C, abdominal pain, and increasing reddened area around the episiotomy. These symptoms may indicate a postpartum or puerperal infection. Normal findings following childbirth include pink (serosanguineous) drainage on the fifth postpartum day, edema, and ecchymosis to the perineal region.

Test-taking strategy: Analyze to determine what information the question asks for, which is symptoms of a puerperal infection. The nurse must accurately consider the amount of time since childbirth and the normal symptoms to be experienced. An elevated temperature over 100.4°F or 38°C is an early indication of infection; the client may have cramping but not pain in the abdominal region; and increasing reddened areas are also indicative of infection. The other symptoms are normal following childbirth. Review symptoms during the postpartum period if you had difficulty answering this question.

Client needs category: Physiological integrity
Client needs subcategory: Physiological adaptation
Cognitive level: Applying

---

16. A postpartum client is experiencing thoughts and behaviors common to the taking-hold phase. Which items are characteristic of this phase? Select all that apply.

☐ **1.** Prefers having the nurse care for her

☐ **2.** Holds new child and breast-feeds without prompting

☐ **3.** Rests to regain physical strength and calm her swirling thoughts

☐ **4.** Expresses a strong interest in taking care of her child

☐ **5.** Gives up fanaticized image of her child and accepts the real one

Answer: 2, 4

🄲 **Rationale:** The taking-in phase occurs in the first 24 hours after birth. The mother is concerned with her own needs and requires support from staff and relatives. She holds her new child with a sense of wonder and rests to gain her physical strength and calm her thoughts. The taking-hold phase occurs when the mother is ready to take responsibility for her care as well as her neonate's care. The letting-go phase begins when the mother accepts her real child and incorporates the neonate into the family unit.

Test-taking strategy: Analyze to determine what information the question asks for, which is characteristics of the taking-hold phase. "Select all that apply" questions require considering each option to decide its merit. Consider the term "taking hold," meaning to take control of the care of herself and her neonate. Consider each option or data that the mother is actively participating in care. Review transitional maternal roles during the postpartum period if you had difficulty answering this question.

Client needs category: Health promotion and maintenance
Client needs subcategory: None
Cognitive level: Analyzing

---

17. The nurse is preparing to perform a fundal massage on a client who is 2 hours postpartum. Order the sequence of events for performing this procedure. All options must be used.

1. Rotate the upper hand to massage the uterus until firm.
2. Place the client in supine position.
3. Gently press the fundus between the hands using slight downward pressure.
4. Place one hand around the top of the fundus.
5. Ask the client to void.
6. Place one hand on the abdomen just above the symphysis pubis.

Answer: 5, 2, 6, 4, 1, 3

🄲 **Rationale:** Fundal massage is performed to promote uterine tone and consistency and to minimize the risk of hemorrhage. First, have the client void to prevent displacement of the bladder and allow an accurate assessment of uterine tone. Then, place the client in proper supine positioning to allow for good visualization. To anchor the lower part of the uterus, place one hand on the abdomen just above the symphysis pubis and then place the other hand around the top of the fundus. Next, rotate the upper hand to massage the uterus until it is firm. Finally, when the uterus is firm, push gently on the fundus, using slight downward pressure against the lower hand.

Test-taking strategy: Analyze to determine what information the question asks for, which is the procedure to perform a fundal massage. Visualize the fundal massage procedure including placement of the hands on the abdomen. Review the fundal massage sequence and the reason for performing maneuvers if you had difficulty answering this question.

Client needs category: Physiological integrity
Client needs subcategory: Reduction of risk potential
Cognitive level: Applying

18. The nurse is assigned to a client who experiences a syncopal episode on her first ambulation after childbirth. Which nursing actions will the nurse delegate to the licensed practical/vocational nurse (LPN/VN)? Select all that apply.

☐ **1.** Obtain orthostatic blood pressures.

☐ **2.** Assist the nurse with ambulating the client back to bed.

☐ **3.** Monitor hemoglobin and hematocrit level.

☐ **4.** Assess pain level on a 0 to 10 pain scale.

☐ **5.** Obtain a cool compress for the head.

☐ **6.** Assist with ambulation on the next trip to the bathroom.

Answer: 2, 5

ⓒ Rationale: The assisting nurse, in this case a licensed practical/vocational nurse (LPN/VN), provides care under the guidance of the assigned registered nurse. When a nurse is caring for a client who has recently given birth to a baby, changing blood levels in the body make the client more susceptible to syncope. It is in the assigned nurse's scope of practice to assess the client and assist her out of bed for at least the first ambulation. Once it is established that the client is safe with the ambulation, the other members of the nursing team can assist the client independently. Until then, the assigned nurse guides care. The registered nurse completes actions that require nursing judgment such as orthostatic blood pressures, assessing pain, and monitoring blood levels.

Test-taking strategy: Analyze to determine what information the question asks for, which is nursing responsibilities when caring for an emergent situation (syncopal episode). Consider that the nurse is always responsible for the care of the assigned client. Skilled assessment is needed in determining the status of the client. Also, utilize the National Council of the State Boards of Nursing (NCSBN) guidelines when determining delegation of duties. Review delegating guidelines if you had difficulty answering this question.

Client needs category: Safe and effective care environment

Client needs subcategory: Management of care

Cognitive level: Analyzing

The neonate

1. The pediatric nurse is being pulled to the nursery for the day. The census is six neonates. Which three neonates are the **best** client care assignment for the pediatric nurse? Select all that apply.

☐ **1.** An 18-hour, postterm, breast-fed neonate with jaundice

☐ **2.** A 2-day-old who has not passed a meconium stool

☐ **3.** A recent admission with Apgar score of 8 and 10

☐ **4.** A 1-day-old with caput succedaneum

☐ **5.** A 4-hour-old with a bluish appearance to the hands and feet

☐ **6.** A 1-day-old with a cleft palate and cleft lip

Answer: 3, 4, 5

ⓓ Rationale: A nurse who is being pulled (reassigned) to a different unit would have a less complicated assignment than the nurse who regularly staffs that unit. The pediatric nurse would be assigned the recent admission with excellent Apgar scores, the 1-day-old with a normal variation of caput succedaneum occurring from swelling of the infant's scalp most commonly from a long labor, and a 4-hour-old with a bluish appearance to the hands and feet. The nurse would identify acrocyanosis as normal in the newborn period and cover the baby to warm. More complicated neonates with specific assessment and parental teaching needs include the breast-fed neonate with jaundice, the 2-day-old who has not had a meconium stool, and the neonate with cleft lip and palate. All neonates will need close observation and increased parental teaching.

Test-taking strategy: Analyze to determine what information the question asks for, which is appropriate assignment for a pulled nurse to the nursery. Analyze each option against the amount of specialized knowledge needed for care. Review common conditions and complications in the neonate if you had difficulty answering this question.

Client needs category: Safe and effective care environment

Client needs subcategory: Management of care

Cognitive level: Analyzing

---

2. A nurse is performing a neurologic assessment on a 1-day-old neonate in the nursery. Which findings would indicate possible asphyxia in utero? Select all that apply.

☐ **1.** The neonate grasps the nurse's finger when put in the palm of the neonate's hand.

☐ **2.** The neonate does stepping movements when held upright with the sole of the foot touching a surface.

☐ **3.** The neonate's toes do not curl downward when the soles of the feet are touched.

☐ **4.** The neonate does not respond when the nurse claps hands.

☐ **5.** The neonate turns toward the nurse's finger when touching the cheek.

☐ **6.** The neonate displays weak, ineffective sucking.

Answer: 3, 4, 6

E **Rationale:** Perinatal asphyxia is an insult to the fetus or newborn because of the lack of oxygen. If the neonate's toes do not curl downward when the soles of the feet are touched and the neonate does not respond to a loud sound, neurologic damage from asphyxia may have occurred. A normal neurologic response would be the downward curling of the toes when touched and extension of the arms and legs in response to a loud noise. Weak, ineffective sucking is another sign of neurologic damage. A neonate would grasp a person's finger when it is placed in the palm of the neonate's hand, do stepping movements when held upright with the sole of the foot touching a surface, and turn toward the nurse's finger when touching the cheek.

Test-taking strategy: Analyze to determine what information the question asks for, which is assessment findings that indicate asphyxia. Recall that the brain is especially susceptible to hypoxia as it has one of the highest oxygen requirement; thus, neurological deficits are common. "Select all that apply" questions require considering each option to decide its merit. When assessing each option, note that all options are neonatal reflexes. Select the options that indicate abnormal findings. Review normal neurologic assessment findings if you had difficulty answering this question.

Client needs category: Health promotion and maintenance

Client needs subcategory: None

Cognitive level: Applying

3. What information would the nurse include when teaching postcircumcision care to the parents of a neonate? Select all that apply.

☐ **1.** The parent must note that the neonate has voided.

☐ **2.** Petroleum jelly or antibiotic ointment would be applied to the glans of the penis with each diaper change.

☐ **3.** The infant can have tub baths while the circumcision heals.

☐ **4.** Any amount of blood noted on the front of the diaper would be reported.

☐ **5.** The circumcision will require care for 2 to 4 days after discharge.

Answer: 1, 2, 5

Ⓒ Rationale: Circumcision is a common surgical procedure when the foreskin of the penis is removed. The infant must void to ensure that the urethra is not obstructed. Parents need to be aware of the first void after circumcision. A lubricating or antibiotic ointment would be applied with each diaper change. Typically, the penis heals within 2 to 4 days, and circumcision care is needed for that period only. To prevent infection, the infant would not have tub baths until the circumcision is healed; sponge baths are appropriate. A small amount of bleeding is expected following a circumcision; parents would report only a large amount of bleeding.

Test-taking strategy: Analyze to determine what information the question asks for, which is postcircumcision care. "Select all that apply" questions require considering each option to decide its merit. Recall that parents need to understand abnormal findings and appropriate care for healing. Also, consider standards of clean technique and infection control. Review teaching guidelines and actions related to circumcision care if you had difficulty answering this question.

Client needs category: Safe and effective care environment

Client needs subcategory: Management of care

Cognitive level: Applying

4. A nurse is caring for a 14-day-old neonate admitted for pyloric stenosis. The health care provider ordered an ultrasound to confirm the diagnosis. When instructing the parents, in which area of the stomach would the nurse stress as the area of concern?

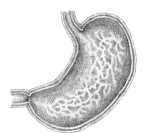

Answer:

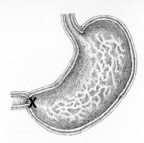

Ⓔ Rationale: Pyloric stenosis is a narrowing of the pylorus, the opening from the stomach into the small intestine. The site of concern is at the pyloric sphincter at the bottom of the stomach where the stomach connects to the small intestine. The pylorus is a muscular valve that holds food in the stomach until it is ready for the next stage in the digestive process. In pyloric stenosis, the pylorus muscles thicken, blocking food from entering the small intestine. Pyloric stenosis can lead to forceful vomiting, dehydration, and weight loss. Neonates with this condition may seem to always be hungry.

Test-taking strategy: Analyze to determine what information the question asks for, which is site of concern for a neonate with pyloric stenosis. Use knowledge of medical terminology to lead to the correct answer (pyloric = located in the stomach and stenosis = narrowing). Review the anatomy of the gastrointestinal system and pathophysiology of pyloric stenosis if you had difficulty answering this question.

Client needs category: Physiological integrity

Client needs subcategory: Physiological adaptation

Cognitive level: Applying

---

5. A nurse is evaluating the return demonstration of cord care by the mother of a neonate. Which actions would the nurse encourage the mother to perform? Select all that apply.

☐ **1.** Placing the diaper below the cord

☐ **2.** Tugging gently on the cord as it begins to dry

☐ **3.** Applying antibiotic ointment to the cord twice daily

☐ **4.** Sponge bathing the infant until the cord falls off

☐ **5.** Cleaning the length of the cord with alcohol several times daily

☐ **6.** Washing the cord with mild soap and water

Answer: 1, 4, 6

E Rationale: The diaper would be positioned below the cord to allow it to air-dry and to prevent urine from getting on the cord. The nurse would instruct the parents to sponge bathe the infant until the cord falls off. Soap and water would be used as a part of cord care. Evidence-based practice states that alcohol is no longer indicated for cord care. Parents would also be instructed to never pull on the cord, but to allow it to fall off naturally. Antibiotic ointments are contraindicated unless there are signs of infection.

Test-taking strategy: Analyze to determine what information the question asks for, which is proper cord care. "Select all that apply" questions require considering each option to decide its merit. Consider that the umbilicus is similar to a scab and must be kept clean and dry so that it is allowed to dry and fall off naturally. Select any option that decreases the risk of infection and promotes healing. Review teaching guidelines and care unique to cord care if you had difficulty answering this question.

Client needs category: Safe and effective care environment

Client needs subcategory: Management of care

Cognitive level: Applying

6. At 5 minutes of age, a neonate is pink with acrocyanosis; has flexed knees, clenched fists, a whimpering cry, and a heart rate of 128 beats/minute; and withdraws the foot when slapped on the sole. What 5-minute Apgar score would the nurse record for this neonate?

SIGN	APGAR SCORE		
	0	**1**	**2**
Heart rate	Absent	<100 beats/minute (slow)	More than 100 beats/minute
Respiratory effort	Absent	Slow, irregular	Good cry
Muscle tone	Flaccid	Some flexion and resistance to extension of extremities	Active motion
Reflex irritability	No response	Grimace or weak cry	Vigorous cry
Color	Pallor, cyanosis	Pink body, blue extremities	Completely pink

☐ **1.** 5.

☐ **2.** 7.

☐ **3.** 8.

☐ **4.** 10.

7. A nurse is administering vitamin K to a neonate following birth. The medication comes in a concentration of 2 mg/ml, and the ordered dose is 0.5 mg to be given subcutaneously. How many milliliters would the nurse administer? Record your answer using two decimal places.

_____ ml

Answer: 3

Ⓓ **Rationale:** The Apgar score provides an assessment of a neonate's health immediately after birth and at 5 minutes of age. Criteria assessed include heart rate, respiratory effort, muscle tone, reflex irritability, and color, each receiving a score from 0 (poor) to 2 (normal). This neonate has a heart rate above 100 beats/minute (score of 2); a weak cry (score of 1); good flexion (score of 2); a good response to a slap on the sole (score of 2); and pink color with acrocyanosis (score of 1). Thus, the total Apgar score is 8.

Test-taking strategy: Analyze to determine what information the question asks for, which is Apgar score using the neonatal data. Match the data provided with scored table data to determine numerical classification. Add the totals from each column to determine the final score. Review the Apgar scale and focus on the data given in the question if you had difficulty answering this question.

Client needs category: Physiological integrity

Client needs subcategory: Physiological adaptation

Cognitive level: Analyzing

Answer: 0.25

Ⓔ **Rationale:** Use the following formula to calculate drug dosages:

$$\text{Dose on hand/quantity on hand} = \text{dose desired}/X$$
$$2 \text{ mg/ml} = 0.5 \text{ mg}/X$$
$$X = 0.25 \text{ ml.}$$

Test-taking strategy: Analyze to determine what information the question asks for, which is calculating the dosage of vitamin K in milliliters using two decimal places. Recall dosage calculations using ratio and proportion and solving for X. Use known data to insert into the calculation. Proofread the math calculation. Be careful to follow decimal instructions. Review dosage calculation if you had difficulty answering this question.

Client needs category: Physiological integrity

Client needs subcategory: Pharmacological and parenteral therapies

Cognitive level: Analyzing

8. A nurse is eliciting reflexes in a neonate during a physical examination. Identify the area that the nurse would touch to elicit a plantar grasp reflex.

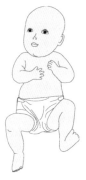

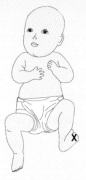

E **Rationale:** To elicit a plantar grasp reflex, the nurse would touch the sole of the foot near the base of the digits, causing flexion or grasping. This reflex disappears at around age 9 months.

Test-taking strategy: Analyze to determine what information the question asks for, which is assessment of the plantar grasp reflex. Use knowledge of medical terminology to lead to the answer (plantar = sole of the feet). Review neonatal reflexes if you had difficulty answering this question.

Client needs category: Health promotion and maintenance
Client needs subcategory: None
Cognitive level: Applying

---

9. A nurse is providing care to a neonate. Place the following steps in the order that the nurse would implement them to properly perform ophthalmia neonatorum prophylaxis. All options must be used.

1. Close and manipulate the eyelids to spread the medication over the eye.

2. Shield the neonate's eyes from direct light, and tilt the head slightly to the side that will receive the treatment.

3. Repeat the procedure for the other eye.

4. Wash hands and put on gloves.

5. Instill the ointment in the lower conjunctival sac.

6. Gently raise the neonate's upper eyelid with the index finger and pull the lower eyelid down with the thumb.

E **Rationale:** Ophthalmia neonatorum prophylaxis involves the instillation of 0.5% erythromycin or 1% tetracycline ointment into a neonate's eyes. This procedure is performed to prevent gonorrheal conjunctivitis. Currently, Canada and the United States mandate that this treatment be given within 1 hour after birth to decrease the risk of permanent eye damage and blindness.

Test-taking strategy: Analyze to determine what information the question asks for, which is procedure to perform ophthalmia neonatorum prophylaxis. When ordering responses, begin with determining the first and last actions to narrow the middle options. Notice that washing hands is a standard first option. The last option would be to conclude the actions of the first eye and move to the next eye. Visualize the procedure to fill in the middle options. Review instilling eye ointment associated with the ophthalmia neonatorum prophylaxis procedure if you had difficulty answering this question.

Client needs category: Physiological integrity
Client needs subcategory: Physiological adaptation
Cognitive level: Applying

10. A nurse is caring for a neonate born addicted to opiates in the special care nursery. The neonate is exhibiting signs of withdrawal. When planning care, which nursing interventions would the nurse expect to be included? Select all that apply.

☐ **1.** Maintain intravenous fluids.

☐ **2.** Administer morphine.

☐ **3.** Swaddle and/or provide a pacifier.

☐ **4.** Feed every 1 to 2 hours.

☐ **5.** Increase environmental stimuli.

☐ **6.** Encourage parental handling.

Answer: 1, 2, 3, 4

Ⓒ Rationale: Neonatal narcotic withdrawal syndrome includes symptoms of irritability, a high-pitched cry, tremors, poor feeding with vomiting and diarrhea, and nasal stuffiness. Nursing interventions include to swaddle and/or offer a pacifier to soothe the neonate, decrease handling and environmental stimuli, and maintain intravenous fluids with regular feeding. The nurse would also administer morphine to ease the withdrawal symptoms and potential seizure activity.

Test-taking strategy: Analyze to determine what information the question asks for, which is nursing interventions for a neonate experiencing withdrawal symptoms. Consider the withdrawal symptoms (stemming from the neurological system) and how to offset those symptoms. Recall the measures used to soothe a neonate. Review the nursing interventions when caring for a neonate addicted to opiates if you had difficulty answering this question.

Client needs category: Physiological integrity

Client needs subcategory: Physiological adaptation

Cognitive level: Applying

---

11. The nurse is caring for a newborn boy of Hispanic heritage. According to the beliefs of this heritage, which would the nurse expect? Select all that apply.

☐ **1.** The maternal elders offer advice to the new mother.

☐ **2.** The neonate will be circumcised by a medicine man.

☐ **3.** The umbilical cord will be kept covered by snug clothing.

☐ **4.** Breast-feeding is common and strongly encouraged.

☐ **5.** The neonate must be bundled at all times.

☐ **6.** The neonate will wear a red or pink bracelet.

Answer: 1, 3, 4, 5, 6

Ⓓ Rationale: Hispanic culture has a strong Catholic faith and deep respect for close family ties. The elder women will advise the younger generation on child rearing. Breast-feeding is strongly encouraged. Long ago, the neonate was thought to breathe air through the umbilical cord so it was kept covered. When the dry umbilical cord stump falls off, snug clothing prevents the belly button from becoming an "outie." American Indians use a medicine man. To protect babies from the evil eye, they are given a red or pink bracelet.

Test-taking strategy: Analyze to determine what information the question asks for, which is expectations when caring for a neonate of Hispanic heritage. Consider characteristics of a heritage such as religion and child-rearing practices. Review cultural practices if you had difficulty answering this question.

Client needs category: Psychosocial integrity

Client needs subcategory: None

Cognitive level: Applying

---

12. A nurse is completing a physical assessment of a neonate following birth. When completing the musculoskeletal assessment, which findings would indicate developmental dysplasia of the hip (DDH)? Select all that apply.

- ☐ **1.** Negative Ortolani test
- ☐ **2.** Positive Barlow test
- ☐ **3.** Asymmetrical leg skin folds
- ☐ **4.** Limitation in adduction of the affected leg
- ☐ **5.** Lengthening of the affected leg

Ⓓ Rationale: Developmental dysplasia (dislocation) of the hip is an abnormal formation of the hip joint in which the ball on the top of the femur is not held firmly in the socket. A neonate with DDH will have a positive Ortolani test, a positive Barlow test, and asymmetrical skin folds in the thigh. The affected leg has limited abduction and appears shorter than the unaffected leg in a neonate with DDH.

Test-taking strategy: Analyze to determine what information the question asks for, which is physical assessment findings that indicate a DDH. "Select all that apply" questions require considering each option to decide its merit. Consider the pathophysiology of the hip (dislocated) and look to the options. Review the characteristics of developmental hip dysplasia if you had difficulty answering this question.

Client needs category: Physiological integrity
Client needs subcategory: Physiological adaptation
Cognitive level: Applying

13. Following the admission assessment of a neonate born at 42 weeks of gestation, the nurse documents which findings as normal? Select all that apply.

- ☐ **1.** A three-vessel umbilical cord
- ☐ **2.** Peeling skin on the feet
- ☐ **3.** Absence of sole creases
- ☐ **4.** Absence of vernix caseosa
- ☐ **5.** Cyanosis of the hands and feet
- ☐ **6.** Large amounts of frothy oral secretions

Ⓓ Rationale: All of the answers are expected findings in a healthy infant at 42 weeks of gestation except for absence of sole creases (creases will be present) and large amounts of frothy oral secretions. Frothy oral secretions are indicative of a tracheoesophageal fistula; it is an abnormal finding in any neonate, regardless of gestational age at the time of birth.

Test-taking strategy: Analyze to determine what information the question asks for, which is normal findings of a postterm neonate. "Select all that apply" questions require considering each option to decide its merit. Consider the effects of remaining in the uterus, within amniotic fluid, past normal gestation. While anatomically the neonates are normal, some postterm neonates have a distinctive appearance as noted above. Review normal assessment findings for full-term neonates and postterm neonates if you had difficulty answering this question.

Client needs category: Health promotion and maintenance
Client needs subcategory: None
Cognitive level: Applying

14. A neonate has been placed on cardiac and apnea monitoring in the neonatal nursery. The nurse notes that the apnea alarm repeatedly triggers. Place the following actions in the order in which they would be completed by the nurse. All options must be used.

1. Silence the alarm to decrease environmental stimuli.

2. Perform a focused assessment on the neonate.

3. Count the respiratory rate for 60 seconds.

4. Document the assessment findings, interventions, and neonate's response.

5. Check all connects on apnea monitor.

Rationale: The priority action is to perform a focused assessment on the neonate. Afterward, the nurse would evaluate the respiratory rate by counting respirations for 60 seconds. Afterward, the nurse would silence the alarm, check all connections on the apnea monitor, and, finally, document the information. Remember to "nurse the client," not the equipment.

Test-taking strategy: Analyze to determine what information the question asks for, which is nursing actions when the apnea monitor repeatedly triggers. Standards of care dictate that the neonate is to be assessed immediately following alarm. Completing a focused assessment including respiratory count ensures neonatal safety. Once it is determined that the neonate is safe, the nurse addresses the apnea monitor and documentation. Recall the ABCs (airway, breathing, and circulation) of care when prioritizing actions if you had difficulty answering this question.

Client needs category: Physiological integrity

Client needs subcategory: Physiological adaptation

Cognitive level: Applying

---

15. A 2-week-old neonate is admitted to the hospital with a diagnosis of possible sepsis. The neonate weighs 3.2 kg. The health care provider prescribes the following orders for the neonate and signs the order sheet. Which order would the nurse question?

Progress notes

08/01/15	Acetaminophen (Tylenol) 10 mg/kg per
1000	rectum, every 4–6 hours prn pain Ampicillin
	200 mg/kg IV every 6 hrs, D₅.45 Normal
	saline IV @ 125 ml/hr. Mom may breastfeed
	ad lib. Draw blood cultures x 3 in A.M. Send
	Urine C & S in A.M.
	—R. Richard, M.D.

☐ **1.** Acetaminophen 10 mg/kg per rectum, every 4 to 6 hours prn pain

☐ **2.** Ampicillin 200 mg/kg intravenously every 6 hours

☐ **3.** Mom may breast-feed ad lib.

☐ **4.** Draw blood cultures × 3 in AM.

Rationale: After the administration of ampicillin, the neonate's blood cultures will be invalid; the cultures would be obtained prior to the administration of the antibiotics. It is the nurse's responsibility to notify the health care provider and seek further clarification before carrying out this order. All of the other health care provider orders are appropriate as written.

Test-taking strategy: Analyze to determine what information the question asks for, which is identification of questionable health care provider order. Questioning a health care provider's order indicates that one of the orders documented is incorrect. Analyze each option for validity. Recall normal protocol for the timing of blood cultures and administration of antibiotics. Note that all other orders are typical for an infant diagnosed with possible sepsis.

Client needs category: Physiological integrity

Client needs subcategory: Pharmacologic and parenteral therapies

Cognitive level: Analyzing

16. The nurse is caring for a neonate who has a suspected neonatal sepsis. The health care provider's order is for ampicillin 100 mg/kg/day to be given in four divided doses. The client weighs 7 lb, 8 oz (3.4 kg). How many milligrams would the nurse give with each dose? Record your answer using a whole number.

_____ mg/dose

Ⓜ Rationale: First, convert the weight to kilograms in the United States:

$$7 \text{ lb, } 8 \text{ oz} = 7.5 \text{ lb}$$
$$1 \text{ lb} = 2.2 \text{ kg}$$
$$7.5 \text{ lb} \div 2.2 \text{ kg} = 3.4 \text{ kg.}$$

Then, multiply the kilograms of body weight by 100 mg (dose given):

$$3.4 \text{ kg} \times 100 \text{ mg} = 340 \text{ mg/kg.}$$

Next, divide 340 mg/kg by four doses per day:

$$340 \div 4 = 85 \text{ mg per dose.}$$

Test-taking strategy: Analyze to determine what information the question asks for, which is medication dose per dose. Consider that there are three steps to this calculation. As usual, weight must be converted to kilograms in the United States. Next, the daily (24-hour) dose is calculated. Lastly, calculate to mg/dose as required in the question. Be sure to carefully read how the dosage is to be reported. Proofread the math calculation. Review conversions and dosage calculations based on body weight if you had difficulty answering this question.

Client needs category: Physiological integrity

Client needs subcategory: Pharmacological and parenteral therapies

Cognitive level: Applying

17. The nurse is caring for a newborn with a heart defect that involves mixing blood from the pulmonary and systemic circulation. Which illustration shows a congenital heart disorder with mixed blood flow?

☐ **1.**

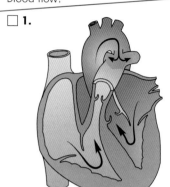

☐ **2.**

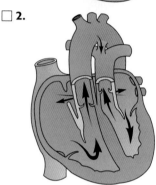

☐ **3.**

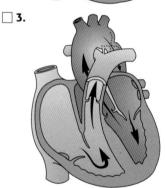

☐ **4.**

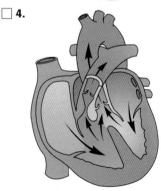

Answer: 2

ⓓ **Rationale:** In transposition of the great arteries (option 2), the aorta arises from the right ventricle instead of the left and the pulmonary artery arises from the left ventricle instead of the right. In most instances, atrial and ventricular defects also occur, making the entire heart have one mixed circulatory system. Option 1 shows patent ductus arteriosus, an increased pulmonary blood flow disorder. Option 3 depicts coarctation of the aorta, an obstruction to blood flow disorder. Option 4 shows tetralogy of Fallot, a decreased pulmonary blood flow disorder.

Test-taking strategy: Analyze to determine what information the question asks for, which is which illustration identifies a congenital heart disorder with mixed blood flow. Mixed blood flow indicates that oxygenated blood is in contact with deoxygenated blood. Consider that this mixing of the blood occurs with blood prior to oxygenation in the lungs. Review the hemodynamic and blood flow patterns of congenital heart disorders if you had difficulty answering this question.

Client needs category: Physiological integrity

Client needs subcategory: Physiological adaptation

Cognitive level: Analyzing

18. A graduate nurse is explaining to the nurse mentor how to assess newborn jaundice and the effects of phototherapy in a dark-skinned neonate. Which statement made by the graduate nurse would need clarification? Select all that apply.

☐ **1.** "It is best to observe for jaundice in the conjunctival sac or oral mucosa."

☐ **2.** "I will monitor the unconjugated bilirubin carefully as it is the dangerous one."

☐ **3.** "I will carefully record the neonate's intake as limiting fluids is helpful."

☐ **4.** "The neonate will be irritable from the elevated bilirubin in the system."

☐ **5.** "Phototherapy treatment can increase the risk of dehydration."

Answer: 3, 4

Ⓜ **Rationale:** The nurse mentor must clarify a graduate nurse's statement relating to limiting fluids. Hydration is crucial for all neonates as they are already at risk for imbalance because of increased body surface area. Intravenous fluids in addition to oral feeding may be necessary. Newborns are typically not irritable because of the bilirubin. Many sleep comfortably throughout their phototherapy treatment. It is correct to observe for the yellowish discoloration of jaundice in the conjunctival sac or oral mucosa in a dark-skinned neonate. In a light-skinned neonate, applying pressure with the thumb over a bony prominence to blanch the skin reveals the yellowish tone. The dangerous bilirubin is the unconjugated, indirect bilirubin. It is measured by subtracting the direct bilirubin level from the total bilirubin level.

Test-taking strategy: Analyze to determine what information the question asks for, which is incorrect statement regarding newborn jaundice needing clarification. Relate different assessment techniques related to a dark-skinned infant. Read each option and analyze for incorrect information. Recall that newborn jaundice is common in neonates and assessed on each infant. Review newborn jaundice assessment techniques if you had difficulty answering this question.

Client needs category: Physiological integrity

Client needs subcategory: Physiological adaptation

Cognitive level: Analyzing

Pediatric nursing

The infant

1. A physician orders an intravenous infusion of dextrose 5% in quarter-normal saline solution (D5.25 NSS) to be infused at 7 ml/kg/hour for a 10-month-old infant. The infant weighs 22 lb (10 kg). How many milliliters of the ordered solution would the nurse infuse each hour? Record your answer using a whole number.

_____ ml/hour

Answer: 70

Ⓔ Rationale: To perform this calculation, the nurse would first convert the infant's weight to kilograms if needed:

$$2.2 \text{ lb/kg} = 22 \text{ lb}/X \text{ kg}$$
$$X = 22/2.2$$
$$X = 10 \text{ kg}.$$

Next, the nurse would multiply the infant's weight by the ordered rate:

$$10 \text{ kg} \times 7 \text{ ml/kg/hour} = 70 \text{ ml/hour}.$$

Test-taking strategy: Analyze to determine what information the question asks for, which is the dose in milliliter per hour. Use knowledge of drug calculations and the calculation method of solving for **X** (see above). Proofread your math calculation for accuracy. Review basic drug calculations and basic conversions if you had difficulty answering this question.

Client needs category: Physiological integrity

Client needs subcategory: Pharmacological and parenteral therapies

Cognitive level: Applying

---

2. A nurse is teaching the parents of a 6-month-old infant about normal growth and development. Which statements regarding infant development are true? Select all that apply.

☐ **1.** A 6-month-old infant has difficulty holding objects.

☐ **2.** A 6-month-old infant can usually roll from prone to supine and supine to prone positions.

☐ **3.** A teething ring is appropriate for a 6-month-old infant.

☐ **4.** Stranger anxiety usually peaks at age 12 to 18 months.

☐ **5.** Head lag is commonly noted in infants at age 6 months.

☐ **6.** Lack of visual coordination usually resolves by age 6 months.

Answer: 2, 3, 6

Ⓓ Rationale: Gross motor skills of the 6-month-old infant include rolling from front to back and back to front. Teething usually begins around age 6 months and, therefore, a teething ring is appropriate. Tooth eruption begins between 6 and 8 months. Visual coordination is usually resolved by age 6 months. At age 6 months, fine motor skills include purposeful grasping and releasing of objects and transferring objects from one hand to another. Stranger anxiety normally peaks at 8 months. The 6-month-old infant also would have good head control and no longer display head lag when pulled up to a sitting position.

Test-taking strategy: Analyze to determine what information the question asks for, which is normal growth and development for a 6-month-old infant. "Select all that apply" questions require considering each option to decide its merit. Memorization of growth and development milestones is a must when answering many pediatric questions. Grouping development into ages may be helpful in recalling milestones on a continuum. Review infant growth and development if you had difficulty answering this question.

3. A nurse is caring for an infant who weighs 8 kg and is ordered to receive ampicillin 25 mg/kg intravenously every 6 hours. How many milligrams would a nurse administer per dose? Record the answer as a whole number.

_____ mg/dose

Answer: 200

Ⓔ Rationale: The nurse would calculate the correct dose by multiplying the infant's weight by the ordered rate:

$$8 \text{ kg} \times 25 \text{ mg/kg} = 200 \text{ mg.}$$

Test-taking strategy: Analyze to determine what information the question asks for, which is the number of milligrams in each dose. Use knowledge of drug calculations to multiply the weight (kg) per milligrams. Proofread your math calculation for accuracy and remember the opportunity to use the drop-down calculator during your NCLEX. Review basic drug calculations if you had difficulty answering this question.

Client needs category: Physiological integrity

Client needs subcategory: Pharmacological and parenteral therapies

Cognitive level: Applying

4. A nurse is conducting a physical examination on a 2-month-old infant at the well-child examination. When measuring chest circumference, identify the standard anatomical landmark used.

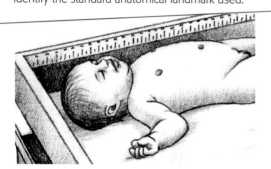

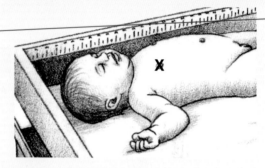

E Rationale: Head circumference and chest size measurements are often taken on newborns and infants to measure growth levels and development. These growth milestones reveal healthy brain growth and development. Chest circumference is most accurately measured by placing the measuring tape around the infant's nipples. Measuring above or below the nipples will yield a false measurement. The measurement would be taken after exhalation.

Test-taking strategy: Analyze to determine what information the question asks for, which is the anatomical site used when measuring chest circumference. When assessing the chest, the nipple line is the most notable landmark on the chest area. This provides a standard reference point for comparison. Chest circumference equals head circumference (within a range of 0.79 inch or 2 cm) at birth. Review assessment of chest circumference if you had difficulty answering this question.

Client needs category: Health promotion and maintenance

Client needs subcategory: None

Cognitive level: Applying

---

5. A healthy 2-month-old infant is being seen in the local clinic for a well-child checkup and initial immunizations. When analyzing the pediatric record, which immunizations would the nurse anticipate administering at this appointment? Select all that apply.

☐ **1.** DTaP (diphtheria, tetanus, and acellular pertussis)

☐ **2.** MMR (measles, mumps, and rubella)

☐ **3.** IPV (inactivated polio vaccine)

☐ **4.** Varicella (chickenpox) vaccine

☐ **5.** Hib (*Haemophilus influenzae* vaccine)

☐ **6.** PCV (pneumococcal vaccine)

Answer: 1, 3, 5, 6

D Rationale: At age 2 months, the American Academy of Pediatrics and Public Health Agency in Canada recommends the administration of DTaP, IPV, (Hep B in the United States), Hib, rotavirus vaccine, and PCV. The MMR and varicella immunizations would be administered at 12 to 15 months.

Test-taking strategy: Analyze to determine what information the question asks for, which is immunizations to be administered at a 2-month well-child check. "Select all that apply" questions require considering each option to decide its merit. Memorization or a working knowledge of the immunization schedule is a necessity in determining the correct immunizations. Consider grouping immunization by months or on a timeline to assist in remembering the schedule. Review the immunization schedule if you had difficulty answering this question.

Client needs category: Health promotion and maintenance

Client needs subcategory: None

Cognitive level: Applying

---

6. The nurse is caring for an emergency room infant who has symptoms of irritability and a high fever. When assessing for increased intracranial pressure using the anterior fontanelle, identify the area where a nurse would palpate.

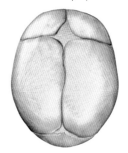

Answer:

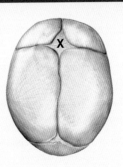

Ⓔ Rationale: The anterior fontanelle is formed by the junction of the sagittal, frontal, and coronal sutures. It is shaped like a diamond and normally measures 4 to 5 cm at its widest point. The posterior fontanelle closes during the first several months of life and the anterior fontanelle closes around 2 years of age. A widened, bulging fontanelle is a sign of increased intracranial pressure.

Test-taking strategy: Analyze to determine what information the question asks for, which is location of the anterior fontanelle for assessment of increased intracranial pressure. The key words are "anterior," meaning before, and "fontanelle," meaning opening covered by a membrane. Look to the illustration to select the opening on the top of the head. Review anterior and posterior fontanelle placement and characteristics if you had difficulty answering this question.

Client needs category: Health promotion and maintenance

Client needs subcategory: None

Cognitive level: Applying

7. A parent is planning to enroll a 9-month-old infant in a day care facility. The parent asks a nurse what to look for as indicators that the facility is adhering to good infection control measures. The nurse identifies which as an indication of meeting proper infection control standards? Select all that apply.

☐ **1.** The facility keeps boxes of gloves in the director's office.

☐ **2.** Soiled diapers are discarded in covered receptacles.

☐ **3.** Toys are kept on the floor for the children to share.

☐ **4.** Disposable papers are used on the diaper-changing surfaces.

☐ **5.** Facilities for hand hygiene are located in every classroom.

☐ **6.** Soiled clothing and cloth diapers are sent home in labeled paper bags.

Answer: 2, 4, 5

Ⓜ Rationale: A parent can assess infection control practices by appraising steps taken by the facility to prevent the spread of disease. Placing soiled diapers in covered receptacles, covering the diaper-changing surfaces with disposable papers, and ensuring that hand sanitizers and sinks are available for personnel to wash their hands after activities are all indicators that infection control measures are being followed. Gloves would be readily available to personnel and, therefore, would be kept in every room—not in an office. Toys typically are shared by numerous children; however, this contributes to the spread of germs and infections. All soiled clothing and cloth diapers would be placed in a sealed plastic bag before being sent home.

Test-taking strategy: Analyze to determine what information the question asks for, which is standard precautions for infection control. "Select all that apply" questions require considering each option to decide its merit. Discriminate between each option to identify how that option meets the criteria for ensuring proper infection control practices. Review infection control practices if you had difficulty answering this question.

Client needs category: Safe and effective care environment

Client needs subcategory: Safety and infection control

Cognitive level: Analyzing

---

8. A pediatric intensive care nurse is performing cardiopulmonary resuscitation (CPR) on an infant. Between cycles of breathing and compressions, place an X where the nurse would assess for a pulse.

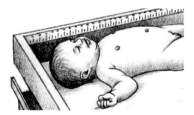

Answer:

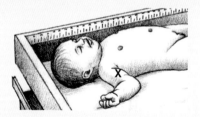

Ⓜ Rationale: The X is placed over the brachial pulse located just above the antecubital of the arm. The brachial pulse is the pulse to assess when performing infant CPR. The carotid pulse, which is used in children and adults, is extremely difficult to locate in an infant because of the infant short neck. For that reason, individuals are to limit time spent on assessing the pulse and move to the compression step.

Test-taking strategy: Analyze to determine what information the question asks for, which is site for pulse assessment during infant CPR. Recall that pulse assessment sites vary according to age of the child and memorize which location corresponds with which age group. Review infant CPR if you had difficulty answering this question.

Client needs category: Physiological adaptation

Client needs subcategory: Physiological integrity

Cognitive level: Understanding

9. A nurse is assessing a 10-month-old infant during a checkup. Which developmental milestones would the nurse expect the infant to display? Select all that apply.

☐ **1.** Holding the head erect

☐ **2.** Self-feeding with a spoon

☐ **3.** Demonstrating good bowel and bladder control

☐ **4.** Sitting on a firm surface without support

☐ **5.** Bearing the majority of weight on legs

☐ **6.** Walking alone

Answer: 1, 4, 5

Ⓒ **Rationale:** By age 4 months, an infant would be able to hold the head erect. By age 9 months, the infant would be able to sit on a firm surface without support and bear the majority of weight on the legs (e.g., walking while holding onto furniture). Self-feeding and bowel and bladder control are developmental milestones of toddlers. By age 12 months, the infant would be able to stand alone and may take the first steps.

Test-taking strategy: Analyze to determine what information the question asks for, which is developmental milestones of a 10-month-old. "Select all that apply" questions require considering each option to decide its merit. Memorization of growth and development milestones is a must when answering many pediatric questions. Grouping development into ages may be helpful in recalling milestones on a continuum. Another helpful point may be to visualize the actions of a child at this age. Review growth and development of infants and toddlers if you had difficulty answering this question.

Client needs category: Health promotion and maintenance

Client needs subcategory: None

Cognitive level: Applying

10. A nurse is conducting an infant nutrition class for parents. Which foods would the nurse tell parents that they may introduce during the first year of life? Select all that apply.

☐ **1.** Bread with honey

☐ **2.** Pureed fruits

☐ **3.** Whole grapes

☐ **4.** Oatmeal cereal

☐ **5.** Strained vegetables

☐ **6.** Fruit drink

Answer: 2, 4, 5

C **Rationale:** The first food provided to a neonate is breast milk or formula. Between ages 4 and 6 months, cereals can be introduced, followed by pureed or strained fruits and vegetables, and then strained or ground meat. Meats, fruits, or any other foods must be chopped or ground before they are fed to an infant to prevent choking. Fruit drinks, many times with added sweeteners, provide no nutritional benefit and would not be encouraged. Honey is not encouraged for an infant because of the risk of botulism.

Test-taking strategy: Analyze to determine what information the question asks for, which is foods to be introduced during the first year of life. "Select all that apply" questions require considering each option to decide its merit. The key words are "during the first year of life." Review each option for introduction into the child's system during the select time frame. If unsure, recall the progression of oral intake. Review infant feeding schedules, including timing and type of solid foods introduced in the first year of life if you had difficulty answering this question.

Client needs category: Health promotion and maintenance

Client needs subcategory: None

Cognitive level: Applying

---

11. A nurse is teaching parents about the developmental milestones of an infant. Place the following developmental activities for an infant in order of occurrence by age from earliest to latest. All options must be used.

| **1.** Crawling on hands and knees |
| **2.** Sitting alone |
| **3.** Turning self from supine to prone |
| **4.** Turning self from prone to supine |
| **5.** Effectively using pincer grasp |

Answer: 4, 3, 2, 1, 5

D **Rationale:** Infants graduate from larger body movements to smaller. In general terms, infants typically roll over before sitting and crawl before they walk. More specifically, infants turn first from prone to supine and then supine to prone by age 3 to 5 months. Sitting alone usually occurs at about age 6 to 7 months. Crawling occurs at around age 8 to 9 months. The use of pincer grasp usually occurs at around 10 to 12 months. The ages are general approximations.

Test-taking strategy: Analyze to determine what information the question asks for, which is identifying the proper progression of developmental milestones. Consider the progression of motor skills from gross to refined. Review infant developmental milestones if you had difficulty answering this question.

Client needs category: Health promotion and maintenance

Client needs subcategory: None

Cognitive level: Applying

12. The nurse is assessing the primitive reflexes of a 1-month-old infant. Of the reflexes shown in the photos, which one would the nurse expect to remain the longest?

☐ **1.**

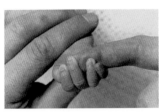

☐ **2.**

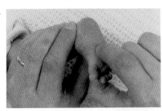

☐ **3.**

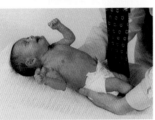

☐ **4.**

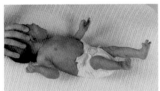

Ⓜ **Rationale:** Option 2 shows the plantar grasp reflex, which is noted to disappear by 8 months. Of the options, this reflex will remain the longest. Option 1 is the palmar grasp, which will disappear around 3 months. Option 3 is the Moro reflex, which will disappear around 4 months. Option 4 is the tonic neck reflex, which will disappear around 3 to 4 months.

Test-taking strategy: Analyze to determine what information the question asks for, which is of the reflexes in the photograph, which reflex remains the longest. Analyze each illustration to identify the reflex that the nurse will be able to assess the longest. It may be helpful to group the primitive reflexes together for remembering. In this case, the plantar grasp is the only reflex out of the 3- to 4-month time frame. Review when each reflex is present and how it is assessed if you have difficulty answering this question.

Client needs category: Physiological integrity

Client needs subcategory: Reduction of risk potential

Cognitive level: Analyzing

---

13. A parent phones the health care provider's office stating that his 13-month-old has had diarrhea for 3 days and he is unsure what fluids to offer. Which suggestions would the nurse provide? Select all that apply.

☐ **1.** Apple juice

☐ **2.** Whole milk

☐ **3.** Ginger ale

☐ **4.** Cola

☐ **5.** Pedialyte®

☐ **6.** Water

Ⓓ **Rationale:** The nurse is correct to instruct on oral rehydration fluids such as Pedialyte®or Lytren®. These solutions rehydrate with fluids and electrolytes and can be offered a teaspoon (5 ml) at a time. Water is also appropriate to provide fluids. The infant may need lactose-free products at this time. Apple juice, ginger ale, and cola have a high osmolality and may cause diarrhea.

Test-taking strategy: Analyze to determine what information the question asks for, which is appropriate fluids for an infant experiencing diarrhea. Consider that diarrhea can cause dehydration; thus, choose drinks that replace fluids and electrolytes. Review oral electrolyte replacements if you had difficulty answering this question.

Client needs category: Physiological integrity

Client needs subcategory: Reduction of risk potential

Cognitive level: Applying

14. A child is brought to the emergency department severely dehydrated after having gastroenteritis for 4 days. The physician orders an intravenous infusion to maintain fluid replacement for this child. If the child weighs 18 kg, what is the hourly flow rate in milliliters? Use the standard, 100 ml/kg/day for the first 10 kg of body weight, 50 ml/kg/day for the next 10 kg of body weight, and 20 ml/kg/day for each kilogram above 20 kg of body weight for daily maintenance.

_____ ml

Answer: 58

Ⓓ Rationale: To find the answer, use the given formula as a guide.

The client is 18 kg meaning that this is a two-step problem.

Step 1: 100 ml/10 kg = 1,000 ml.

Step 2: 50 ml × 8 kg = 400 ml.

Total: 1,400 ml of daily maintenance fluids

Next, to find the hourly flow rate, divide by 24:

1,400 ml divided by 24 = 58.3 ml.

Test-taking strategy: Analyze to determine what information the question asks for, which is calculation of hourly fluid maintenance. Look for key information in the problem to place in the standard equation and calculate. Make sure that the answer provided answers the intended question, as in this question it was not daily amount but hourly. Proofread the math calculation. Review fluid maintenance calculations if you had difficulty answering this question.

Client needs category: Physiological integrity

Client needs subcategory: Pharmacological and parenteral therapies

Cognitive level: Applying

15. The nurse is caring for an infant who exhibits the following characteristics:

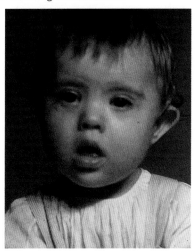

From Bickley LS and Szilagyi P. *Bates' Guide to Physical Examination and History Taking*, 8th ed. Philadelphia, PA: Lippincott Williams & Wilkins; 2003.

When planning care, which would be the **best** long-term client goal?

☐ **1.** The client will feed himself/herself independently.

☐ **2.** The client will reach his/her optimal level of functioning.

☐ **3.** The client will care for himself/herself without supervision.

☐ **4.** The client will express his/her thoughts and feelings.

Answer: 2

ℰ Rationale: Down's syndrome results from trisomy of chromosome 21 and is evidenced by various physical and cognitive impairments. Common physical characteristics include a flat, broad nasal bridge, inner epicanthal folds, slanted eyes, a protruding tongue, a short neck, hypotonia, and a palmar crease. Nursing interventions include supporting the parents through the diagnostic process, monitoring for cardiac or respiratory problems with a long-term goal to help to assist the client to reach his/her optimal level of functioning. Specific goals include feeding, personal care, and communication skills.

Test-taking strategy: Analyze to determine what information the question asks for, which is identification of a long-term goal. Analyze each option for a long-term comprehensive goal appropriate for a wide variety of potential characteristics. Option 2 is the most general and broad option for the future when unsure of a client's ability. Review nursing goals appropriate for a client with Down's syndrome if you had difficulty answering this question.

Client needs category: Health promotion and maintenance

Client needs subcategory: None

Cognitive level: Applying

16. The nurse is caring for the following infant after surgery. Which short-term goal is the **priority**?

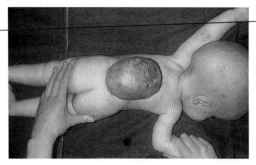

Reprinted with permission from Pillitteri A. *Maternal and child health nursing*, 5th ed. Philadelphia, PA: Wolters Kluwer; 2008.

☐ **1.** The infant will continue breast-feeding 3 to 5 times daily.

☐ **2.** The infant will bond with parents by holding and cuddling during each visit.

☐ **3.** The infant will remain infection-free in the postoperative period.

☐ **4.** The infant will maintain 5 to 7 moderately wet diapers daily.

Answer: 3

E **Rationale:** The client has spina bifida with a myelomeningocele (protrusion of the spinal cord and meninges). Surgery is completed within the first days of life. Following surgery and in the recovery period, it is most important to maintain meticulous care to the incision to reduce the potential for infection. Infection can spread through the incision and up the spinal tract to the brain. All other goals are important but not as great a priority as infection.

Test-taking strategy: Analyze to determine what information the question asks for, which is postoperative short-term goal. First, identify that the client has a myelomeningocele and relate the need for surgical treatment. Also realize the open tract established from the nonclosure of the spinal column. Consider the highest priority to maintain client healing postoperatively. Review surgical treatment of a myelomeningocele and nursing goals if you had difficulty answering this question.

Client needs category: Physiological integrity
Client needs subcategory: Reduction of risk potential
Cognitive level: Analyzing

The toddler

1. A nurse is preparing a dose of amoxicillin for a 3-year-old with acute otitis media. The child weighs 33 lb (15 kg). The dosage prescribed is 50 mg/kg/day in divided doses for every 8 hours. The concentration of the drug is 250 mg/5 ml. How many milliliters would the nurse administer? Record your answer using a whole number.

_____ ml

Answer: 5

M **Rationale:** To calculate the child's weight in kilograms as listed, the nurse would use the following formula:

$$2.2 \text{ lb}/1 \text{ kg} = 33 \text{ lb}/X \text{ kg}$$
$$X = 33 \div 2.2$$
$$X = 15 \text{ kg.}$$

Next, the nurse would calculate the daily dosage for the child:

$$50 \text{ mg/kg/day} \times 15 \text{ kg} = 750 \text{ mg/day.}$$

To determine divided daily dosage, the nurse would know that "every 8 hours" means three times per day. So, the nurse would perform the calculation in this way:

Total daily dosage ÷ 3 times per day = divided daily dosage

Total daily dosage ÷ 3 times per day = divided daily dosage
$$750 \text{ mg/day} \div 3 = 250 \text{ mg.}$$

The drug's concentration is 250 mg/5 ml, so the nurse would administer 5 ml.

Test-taking strategy: Analyze to determine what information the question asks for, which is milliliters of medication to be administered per dose. Follow the steps above thinking through the process of determining kilograms (if needed) and then calculating daily dose and then each dose. Lastly, use the known concentration to determine the milliliters to be administered. Proofread the math calculations. Review multistep dosage calculations if you had difficulty answering this question.

Client needs category: Physiological integrity

Client needs subcategory: Pharmacological and parenteral therapies

Cognitive level: Applying

---

2. Which nursing interventions are important when caring for a hospitalized toddler? Select all that apply.

☐ **1.** Provide thorough explanation to the toddler prior to a procedure.

☐ **2.** Instruct parent that regression commonly occurs.

☐ **3.** Encourage use of a security object from home.

☐ **4.** Allow client autonomy by offering select choices.

☐ **5.** Maintain the toddler's routine when able.

☐ **6.** Discourage parents' participation in client care.

Answer: 2, 3, 4, 5

C **Rationale:** Hospitalization is a stressful time for both the toddler and the parents. Important nursing interventions decrease the stress level. Toddler inventions include allowing security objects from home, maintaining the usual routine, and providing autonomy by allowing select or appropriate choices. Parental interventions include instruction on common regression behavior and allowing participation in the toddler's care. Brief, age-appropriate explanations to a toddler immediately prior to a procedure are best.

Test-taking strategy: Analyze to determine what information the question asks for, which is nursing interventions for a hospitalized toddler. Always think "developmental level" when considering each option. Consider each option related to the benefits to the client and parent. Realize that helping the parent through communication of knowledge will empower the parents to care for the toddler. Review growth and development and nursing interventions of hospitalized toddlers if you had difficulty answering this question.

Client needs category: Safe and effective care environment

Client needs subcategory: Management of care

Cognitive level: Applying

3. A 3-year-old is to receive 500 ml of dextrose 5% in normal saline solution (D_5NSS) over 8 hours. At what rate (in milliliters per hour) would a nurse set the infusion pump? Round your answer to a whole number.

_____ ml/hour

Answer: 63

E **Rationale:** To calculate the rate per hour for the infusion, the nurse would divide 500 ml by 8 hours: 500 ml ÷ 8 hours = 62.5 ml/hour (63 ml/hour).

Test-taking strategy: Analyze to determine what information the question asks for, which is infusion rate in milliliters per hour. Recall that there are two types of infusion calculations: (1) looking at quantity in milliliter per hour and (2) drip factor rates in gtts per minute. Quantity of fluid (ml/hour) calculations divides the amount of fluid by the number of hours to be infused. Proofread all mathematical calculations. Review dosage calculations for hourly flow rates if you had difficulty answering this question.

Client needs category: Physiological integrity

Client needs subcategory: Pharmacological and parenteral therapies

Cognitive level: Applying

4. A 2-year-old is being treated for pneumonia. After reviewing the respiratory section of the client care flow sheet (shown below), the nurse concludes that which position is **most** beneficial to maximize oxygenation?

Flow Sheet

Date: 4/2/16	2300–0700	0700–1500	1500–2300
Breath sounds	Diminished BS LLL	Diminished BS LLL	Crackles LLL
Treatment/ results	——	Chest physiotherapy (CPT) and postural drainage	CPT and postural drainage
Cough/results	Nonproductive	Nonproductive	Yellow sputum
Oxygen therapy	Via humidified mask	Via humidified mask	Via humidified mask

☐ **1.** Left-side lying

☐ **2.** Right-side lying

☐ **3.** Semi-Fowler

☐ **4.** Supine with the head of the bed elevated 30°

Answer: 2

C **Rationale:** The client would be positioned on the right side. Gravity will help mobilize secretions from the affected (left) lung, thereby allowing for improved blood flow and oxygenation. Elevating the head of the bed does not facilitate drainage removal.

Test-taking strategy: Analyze to determine what information the question asks for, which is the analysis of the nurse's note to determine the status of the client and progression of symptoms. Identify that breath sounds, cough results, and treatment results provide data that secretion status is a priority. Determine which position would eliminate secretions from the lung fields. Review respiratory data and postural drainage treatment if you had difficulty answering this question.

Client needs category: Physiological integrity

Client needs subcategory: Physiological adaptation

Cognitive level: Analyzing

5. A 15-month-old has just received routine immunizations, including DTaP, IPV, and MMR. What information would the nurse give to the parents before they leave the office? Select all that apply.

- ☐ **1.** Minor symptoms can be treated with acetaminophen.

- ☐ **2.** Minor symptoms can be treated with aspirin.

- ☐ **3.** Call the office if the toddler develops a fever above 103°F (39.4°C), seizures, or difficulty breathing.

- ☐ **4.** Discomfort at the immunization site and mild fever are common.

- ☐ **5.** The immunizations prevent the toddler from contracting their associated diseases.

- ☐ **6.** The parents would restrict toddler activity for the remainder of the day.

C Rationale: Minor symptoms, such as soreness at the immunization site and mild fever, can be treated with acetaminophen or ibuprofen. Aspirin would be avoided in children because of its association with Reye's syndrome. The parents would notify the clinic if serious complications (such as a fever above 103°F [39.4°C], seizures, or difficulty breathing) occur. Minor discomforts, such as soreness and mild fever, are common after immunizations. Immunizing the child decreases the health risks associated with contracting certain diseases; it does not prevent the toddler from acquiring them. Although the child may prefer to rest after immunizations, it is not necessary to restrict activity.

Test-taking strategy: Analyze to determine what information the question asks for, which is parent teaching following immunizations. "Select all that apply" questions require considering each option to decide its merit. Note routine standards that can be eliminated for inaccurate information such as providing aspirin to a child and immunizations preventing diseases. Recall the rationale for immunizations and side effects that can occur if you had difficulty answering this question.

Client needs category: Health promotion and maintenance

Client needs subcategory: None

Cognitive level: Applying

6. The emergency room nurse documents the following in the note:

Progress notes

8/11/15	2-year-old brought to the emergency
0800	department by maternal grandparents,
	concerned about multiple physical injuries.
	Grandparents report that toddler has
	multiple bruises on torso and arms which
	were reported as injuries from a recent
	fall by parents.
	—— S. Brown, RN

When completing the documentation, which information would be included? Select all that apply.

☐ **1.** Diagram of site of injuries

☐ **2.** Information about the parent's mental health

☐ **3.** Description, including color and measurement, of injuries

☐ **4.** Quotes from the toddler of what happened

☐ **5.** Documentation of notifying Children and Youth Services

☐ **6.** Objective findings from a thorough head to toe assessment

---

Answer: 1, 3, 6

Ⓓ **Rationale:** The nurse's documentation would include only facts reported in an objective manner. This includes a diagram of the injuries, which includes color and size. The nurse would also include a thorough assessment of all body systems noting any pain or discomfort. Quotes from the grandparent would be included; however, it is not anticipated that a 2-year-old would be able to effectively communicate reliable data. Information regarding the parent's mental health status is not determined to be accurate without personal contact with the parents so that an objective assessment can be made. Hospital social services are typically notified when an issue with potential abuse arises. It is not determined at this time if an abuse has occurred.

Test-taking strategy: Analyze to determine what information the question asks for: which documentation is needed when there are suspicions of abuse? Consider the legal, descriptive documentation needed, which would provide the detail to support or reject a claim of abuse. Rely on standards of care and the Code of Ethics for Nurses for guidance on nonjudgmental documentation. Review how to document suspicions of abuse if you had difficulty answering this question.

Client needs category: Safety and infection control
Client needs subcategory: Management of care
Cognitive level: Applying

---

7. A nurse is assessing the apical impulse of a 28-month-old child. Identify the area where the nurse would locate the apical impulse.

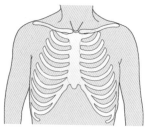

Answer:

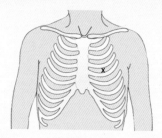

Ⓜ **Rationale:** The heart's apex for a toddler is located at the fourth intercostal space, immediately to the left of the midclavicular line. It is one or two intercostal spaces above what is considered normal for an adult because the heart's position in a child of this age is more horizontal and larger in diameter than that of an adult.

Test-taking strategy: Analyze to determine what information the question asks for, which is anatomical location for the apical pulse. First, identify the point of maximal impulse and then count the number of ribs to identify the intercostal spaces. Review procedure for obtaining an apical pulse if you had difficulty answering this question.

Client needs category: Health promotion and maintenance

Client needs subcategory: None

Cognitive level: Applying

---

8. A nurse is caring for a 3-year-old diagnosed with viral meningitis. Which signs and symptoms would the nurse expect to find during the admission assessment? Select all that apply.

☐ **1.** Bulging anterior fontanelle

☐ **2.** Fever

☐ **3.** Nuchal rigidity

☐ **4.** Petechiae

☐ **5.** Irritability

☐ **6.** Photophobia

Answer: 2, 3, 5, 6

ⓒ Rationale: Common signs and symptoms of viral meningitis include fever, nuchal rigidity, irritability, and photophobia. A bulging anterior fontanelle is a sign of hydrocephalus, which is not likely to occur in a toddler because the anterior fontanelle typically closes by age 24 months. A petechial, purpuric rash may be seen with bacterial meningitis.

Test-taking strategy: Analyze to determine what information the question asks for, which is signs and symptoms associated with viral meningitis. "Select all that apply" questions require considering each option to decide its merit. When determining pediatric assessment questions, always note the child's age to ensure that the symptoms compare with the age. Also, if unsure, use knowledge of terminology to break the word apart (meninges = layer of the brain; itis = inflammation). Review the clinical findings of viral meningitis if you had difficulty answering this question.

Client needs category: Physiological integrity

Client needs subcategory: Physiological adaptation

Cognitive level: Applying

9. The nurse is caring for a 3-year-old client being treated for severe status asthmaticus. After comparing clinical manifestations with laboratory results (reported below), a nurse determines evidence that this client has progressed to which condition?

Progress notes

4/5/16	Client was acutely restless, diaphoretic, and
0600	with SOB at 0530. Dr. T. Smith notified
	and ordered ABG analysis. ABG drawn from
	R radial artery. Stat results as follows: pH
	7.28, PaCO₂ 55 mm Hg (7.3 kPa), HCO₃⁻
	26 mEg/L (26 mmol/L). Dr. Smith with
	client now. ———————— J. Collins, RN.

☐ **1.** Metabolic acidosis

☐ **2.** Respiratory alkalosis

☐ **3.** Respiratory acidosis

☐ **4.** Metabolic alkalosis

Answer: 3

Ⓔ Rationale: A pH less than 7.35 and a partial pressure of arterial carbon dioxide (PaCO₂) greater than 45 mm Hg (6.0 kPa) indicate respiratory acidosis. Status asthmaticus is a medical emergency characterized by respiratory distress. At first, the client hyperventilates; then respiratory alkalosis occurs, followed by metabolic acidosis. If treatment is ineffective or has not begun, symptoms can progress to hypoventilation and respiratory acidosis, both of which are life threatening. A client with respiratory alkalosis would have a pH greater than 7.45 and a PaCO₂ less than 35 mm Hg (4.7 kPa). Metabolic acidosis is characterized by a pH less than 7.35 and a bicarbonate (HCO₃⁻) level less than 22 mEq/L (22 mmol/L). Metabolic alkalosis is characterized by a pH greater than 7.45 and HCO₃⁻ above 26 mEq/L (26 mmol/L).

Test-taking strategy: Analyze to determine what information the question asks for, which is the selection of correct metabolic state coordinating with reported data. Use the data provided and reference ranges to analyze blood gases. If unsure, recall the normal range for blood gas values to determine either acidosis or alkalosis and that the admission disease process is respiratory in nature. Review analysis techniques of ABG (arterial blood gas) values if you had difficulty answering this question.

Client needs subcategory: Physiological integrity

Client needs subcategory: Physiological adaptation

Cognitive level: Analyzing

10. A 30-month-old toddler is being evaluated for a ventricular septal defect (VSD). When teaching the parents about the condition, identify the area where a VSD occurs.

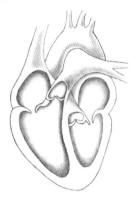

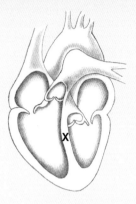

Ⓜ **Rationale:** A VSD is a small hole between the right and left ventricles that allows blood to shunt between them, causing right ventricular hypertrophy and, if left untreated, biventricular heart failure. It is a common congenital heart defect and accounts for approximately 20% to 30% of all heart lesions.

Test-taking strategy: Analyze to determine what information the question asks for, which is anatomical location where a VSD occurs. *Use knowledge of medical terminology to guide to the location (ventricular = ventricles; septal = septum or wall defect or between the two ventricles).* Review congenital heart defects and how blood flow is altered by each defect if you had difficulty answering this question.

Client needs category: Physiological integrity

Client needs subcategory: Physiological adaptation

Cognitive level: Applying

11. A child weighing 44 lb (20 kg) is to receive 45 mg/kg/day of penicillin V potassium oral suspension in four divided doses for every 6 hours. The suspension that is available is penicillin V potassium 125 mg/5 ml. How many milliliters would the nurse administer for each dose? Record your answer using a whole number.

_____ ml

Answer: 9

Ⓔ **Rationale:** First, convert the child's weight to kilograms if not already done:

$$44 \text{ lb} \div 2.2 \text{ kg/lb} = 20 \text{ kg}.$$

Next, determine the daily dose:

$$45 \text{ mg} : 1 \text{ kg} = X \text{ mg} : 20 \text{ kg}$$
$$45 \times 20 = 1 \times X$$
$$900 = X.$$

Then, determine the dose to administer every 6 hours (four doses):

$$900 \text{ mg} \div 4 = 225 \text{ mg}.$$

Finally, determine the volume to be given at each dose:

$$225 \text{ mg} : X = 125 \text{ mg} : 5 \text{ ml}$$
$$1,125 \text{ mg/ml} = 125 \text{ mg}/X$$
$$9 \text{ ml} = X.$$

Test-taking strategy: Analyze to determine what information the question asks for, which is milliliters to be administered per dose. First, recall the conversion of pounds to kilograms. Next, follow the steps above to determine daily dose and then single dose. Use caution to ensure that the question is answered in the proper measuring units such as milliliter per dose administered. Proofread math calculations. Review drug dose calculations if you had difficulty answering this question.

Client needs category: Physiological integrity

Client needs subcategory: Pharmacological and parenteral therapies

Cognitive level: Applying

---

12. A nurse is caring for a 34-month-old who is hospitalized for a lengthy illness. Which behaviors would the nurse identify as examples of expected developmental regression for the child's age group? Select all that apply.

☐ **1.** Enuresis

☐ **2.** Encopresis

☐ **3.** One- to two-word expressions

☐ **4.** Altered gait

☐ **5.** Loss of fine motor skills

Answer: 1, 2, 3

Ⓓ **Rationale:** Enuresis (uncontrolled voiding) and encopresis (uncontrolled stooling) are often seen in toddlers who were previously toilet trained and return to diapers during hospitalization. Language regression with one- to two-word expressions ("baby talk") is often observed during hospitalization. Altered gait and loss of fine motor skills are not typical regressive behaviors; when seen in a child, they may indicate musculoskeletal or neurological problems.

Test-taking strategy: Analyze to determine what information the question asks for, which is behaviors that are characteristic of developmental regression. "Select all that apply" questions require considering each option to decide its merit. Consider each option listed against current age of the child to decide if that milestone has been previously reached. Review the developmental milestones of toddlers, which may regress if hospitalized, if you had difficulty answering this question.

Client needs category: Health promotion and maintenance

Client needs subcategory: None

Cognitive level: Applying

---

13. A nurse is caring for a group of toddlers in a large urban hospital. When considering providing care, which clients require contact precautions? Select all that apply.

☐ **1.** A toddler with scabies

☐ **2.** A toddler with mumps

☐ **3.** A toddler with streptococcal pharyngitis

☐ **4.** A toddler with pulmonary tuberculosis

☐ **5.** A toddler with a multidrug-resistant organism

Answer: 1, 5

Ⓜ Rationale: According to the Centers for Disease Control and Infection Prevention and Control Canada, in addition to standard precautions, contact isolation precautions are used for clients with known or suspected infections. Scabies is a skin infection and requires contact precautions. Multidrug-resistant infection also requires contact precautions because of potential contamination. A toddler with mumps or streptococcal pharyngitis requires droplet precautions. Pulmonary tuberculosis requires airborne precautions.

Test-taking strategy: Analyze to determine what information the question asks for, which is determining conditions that need to be placed in contact isolation. "Select all that apply" questions require considering each option to decide its merit. Recall that contact isolation means that the client is preferred to be in a private room with disposable equipment if possible, and gowns and gloves are required and removed prior to leaving the room. Review the pathophysiology of the listed diseases and transmission-based precautions if you had difficulty answering this question.

Client needs category: Safe and effective care environment

Client needs subcategory: Safety and infection control

Cognitive level: Applying

14. A nurse, on the pediatric unit, received shift handoff on a 15-month-old with the following needs. Using Maslow's hierarchy framework, prioritize the following nursing care activities for the toddler. All options must be used.

1. Progressing the diet after surgery

2. Clearing the airway of thick secretions

3. Changing a soiled diaper

4. Administering antipyretics for an axillary temperature of 103°F (39.4°C)

5. Notifying the practitioner about suspected compartment syndrome

Answer: 2, 5, 3, 4, 1

D **Rationale:** According to Maslow's hierarchy framework, the five categories, or hierarchy of needs in order of priority, are as follows: physiologic needs, safety, love, esteem, and self-actualization. Within the physiologic needs category are the essentials for existence: air, nutrition, water, elimination, sleep and rest, thermoregulation, and sex. Therefore, maintaining a patent airway is the first priority, followed by notifying the practitioner of suspected compartment syndrome because of the risk of loss of limb. Changing a soiled diaper would be next because this is necessary to prevent skin breakdown. Administering antipyretics for fever primarily provides comfort to the child. The lowest priority, although important, is progressing the child's diet following surgery.

Test-taking strategy: Analyze to determine what information the question asks for, which is prioritizing the care of a toddler. Recall Maslow's hierarchy of needs and the levels that guide decision making about care. Consider that clearing an airway is typically a top priority, followed by potential safety concerns. Review Maslow's hierarchy of needs associated with a variety of client scenarios if you had difficulty answering this question.

Client needs category: Safe and effective care environment

Client needs subcategory: Management of care

Cognitive level: Applying

15. The nurse is preparing to insert an intravenous catheter into an acutely ill toddler. Place the following steps in the order the nurse would follow. All options must be used.

1. Wash hands and gather supplies.

2. Prepare the equipment.

3. Inform the toddler of the procedure.

4. Inform the parents of the procedure.

5. Select and prep the appropriate site.

6. Insert the intravenous catheter and secure it appropriately.

Answer: 4, 1, 2, 3, 5, 6

C **Rationale:** It is important to inform the parents and gain their support for the procedure first, especially if the child is acutely ill. A toddler does not understand the concept of time, so the nurse would not inform the toddler until very shortly before the catheter insertion. Next, the nurse would wash hands and prepare the supplies and equipment, keeping them out of the child's sight to decrease anxiety. Finally, the nurse would inform the toddler of what is about to happen and then perform the procedure by selecting and prepping the site, inserting the catheter, and securing it.

Test-taking strategy: Analyze to determine what information the question asks for, which is considerations when performing a procedure on a toddler. Use knowledge of growth and development and psychosocial skills to plan care realizing that skill and efficiency are important. For any invasive procedure, informed consent, which would be provided by the parents, is completed first. Next, the efficient nurse prepares and gathers all supplies. Lastly, the child is told and the procedure completed. Review prioritizing nursing actions for a toddler if you had difficulty answering this question.

Client needs category: Physiological integrity

Client needs subcategory: Basic care and comfort

Cognitive level: Applying

The preschooler

1. A 4½-year-old is ordered to receive 25 ml/hour of intravenous solution. The nurse is using a pediatric microdrip chamber (60 gtts/min) to administer the medication. For how many drops per minute would the microdrip chamber be set? Record your answer using a whole number.

_____ drops/minute

Answer: 25

Ⓜ **Rationale:** When using a pediatric microdrip chamber (60 gtts/minute), the number of milliliters per hour equals the number of drops per minute. If 25 ml/hour is ordered, the solution would infuse at 25 drops/minute.

For example:

$$\frac{\text{Volume} \times \text{drip factor}}{\text{Minutes}} = \text{gtts/minute}.$$

Thus, if the drip factor on a microdrip tubing is 60 and the infusion time is 60 minutes, these cancel and the answer is the volume (ml).

Test-taking strategy: Analyze to determine what information the question asks for, which is the number of drops per minute. Use the math calculation above and quick check to provide the answer. Be sure that the tubing is a microdrip set to be able to use the quick check of canceling the microdrip and time per hour. Review intravenous infusion rates if you had difficulty answering this question.

Client needs category: Physiological integrity

Client needs subcategory: Pharmacological and parenteral therapies

Cognitive level: Applying

2. While assessing a child experiencing respiratory distress, the nurse notes subcostal retractions. Which graphic highlights (in blue) the area where subcostal retractions are seen?

☐ **1.**

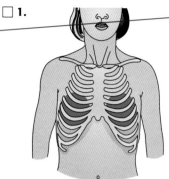

☐ **2.**

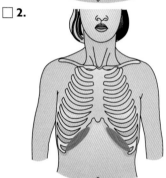

☐ **3.**

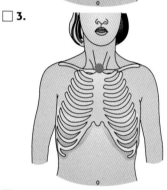

☐ **4.**

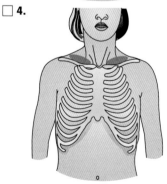

Answer: 2

ⓔ Rationale: Subcostal retractions are retractions seen below the lower costal margin of the rib cage. Option 2 highlights the area where subcostal retractions are seen. Option 1 shows the areas where intercostal retractions would be seen. Option 3 shows the area for suprasternal retraction. Option 4 shows the areas for clavicular retractions.

Test-taking strategy: Analyze to determine what information the question asks for, which is location of subcostal retractions. Use knowledge of medical terminology to guide to the location (sub = below; costal = ribs). Review the definition of retractions and the anatomical landmarks associated if you had difficulty answering this question.

Client needs category: Physiological integrity
Client needs subcategory: Physiological adaptation
Cognitive level: Applying

3. A nurse is completing a screening tool on a 4½-year-old child. To be consistent with others at this age, what behaviors would the nurse expect the child to demonstrate? Select all that apply.

- ☐ **1.** The child balances on each foot for at least 6 seconds.
- ☐ **2.** The child copies a circle that is closed or very nearly closed.
- ☐ **3.** The child speaks clearly.
- ☐ **4.** The child draws a person with at least three body parts.
- ☐ **5.** The child is able to follow one basic instruction through completion.

Answer: 2, 3, 4, 5

ⓓ Rationale: By age 4½, a child would be able to copy a circle, speak clearly, and draw a person with at least three body parts. If given an appropriate task, the child is able to follow an instruction through completion. The majority of children do not achieve balancing on each foot for 6 seconds until about age 5½.

Test-taking strategy: Analyze to determine what information the question asks for, which is anticipated behaviors of a 4½-year-old. "Select all that apply" questions require considering each option to decide its merit. Recall that cognitive growth is substantial during these years, and each year during this period marks a major step forward in cognitive, gross motor, fine motor, and language development. If unsure, consider that preschoolers draw circles and stick figures and are able to communicate through speaking but are uncoordinated at this age. Review the growth and development for preschoolers if you had difficulty answering this question.

Client needs category: Health promotion and maintenance

Client needs subcategory: None

Cognitive level: Analyzing

---

4. The nurse is caring for a 4-year-old recently diagnosed with acute lymphocytic leukemia (ALL). Which statement, made by the parents, indicates the effectiveness of teaching? Select all that apply.

- ☐ **1.** "I read that ALL is a rare form of childhood leukemia."
- ☐ **2.** "I understand that ALL affects all blood-forming organs and systems throughout the body."
- ☐ **3.** "Because of the increased risk of bleeding, I will eliminate evening teeth brushing."
- ☐ **4.** "I realize that the adverse effects of chemo-therapy include sleepiness, alopecia, and stomatitis."
- ☐ **5.** "I am glad that there's a 95% chance of obtaining a first remission with treatment."
- ☐ **6.** "I will not discipline my child during this dif-ficult time."

Answer: 2, 4, 5

ⓓ Rationale: Acute lymphocytic leukemia (ALL) is the most common form of leukemia. In ALL, immature white blood cells (WBCs) crowd out healthy WBCs, red blood cells, and platelets in the bone marrow. These abnormal WBCs affect all blood-forming organs and systems. Common adverse effects of chemotherapy and radiation include nausea, vomiting, diarrhea, sleepiness, alopecia, anemia, stomatitis, pain, and increased susceptibility to infection. A first remission occurs in about 95% of cases. Brushing teeth does not result in increased or abnormal bleeding. A child with leukemia still needs appropriate discipline and limits because a lack of consistent parenting may lead to negative behaviors and fear.

Test-taking strategy: Analyze to determine what information the question asks for, which is accurate statements, made by the parent, regarding issues of ALL. "Select all that apply" questions require considering each option to decide its merit. Consider each option for a correct statement. Review the pathophysiology of ALL and parent teaching guidelines if you had difficulty answering this question.

Client needs category: Physiological integrity

Client needs subcategory: Reduction of risk potential

Cognitive level: Applying

---

5. A 5-year-old is admitted to the pediatric unit with diagnosis of possible intussusception. Which assessment data supports this diagnosis? Select all that apply.

☐ **1.** Currant jelly stools

☐ **2.** Diarrhea

☐ **3.** Abdominal pain

☐ **4.** Tarry, black stools

☐ **5.** Abdominal distention

Answer: 1, 3, 5

Ⓜ **Rationale:** Intussusception is when a portion of the intestine telescopes into another part of the intestine causing the walls of the intestine to press against each other. Inflammation, edema, and hemorrhage occur leading to abdominal symptoms of currant jelly stools (a combination of blood and mucus); abdominal pain, which is sharp at times; and abdominal distention. Constipation, not diarrhea, is also common from the swelling and obstructive flow of stool. Tarry, black stools are common in intestinal bleeding and ulcers.

Test-taking strategy: Analyze to determine what information the question asks for, which is symptoms characteristic of intussusception. Relate intussusception and telescoping limiting blood flow. Review the pathophysiology and signs and symptoms of intussusception if you had difficulty answering this question.

Client needs category: Physiological integrity

Client needs subcategory: Physiological adaptation

Cognitive level: Applying

---

6. A critically ill 4-year-old is in the pediatric intensive care unit. Telemetry monitoring reveals junctional tachycardia. Identify where this arrhythmia originates.

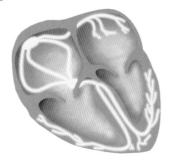

Answer:

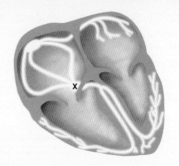

Ⓜ **Rationale:** In junctional tachycardia, the atrioventricular node fires rapidly. The atria are depolarized by retrograde conduction; however, conduction through the ventricles remains normal.

Test-taking strategy: Analyze to determine what information the question asks for, which is site for the origination of junctional tachycardia. Recall that tachycardia is an increase in the heart rate as controlled by the atrioventricular node or the electrical control system of heart contractions. Review the heart's anatomy, physiology, and conduction system if you had difficulty answering this question.

Client needs category: Physiological integrity

Client needs subcategory: Physiological adaptation

Cognitive level: Applying

7. A school nurse is gathering registration data for a child entering first grade. Which immunizations would the school nurse verify that the child has had? Select all that apply.

☐ **1.** Influenza vaccine

☐ **2.** Diphtheria–tetanus–pertussis series

☐ **3.** *H. influenzae* type b series

☐ **4.** Varicella vaccine

☐ **5.** Pneumonia vaccine

☐ **6.** Oral polio series

Ⓓ **Rationale:** The exact immunization schedule differs between the United States and Canadian provinces, but there are many similarities. Diphtheria–tetanus–pertussis series, *H. influenzae* type b series, varicella, and inactivated (not oral) polio series are the immunizations that the child would receive before entering first grade. The oral polio vaccine was discontinued; the safer IPV is now used. Pneumonia vaccine is not required or routinely given to children.

Test-taking strategy: Analyze to determine what information the question asks for, which is immunizations needed to begin school. "Select all that apply" questions require considering each option to decide its merit. Consider immunization received in childhood as the basis of those needed prior to school. These vaccines are typically those administered from birth, as infants and then in preschool years. Review immunization and infection control recommendations provided by the American Academy of Pediatrics, Centers for Disease Control and Prevention, and the Canadian Public Health Agency if you had difficulty answering this question.

Client needs category: Physiological integrity

Client needs subcategory: Physiological adaptation

Cognitive level: Analyzing

8. A 4-year-old child is brought to the emergency department in cardiac arrest. During CPR, identify the area where the child's pulse would be assessed.

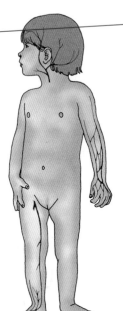

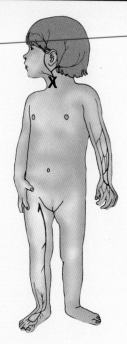

Ⓜ Rationale: The carotid artery would be used to assess for a pulse when performing CPR on children and adults. The brachial pulse would be used when performing CPR on an infant.

Test-taking strategy: Analyze to determine what information the question asks for, which is site for assessment of a pulse during the child's CPR. Consider that children have the same assessment site for a pulse as do adults. The rationale for the change in pulse site for infants is because of the shortness of the neck. Review the recommendations for CPR in infants, children, and adults if you had difficulty answering this question.

Client needs category: Physiological integrity
Client needs subcategory: Physiological adaptation
Cognitive level: Understanding

9. A nurse is caring preoperatively for a preschooler scheduled for a Wilms' tumor removal. When explaining the location of the tumor to the parents, identify the area of the urinary system impacted.

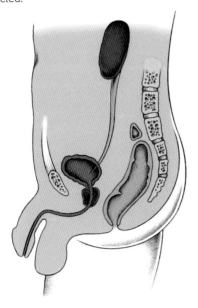

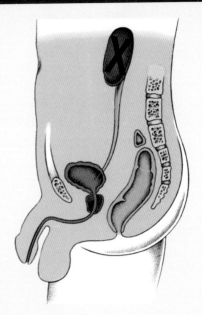

Ⓜ Rationale: Wilms' tumor, also known as a nephroblastoma, is located on the kidney. The most common intra-abdominal tumor in children, Wilms' tumor, usually affects children aged 6 months to 4 years and favors the left kidney.

Test-taking strategy: Analyze to determine what information the question asks for, which is location of a Wilms' tumor. Since this is a common pediatric tumor, memorization of the location, signs and symptoms, and nursing actions is important. Review the anatomy of the urinary system and the pathophysiology of Wilms' tumor if you had difficulty answering this question.

Client needs category: Physiological integrity

Client needs subcategory: Physiological adaptation

Cognitive level: Applying

10. A nurse is caring for a 5-year-old child who is in the terminal stages of cancer. Which statements about the child's impending death are **most** likely to be true? Select all that apply.

☐ **1.** The parents may be at different stages of grief in dealing with the child's impending death.

☐ **2.** The child is thinking about the future and knows he/she may not be able to participate.

☐ **3.** The dying child may become clingy and act like a toddler.

☐ **4.** Whispering in the child's room will help the child to cope.

☐ **5.** The death of a child may have long-term disruptive effects on the family.

☐ **6.** The child does not fully understand the concept of death.

Answer: 1, 3, 5, 6

Ⓒ Rationale: When dealing with a dying child, parents may be at different stages of grief at different times. The child may regress in behaviors. The stress of a child's death commonly results in divorce of parents and behavioral problems in siblings. Preschoolers see illness and death as a form of punishment. They fear separation from parents and might worry about who will provide care for them. Preschoolers have only a rudimentary concept of time; thinking about the future is typical of an adolescent facing death, not a preschooler. Whispering in front of the child only increases fear of death.

Test-taking strategy: Analyze to determine what information the question asks for, which is correct statements about a child's impending death. "Select all that apply" questions require considering each option to decide its merit. Recall the stages of the grief process (adults and children) and developmental stage of preschoolers when selecting an option. Review psychosocial concepts associated with childhood death if you had difficulty answering this question.

Client needs category: Psychosocial integrity

Client needs subcategory: None

Cognitive level: Analyzing

---

11. A 3-year-old boy has arrived in the emergency department. The nurse documents the following assessment findings in the client's chart, knowing that they are consistent with which disease process?

Progress notes	
5/15/15 1100	Client admitted to ER with T. 103.6° F (39.8° C), HR 100, RR 24. Respirations are shallow, and breath sounds are decreased, with rales auscultated on the right side. Client has a harsh cough and mother states he has had a discolored productive cough at home.————————S. Jones, RN

☐ **1.** Bronchiolitis

☐ **2.** Pneumonia

☐ **3.** Asthma

☐ **4.** Cystic fibrosis

Answer: 2

Ⓜ Rationale: The elevated fever, shallow respirations, decreased breath sounds, rales, harsh cough, and productive mucus are findings associated with pneumonia. Typically, there is no fever with asthma and cystic fibrosis, and bronchiolitis presents with a low-grade fever. Wheezing is associated with asthma and bronchiolitis; however, this was not found upon physical examination of this client. Bronchiolitis produces a dry cough, and pneumonia causes a productive, harsh cough. The client with cystic fibrosis typically presents with wheezing, rhonchi, and thick, tenacious mucus.

Test-taking strategy: Analyze to determine what information the question asks for, which is assessment findings associated with a respiratory disease process. Compare and contrast the clinical findings as documented to the findings associated with the illness. Focus on specific details such as temperature and breath sounds that either confirm or disprove a disease process. Review disorders of the respiratory tract if you had difficulty answering this question.

Client needs category: Physiological integrity

Client needs subcategory: Physiological adaptation

Cognitive level: Analyzing

12. A 4-year-old postoperative child is found unresponsive. Place the following actions in the correct sequence to perform CPR after the child has been assessed for responsiveness and help has been called. All options must be used.

1. Open the airway.

2. Feel for the carotid pulse.

3. Check for breathing.

4. Perform 30 compressions.

5. Provide 2 rescue breaths.

D Rationale: Following the 2015 American Heart Association guidelines for CPR, the rescuer would activate the emergency response system and get an automatic external defibrillator (AED) or appoint another person to do this. The next step is to check the pulse for no more than 10 seconds. If no pulse is detected, the rescuer gives 30 chest compressions. Next, the rescuer opens the airway with the head tilt–chin lift or jaw thrust maneuver and checks for breathing. If breathing is not detected, the rescuer gives 2 rescue breaths and immediately resumes chest compressions at a cycle of 30 compressions to 2 breaths. The rescuer would use the AED as soon as it arrives.

Test-taking strategy: Analyze to determine what information the question asks for, which is the sequence for CPR on a child. Visualize the steps in the process by first determining the need for CPR, then circulating blood through manual compressions, and lastly providing breaths. Review the CPR steps and checking the ABCs (airway, breathing, and circulation) if you had difficulty answering this question.

Client needs category: Physiological integrity

Client needs subcategory: Physiological adaptation

Cognitive level: Applying

13. A nurse is caring for a 4-year-old child who developed acute renal failure after a traumatic injury with hemorrhaging. Place the following events in the order in which they most likely occurred during progression of the severe renal deterioration. All options must be used.

1. Acidosis

2. Severe hypocalcemia

3. Azotemia

4. Oliguria

D Rationale: The first symptom of acute renal failure is oliguria (urine output less than 1 ml/kg of the child's body weight per hour). The inability to produce urine causes azotemia, an accumulation of nitrogen waste in the bloodstream, which leads to rising blood urea nitrogen levels. This leads to acidosis because of the body's inability to excrete H^+ ions. The acidotic state results in hyperphosphatemia (high phosphorus levels), which in turn causes hypocalcemia (low calcium levels). When hypocalcemia is severe, muscle twitching and tetany can occur.

Test-taking strategy: Analyze to determine what information the question asks for, which is sequence of events during acute renal failure. Consider the definition of each term and place from simple to complex. Note that as the disease process continues, more symptoms become involved. Review the pathophysiology of acute renal failure if you had difficulty answering this question.

Client needs category: Physiological integrity

Client needs subcategory: Physiological adaptation

Cognitive level: Analyzing

The school-aged child

1. A 7-year-old child is admitted to the hospital for a course of intravenous antibiotics. What actions would the nurse take before inserting the peripheral intravenous catheter? Select all that apply.

☐ **1.** Explain the procedure to the child immediately before the procedure.

☐ **2.** Apply a topical anesthetic to the I.V. site before the procedure.

☐ **3.** Ask the child which hand he/she uses for drawing.

☐ **4.** Explain the procedure to the child using abstract terms.

☐ **5.** Do not let the child see the equipment to be used in the procedure.

☐ **6.** Tell the child that the procedure will not hurt.

Answer: 2, 3

Ⓒ Rationale: Topical anesthetics reduce the pain of a venipuncture. The cream would be applied about 1 hour before the procedure and requires a health care provider's order. The intravenous catheter would be inserted into the hand opposite the one the child identifies as his/her drawing hand. The procedure would be explained to the child in simple, concrete words well before it takes place so that he/she has time to ask questions. Unfamiliar terms would be defined. To help ease anxiety, the child would be shown the equipment that will be used for the procedure. The use of dolls for role-play can also be utilized. Although the topical anesthetic will relieve some pain, there is usually some pain or discomfort involved in venipuncture, so the child would not be told otherwise.

Test-taking strategy: Analyze to determine what information the question asks for, which is nursing actions related to peripheral intravenous catheter insertion. "Select all that apply" questions require considering each option to decide its merit. Visualize the steps in placing an intravenous catheter and then consider the age-appropriate adjustments needed for a school-aged pediatric client. Recall that the cognitive development of a school-aged child is concrete operational thinking. Review the nursing process for administration of intravenous fluids to a school-aged child if you had difficulty answering this question.

Client needs category: Health promotion and maintenance
Client needs subcategory: None
Cognitive level: Applying

2. A mother brings her child to the health care provider's office for evaluation of chronic stomach pain. The mother states that the pain seems to go away when she keeps the child home from school. The health care provider diagnoses school phobia. Which other behaviors or symptoms may the child exhibit? Select all that apply.

☐ **1.** Nausea

☐ **2.** Headaches

☐ **3.** Weight loss

☐ **4.** Dizziness

☐ **5.** Fever

ⓒ Rationale: Children with school phobia commonly complain of vague symptoms, such as stomachaches, nausea, headaches, and dizziness, to avoid going to school. These symptoms typically do not occur on weekends. A careful history must be taken to identify a pattern of school avoidance. Weight loss and fever are more likely to have a physiological cause and are uncommon in children with school phobia.

Test-taking strategy: Analyze to determine what information the question asks for, which is symptoms of school phobia. "Select all that apply" questions require considering each option to decide its merit. Relate school phobia to symptoms of anxiety as the children are anxious about going to school. Recall that anxiety and fears manifest with acute episodes of symptoms (such as gastrointestinal problems). Review symptoms associated with school phobia if you had difficulty answering this question.

Client needs category: Psychosocial integrity

Client needs subcategory: None

Cognitive level: Applying

3. A child with sickle cell anemia is being discharged after treatment for a crisis. Which instructions for avoiding future crises would the nurse provide to the child and family? Select all that apply.

☐ **1.** Avoid foods high in folic acid.

☐ **2.** Drink plenty of fluids.

☐ **3.** Use cold packs to relieve joint pain.

☐ **4.** Report a sore throat to an adult immediately.

☐ **5.** Restrict activity to quiet board games.

☐ **6.** Wash hands before meals and after playing.

Answer: 2, 4, 6

Ⓜ **Rationale:** Sickle cell anemia is an autosomal recessive genetic disease passed down through families in which red blood cells form an abnormal sickle or crescent shape. Fluids would be encouraged to prevent stasis in the bloodstream, which can lead to sickling. Sore throats and all other cold symptoms would be reported promptly because they may indicate an infection, which can precipitate a crisis (red blood cells sickle and obstruct blood flow to tissues). Children with sickle cell anemia would learn appropriate measures to prevent infection, such as proper hand-washing techniques and good nutrition. Folic acid intake would be encouraged to help support new cell growth; new cells replace fragile sickled cells. Warm packs would be applied to promote comfort and relieve pain; cold packs cause vasoconstriction. The child would maintain an active, normal life but would avoid excessive exercise, which can precipitate an attack. When the child experiences a crisis, he/she will typically limit his/her own activity according to the pain level.

Test-taking strategy: Analyze to determine what information the question asks for, which is nursing instructions helpful to avoid a sickle cell crisis. "Select all that apply" questions require considering each option to decide its merit. Recall that infants and children are at an increased risk for a crisis because of exposure to various bacterial infections, which could cause dehydration and infection. Daily penicillin therapy may be prescribed. Also, encouraging fluids such as water is important as a daily routine, especially during the summer when outside playing. Review the events that may trigger a sickle cell crisis if you had difficulty answering this question.

Client needs category: Physiological integrity

Client needs subcategory: Reduction of risk potential

Cognitive level: Applying

---

4. A nurse is preparing to administer intravenous methylprednisolone sodium succinate to a child who weighs 42 lb. The order is for 0.03 mg/kg intravenously daily. How many milligrams would the nurse prepare? Record your answer using one decimal place.

_____ mg

Answer: 0.6

Ⓔ **Rationale:** To perform this dosage calculation, the nurse would first convert the child's weight to kilograms:

$$44 \text{ lb} \div 2.2 \text{ kg/lb} = 20 \text{ kg}.$$

Then, the nurse would use this formula to determine the dose:

$$20 \text{ kg} \times 0.03 \text{ mg/kg} = X \text{ mg}$$
$$X = 0.6 \text{ mg}.$$

Test-taking strategy: Analyze to determine what information the question asks for, which is dosage of methylprednisolone sodium succinate. First, recall the conversion of pounds to kilograms. Next, follow the steps above to determine the single dose. Use caution to ensure that the question is answered in the proper measuring units such as milligram per dose administered. Proofread math calculations. Review drug dose calculations if you had difficulty answering this question.

Client needs category: Physiological integrity

Client needs subcategory: Pharmacological and parenteral therapies

Cognitive level: Applying

---

5. A nurse is caring for an 8-year-old postoperative tonsillectomy client. When performing a postoperative assessment, which signs and symptoms of bleeding would be monitored for by the nurse? Select all that apply.

☐ **1.** Frequent clearing of the throat

☐ **2.** Breathing through the mouth

☐ **3.** Frequent swallowing

☐ **4.** Sleeping for long intervals

☐ **5.** Pulse rate of 98 beats/minute

☐ **6.** Blood red vomitus

Answer: 1, 3, 6

Ⓜ Rationale: A classic sign of bleeding after tonsillectomy is frequent swallowing; this occurs because blood drips down the back of the throat, tickling it. Other signs include frequent clearing of the throat and vomiting of bright red blood. Vomiting of dark blood may occur if the child swallowed blood during surgery, but this does not indicate postoperative bleeding. Breathing through the mouth is common because of dried secretions in the nares. Sleeping for long intervals is normal after receiving sedation and anesthesia. A pulse rate of 98 beats/minute is in the normal range for this age group.

Test-taking strategy: Analyze to determine what information the question asks for, which is signs of postoperative tonsillectomy bleeding. "Select all that apply" questions require considering each option to decide its merit. Consider the location of the tonsils and what sign may be present if there was bleeding. Bleeding at the rear of the oral cavity would lead to clearing of the throat, swallowing, and bright red bleeding down the gastrointestinal tract. Review the postoperative management of a child after a tonsillectomy and the signs and symptoms of complications if you had difficulty answering this question.

Client needs category: Physiological integrity

Client needs subcategory: Reduction of risk potential

Cognitive level: Applying

6. A 6-year-old child who reports fever, malaise, and anorexia is diagnosed with varicella (chickenpox). The nurse explains to the parents how skin lesions will develop. Place the following descriptions in the order that they will occur as the disease progresses. All options must be used.

1. As initial lesions progress through stages, new lesions form on the trunk and extremities.

2. Papules develop into clear vesicles on an erythematous base.

3. Itchy red macules on the face, scalp, and trunk progress to papules.

4. Vesicles become cloudy and break easily.

5. Scabs form.

Answer: 3, 2, 4, 5, 1

D **Rationale:** Varicella (chickenpox) is a common childhood illness, which is usually mild but can be serious. Fever, malaise, and anorexia occur 24 to 48 hours before a rash develops. The rash begins as itchy red macules on the face, scalp, and trunk. These macules progress to papules, which develop into clear vesicles on an erythematous base. The vesicles become cloudy and break, forming scabs. New lesions continue to form on the trunk and extremities.

Test-taking strategy: Analyze to determine what information the question asks for, which is sequence of chickenpox. If unsure, identify the first and last option to narrow the middle options. Consider the development of the clear to cloudy vesicles before being scabbed. Review the pathophysiology of varicella and characteristics of lesions if you had difficulty answering this question.

Client needs category: Physiological integrity
Client needs subcategory: Basic care and comfort
Cognitive level: Analyzing

---

7. The school nurse is assessing the chest of a first-grade child and notes a pectus excavatum. Which graphic depicts this abnormality?

☐ **1.**
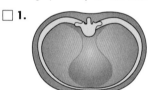

☐ **2.**
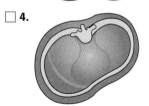

☐ **3.**
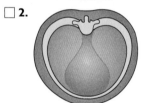

☐ **4.**
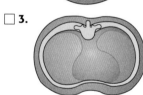

Answer: 3

M **Rationale:** Pectus excavatum is an indentation of the lower portion of the sternum (option 3). Option 1 shows a normal chest contour. Option 2 shows a barrel chest contour. Option 4 shows a thoracic scoliosis chest contour.

Test-taking strategy: Analyze to determine what information the question asks for, which is the graphic that denotes a pectus excavatum. Use knowledge of medical terminology (pectus = chest, excavatum = hollow) to determine the type of abnormality and then compare with the illustration. Review disorders of the thoracic region if you had difficulty answering this question.

Client needs category: Physiological integrity
Client needs subcategory: Reduction of risk potential
Cognitive level: Applying

8. A 10-year-old child visits the pediatrician's office for an annual sports examination. When a nurse asks how he is doing, he becomes quiet and states that his grandmother died last week. Which statements by the child show that he understands the concept of death? Select all that apply.

- ☐ **1.** "I am mad that she is gone."
- ☐ **2.** "All people must die."
- ☐ **3.** "My grandmother's death has been hard to understand."
- ☐ **4.** "My grandmother died because she was sick and nothing could make her better."
- ☐ **5.** "My grandmother is dead, but she'll come back."
- ☐ **6.** "My grandmother died because someone in the family did something bad."

Answer: 1, 3, 4

Ⓜ **Rationale:** By age 10, most children understand the reality of death and know that death is irreversible and final. However, a child may still have difficulty understanding the death of a specific loved one or understanding that children can die. School-aged children should be able to identify cause-and-effect relationships, such as when a terminal illness causes someone to die. Adolescents, not school-aged children, understand that death is a universal process. Preschoolers see death as temporary and may think of it as a punishment. Different cultures prepare children on death differently.

Test-taking strategy: Analyze to determine what information the question asks for, which is a 10-year-old's concept of death. "Select all that apply" questions require considering each option to decide its merit. Recall the cognitive stages of development for a school-aged child as having a more realistic understanding of death. They may be curious about the physical process of death and what happens after a person dies. Review children's concept of death at various ages if you had difficulty answering this question.

Client needs category: Psychosocial integrity
Client needs subcategory: None
Cognitive level: Analyzing

---

9. The nurse is caring for an 11-year-old client experiencing status epilepticus. When providing and delegating immediate nursing care, which nursing actions would be completed? Select all that apply.

- ☐ **1.** Administer oxygen via nasal cannula.
- ☐ **2.** Pad side rails with pillows.
- ☐ **3.** Instruct the nursing assistant to obtain the crash cart.
- ☐ **4.** Place the bed in the lowest position and restrain all extremities.
- ☐ **5.** Instruct the licensed practical/vocational nurse (LPN/VN) to obtain vital signs.
- ☐ **6.** Open clenched mouth to place an oral airway.

Answer: 1, 2, 5

Ⓒ **Rationale:** The nurse caring for a client experiencing status epilepticus is focused on safety and client stabilization. Client safety is ensured with padded side rails, so the client has little possibility of falling or hitting the body during the seizure activity. Vital signs are an important assessment tool. Oxygen is administered via nasal cannula placement. CPR is not anticipated during seizure activity. Neither restraining the client nor opening a clenched mouth is acceptable nursing care, and these may further injure the client.

Test-taking strategy: Analyze to determine what information the question asks for, which is immediate nursing actions during a status epilepticus event. Consider priority ABCs of emergency situations and/or Maslow's hierarchy of needs. Both identify maintaining the airway and oxygenation. Recall that seizure activity requires increased oxygen demand because of the physical nature of muscle contraction. Safety is also a priority and an essential portion of Maslow's hierarchy of needs. Review priority nursing actions during status epilepticus if you had difficulty answering this question.

Client needs category: Physiological integrity
Client needs subcategory: Physiological adaptation
Cognitive level: Applying

10. A child with sickle cell anemia is being treated for sickle cell crisis. The physician orders morphine sulfate 2 mg intravenously. The concentration of the vial is 10 mg/1 ml of solution. How many milliliters of solution would the nurse administer? Record your answer using one decimal place.

_____ ml

E **Rationale:** The nurse would calculate the volume to be given using this ratio and proportion equation and solving for *X*:

$$2 \text{ mg}/X \text{ ml} = 10 \text{ mg}/1 \text{ ml}$$

$$\frac{10 \text{ mg} \times X}{10 \text{ mg}} = \frac{2 \text{ mg} \times 1 \text{ ml}}{10 \text{ mg}}$$

$$X = 0.2 \text{ ml.}$$

Test-taking strategy: Analyze to determine what information the question asks for, which is the amount of milliliters of medication to be administered to the client. Use the ratio proportion equation above. Make sure that the milligram per milliliter matches between the known proportions and unknown on both sides of the equation. Proofread the math calculation. Review the unit doses for medications and how to calculate fractional doses if you had difficulty answering this question.

Client needs category: Physiological integrity

Client needs subcategory: Pharmacological and parenteral therapies

Cognitive level: Applying

11. The pediatric cardiac nurse is assessing the heart sounds of a 3-year-old child with a mitral valve regurgitation. Which graphic shows the area where the nurse would assess the site of the insufficiency?

☐ **1.**

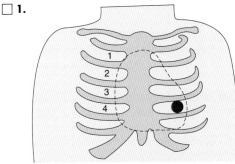

☐ **2.**

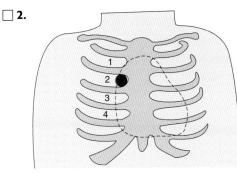

☐ **3.**

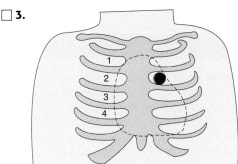

☐ **4.**

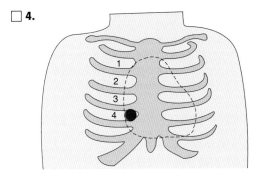

Ⓜ **Rationale:** Mitral valve regurgitation or insufficiency is a heart disorder where the mitral valve does not close properly when the heart pumps out blood, thus causing an abnormal leaking of blood from the left ventricle through the mitral valve and into the left atrium. The mitral valve is heard best at the fourth left intercostal space at the nipple line (option 1). The aortic valve is heard best at the second intercostal space to the right of the sternum (option 2). The pulmonic valve is heard best at the second intercostal space to the left of the sternum (option 3). The tricuspid valve is heard best in the fourth intercostal space to the right of the sternum (option 4).

Test-taking strategy: Analyze to determine what information the question asks for, which is the location of the mitral valve. Recall that the mitral valve is like a one-way gate helping blood flow in one direction through the heart. Recall that the mitral valve is on the left side of the heart and allows blood flow from the upper to the lower chambers. Review where each heart valve is located if you had difficulty answering this question.

Client needs category: Physiological integrity

Client needs subcategory: Reduction of risk potential

Cognitive level: Analyzing

12. An 11-year-old girl comes into the health care provider's office stating dysuria. The nurse suspects a urinary tract infection. Which finding on the laboratory report is consistent with a urinary tract infection?

Laboratory Results

Test: Urinalysis
Date: 07/16/15   **Time collected:** 0700

Parameter	Results
Color	Pale yellow
Turbidity	Clear
pH	7.8
Specific gravity	1.015
Protein	Negative
Glucose	Positive
Ketones	Positive
Red blood cells	<1 per high-power field
White blood cells	20 per high-power field
Casts	None

☐ **1.** WBCs: 20 per high-power field

☐ **2.** pH 7.8

☐ **3.** Ketones: positive

☐ **4.** Glucose: positive

Answer: 1

Rationale: Urinary tract infections are more common in school-aged girls than in school-aged boys. A normal urinalysis would show less than 5 WBCs per high-power field. An elevated WBC count of 20 is an indication of bacteria and urinary tract infection. The normal range of urinary pH is 4.6 to 8.0. The presence of glucose or ketones in the urine does not indicate a urinary tract infection but may indicate diabetes mellitus.

Test-taking strategy: Analyze to determine what information the question asks for, which is laboratory evidence of a urinary tract infection. Discriminate through the lab report for abnormal results and then identify if that result would indicate a urinary tract infection. Review the normal and abnormal findings for a urinalysis if you had difficulty answering this question.

Client needs category: Physiological integrity
Client needs subcategory: Reduction of risk potential
Cognitive level: Analyzing

---

13. A 10-year-old child is admitted to the hospital with a temperature of 104°F (40°C) and is difficult to arouse. The child has a history of varicella 2 weeks ago. Reye's syndrome is suspected. Which objective data are supportive of the diagnosis? Select all that apply.

☐ **1.** Dysuria

☐ **2.** An abnormal liver biopsy

☐ **3.** Vomiting

☐ **4.** Client states, "I have a headache"

☐ **5.** Coma

☐ **6.** Disorientation

Answer: 2, 3, 5, 6

Rationale: Reye's syndrome is an acute multisystem disorder that causes encephalopathy and predominately affects school-aged children. Symptoms develop within a few days to weeks after a viral infection (varicella), beginning with vomiting, sleepiness, and liver dysfunction. About 24 to 48 hours after onset of symptoms, the child's condition rapidly deteriorates, causing disorientation, hallucinations, and sometimes a coma with decorticate posturing. The coma may progress to a deepened coma with decerebrate posturing and, eventually, flaccid paralysis. The majority of children who survive the acute stage of illness completely recover. A client statement is subjective data.

Test-taking strategy: Analyze to determine what information the question asks for, which is objective data indicating Reye's syndrome. Recall that symptoms begin quickly after a viral infection and quickly deteriorate with significant neurological findings. Also, recall that a change in liver mitochondria confirmed by a liver biopsy provides definitive diagnosis. Review the clinical findings of Reye's syndrome if you had difficulty answering this question.

Client needs category: Physiological integrity

Client needs subcategory: Reduction of risk potential

Cognitive level: Analyzing

The adolescent

1. A nurse is caring for an adolescent who was admitted to the hospital's medical unit after attempting suicide by ingesting acetaminophen. Which interventions would the nurse incorporate into the client's care plan? Select all that apply.

☐ **1.** Limit care until the client initiates a conversation.

☐ **2.** Ask the client's parents if they keep firearms in their home.

☐ **3.** Ask the client if he/she is currently having suicidal thoughts.

☐ **4.** Assist the client with bathing and grooming as needed.

☐ **5.** Inspect the client's mouth after giving oral medications.

☐ **6.** Assure the client that anything said will be held in strict confidence.

Answer: 2, 3, 4, 5

Ⓓ Rationale: Safety is the primary consideration when caring for suicidal clients. Because firearms are the most common method used in suicides, the client's parents would be taught to lock firearms and ammunition in separate locations and not give the client access to the keys. Safety also includes assessing for current suicidal ideation. Many suicidal people are depressed and do not have the energy to care for themselves, so the client may need assistance with bathing and grooming. Because depressed and suicidal clients may hide pills in their cheeks, the nurse would inspect the client's mouth after giving oral medications. Rather than limit care, the nurse should try to establish a trusting relationship through nursing interventions and therapeutic communication. The client cannot be guaranteed confidentiality when self-destructive behavior is an issue.

Test-taking strategy: Analyze to determine what information the question asks for, which is nursing interventions for a client who attempted suicide. "Select all that apply" questions require considering each option to decide its merit. Consider the nursing care of the suicidal adolescent with emphasis that safety is the priority. Review care of the client who attempted suicide if you had difficulty answering this question.

Client needs category: Physiological integrity

Client needs subcategory: Reduction of risk potential

Cognitive level: Applying

2. A nurse is teaching a 16-year-old female client with inflammatory bowel disease about corticosteroid treatment. Which adverse effects are likely to be concerns for this client? Select all that apply.

- ☐ **1.** Acne
- ☐ **2.** Hirsutism
- ☐ **3.** Mood swings
- ☐ **4.** Osteoporosis
- ☐ **5.** Growth spurts
- ☐ **6.** Adrenal suppression

Answer: 1, 2, 3, 4, 6

Ⓓ Rationale: Adverse effects of corticosteroids include acne, hirsutism, mood swings, osteoporosis, and adrenal suppression. Steroid use in children and adolescents may cause delayed growth, not growth spurts.

Test-taking strategy: Analyze to determine what information the question asks for, which is adolescent concerns about corticosteroid use. "Select all that apply" questions require considering each option to decide its merit. Consider side effects of the corticosteroid use that may impact typical growth and development issues in adolescents. Since adolescents place great influence on relationships with peers, appearance and mood swings are of particular concern. Review the pharmacology of corticosteroids and how the adverse effects of corticosteroids relate to adolescents if you had difficulty answering this question.

Client needs category: Physiological integrity

Client needs subcategory: Pharmacological and parenteral therapies

Cognitive level: Applying

---

3. The nurse is caring for a 15-year-old client with myelogenous leukemia whose platelet count is 26,000/mcl. Which nursing interventions would be included in the plan of care? Select all that apply.

- ☐ **1.** Instruct the client not to use a razor for shaving.
- ☐ **2.** Plan to infuse packed red blood cells.
- ☐ **3.** Encourage the client to eat foods high in iron.
- ☐ **4.** Assess the client for pain in the joints.
- ☐ **5.** Encourage vigorous exercise to muscle strength.

Answer: 1, 4

Ⓓ Rationale: Leukemia is a cancer of the blood-forming tissues including bone marrow and the lymphatic system. Myelogenous leukemia affects the myeloid cells, which give rise to red blood cells, white blood cells, and platelet-producing cells. Since the platelet count is significantly low, bleeding is a concern. Instruction to prevent bleeding, such as not using a razor for shaving and assessing active bleeding (pain) in movable joints, is important. The nurse would infuse platelets not red blood cells. Eating foods high in iron is helpful for clients with anemia. Vigorous exercise is not encouraged because of the risk of bleeding.

Test-taking strategy: Analyze to determine what information the question asks for, which is nursing interventions for a client with myelogenous leukemia and a low platelet count. "Select all that apply" questions require considering each option to decide its merit. When identifying a low platelet count, think "bleeding." Include nursing interventions that address safety and bleeding. Review nursing considerations for a client with myelogenous leukemia if you had difficulty answering this question.

Client needs category: Physiological integrity

Client needs subcategory: Physiological adaptation

Cognitive level: Applying

4. A nurse is caring for a 17-year-old female client with cystic fibrosis who has been admitted to the hospital for administration of intravenous antibiotics and respiratory treatment for exacerbation of a lung infection. The client states, "I have a number of questions about my future and the consequences of this disease." Which statements about the course of cystic fibrosis are true? Select all that apply.

☐ **1.** Breast development is commonly delayed.

☐ **2.** The client is at risk for developing diabetes.

☐ **3.** Pregnancy and childbearing are not affected.

☐ **4.** Normal sexual relationships can be expected.

☐ **5.** Only males carry the gene for the disease.

☐ **6.** By age 20, the client is able to decrease the frequency of respiratory treatments.

Answer: 1, 2, 4

Ⓓ Rationale: Cystic fibrosis delays growth and the onset of puberty. Children with cystic fibrosis tend to be smaller than the average size and develop secondary sex characteristics later in life. In addition, they are at risk for developing diabetes mellitus because the pancreatic duct becomes obstructed as pancreatic tissues are destroyed. Clients with cystic fibrosis can expect to have normal sexual relationships, but thick secretions that obstruct the cervix and block sperm entry may impair fertility. Males and females carry the gene for cystic fibrosis. Pulmonary disease commonly progresses as the client ages, requiring additional respiratory treatment, not less.

Test-taking strategy: Analyze to determine what information the question asks for, which is providing accurate information about the disease process as it relates to a young adult. "Select all that apply" questions require considering each option to decide its merit. Consider that cystic fibrosis has metabolic consequences that impact every stage of development because of the metabolic effects on body systems. Review the pathophysiology of cystic fibrosis and its effects on sexual development and reproduction if you had difficulty answering the question.

Client needs category: Physiological integrity

Client needs subcategory: Physiological adaptation

Cognitive level: Analyzing

5. The nurse is caring for an adolescent with diabetes who admits to consuming many simple sugars and carbohydrates at a graduation party. The parents brought the client to the emergency room with unusual behavior. The serum glucose level was 375 mg/dl (20.8 mmol/L).

The physician provided a coverage schedule:

150 to 200 mg/dl (8.3 to 11.1 mmol/L)—
    2 units of Humulin R

201 to 250 mg/dl (11.1 to 13.9 mmol/L)—
    4 units of Humulin R

251 to 300 mg/dl (13.9 to 16.7 mmol/L)—
    6 units of Humulin R

301 to 350 mg/dl (16.7 to 19.4 mmol/L)—
    8 units of Humulin R

351 to 399 mg/dl (19.5 to 22.1 mmol/L)—
    10 units of Humulin R

Over 400 mg/dl 22.2 (mmol/L)—
    call the physician.

Indicate with and draw a line on the low-dose insulin syringe, which amount of insulin would be drawn into the syringe.

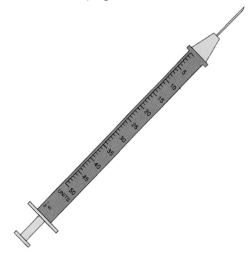

Answer:

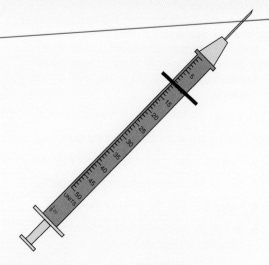

Ⓔ Rationale: The adolescent's blood sugar is 375 mg/dl (20.8 mmol/L), thus falling within the 10-unit range. The nurse would draw up 10 units of Humulin R to administer as per health care provider's orders.

Test-taking strategy: The key words are "blood sugar of 375." The nurse must obtain the blood sugar and then compare with the sliding schedule to determine the correct amount of coverage. Recall that the low-dose syringe uses 1 unit increments to document amounts. Review types of insulin syringes and the use of insulin sliding scales if you had difficulty answering this question.

Client needs category: Physiological integrity

Client needs subcategory: Pharmacological and parenteral therapies

Cognitive level: Applying

6. A nurse is caring for a 14-year-old boy who arrives in the office stating abdominal pain with nausea and vomiting for the past 24 hours. The mother reports the client experiencing sharp pain when hitting a pothole along the road. The vital signs are temperature, 101.6°F (37.8°C); pulse, 92 beats/minute; respirations, 24 breaths/minute; and blood pressure, 142/82 mm Hg. As the nurse is collecting all data, in which location of the abdomen will the nurse obtain definitive assessment data?

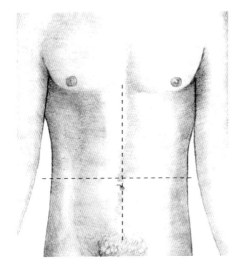

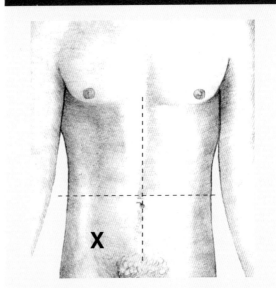

Ⓜ Rationale: The X is placed in the right lower quadrant. All of the data provided (abdominal pain, nausea with vomiting, elevated temperature, and rebound tenderness when hitting a pothole) indicate a potential appendicitis. Appendicitis typically begins with anorexia, nausea, and vomiting for the first 12 to 24 hours. Abdominal pain, a late sign, is usually diffuse at first and gradually localizes to the right lower quadrant. The sharpest pain would be noted at McBurney's point, which is one third of the way between the anterior and superior iliac crest and the umbilicus.

Test-taking strategy: Analyze to determine what information the question asks for, which is site for abdominal assessment of a potential appendicitis. Use the data listed to focus on an abdominal disease process. Once appendicitis is selected, recall the classic assessment point (McBurney's point) and assessment finding (rebound tenderness) in the right lower quadrant. Review the anatomy of the gastrointestinal system and the organs within each of the abdominal quadrants if you had difficulty answering this question.

Client needs category: Physiological integrity

Client needs subcategory: Reduction of risk potential

Cognitive level: Analysis

7. A 17-year-old client confides in the school nurse that he/she is interested in understanding safe sex practices. In instructing the client on how to correctly use a condom, which information would be stressed? Select all that apply.

☐ **1.** The condom only needs to be placed on the penis immediately before ejaculation.

☐ **2.** Condoms should be stored in a cool, dry place to prevent damage.

☐ **3.** A condom would be applied to the penis before it becomes fully erect.

☐ **4.** Leave a ½ inch space at the end of the condom.

☐ **5.** Never reuse a condom.

☐ **6.** The condom would be applied on an erect penis.

Answer: 2, 4, 5, 6

ℰ Rationale: Condoms can be a reliable method of birth control offered with proper instruction. Condoms would be stored in a cool, dry place to prevent heat damage. A ½-inch space would be left at the tip of the condom to allow for collection of the ejaculate and to prevent tearing of the condom. A condom is applied after the penis is erect. A condom would not be reused.

Test-taking strategy: Analyze to determine what information the question asks for, which is instruction for proper use of a condom. "Select all that apply" questions require considering each option to decide its merit. Recall that maintaining the integrity of the condom is key in proper use and to prevent pregnancy and sexually transmitted diseases. Review the proper use of condoms if you had difficulty answering this question.

Client needs category: Health promotion and maintenance

Client needs subcategory: None

Cognitive level: Applying

8. The nurse is examining an adolescent boy. The nurse classifies his sexual maturity as Tanner stage 3. Which graphic depicts this stage?

☐ **1.**

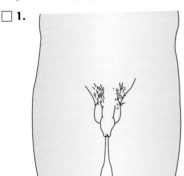

☐ **2.**

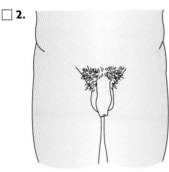

☐ **3.**

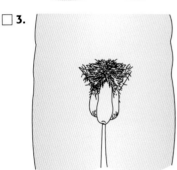

☐ **4.**

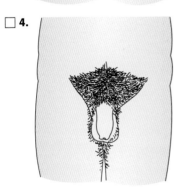

Ⓜ **Rationale:** Because the onset and progression of puberty is variable, the Tanner stage is a widely acceptable scale to describe progression. In Tanner stage 3, pubic hair extends across the pubis. The testes and scrotum begin to enlarge more, and the penis increases in length. Option 1 shows Tanner stage 2, option 3 shows Tanner stage 4, and option 4 shows Tanner stage 5. Tanner also has a scale for females.

Test-taking strategy: Analyze to determine what information the question asks for, which is proper classification of sexual development using Tanner stages. Recall that Tanner stage 1 begins in the preadolescent period and Tanner stage 5 progresses to the adult. Tanner stage 3 is in the middle, where hair is located across the pubis. Review secondary sex changes in male adolescents (genital and pubic hair development) and the Tanner stages 1 to 5 if you had difficulty answering this question.

Client needs category: Physiological integrity

Client needs subcategory: Reduction of risk potential

Cognitive level: Analyzing

9. The nurse is caring for an adolescent with the following skin disorder.

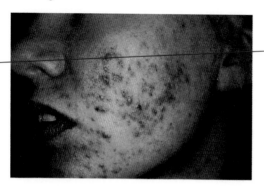

Which client statement indicates a need for further teaching?

☐ **1.** "My breakouts are exacerbated by eating fatty foods."

☐ **2.** "I wash my face with soap and water every morning and night."

☐ **3.** "I use topical retinoids as prescribed at night on my skin."

☐ **4.** "Stress and hormones worsen my breakouts."

Ⓜ **Rationale:** The common skin condition on the adolescent is acne. Acne is a skin condition that occurs when hair follicles become plugged with oil and dead skin cells. Acne is not exacerbated by eating fatty foods. This information would need clarification. Treatment for acne is washing the face with soap and water and using topical retinoids. Stress and fluctuating hormones can cause acne breakouts.

Test-taking strategy: Analyze to determine what information the question asks for, which is identifying the client statement that needs clarification. First, identify that the adolescent's skin condition is acne. Next, analyze each statement for accuracy. Select which statement is incorrect. Review the pathophysiology and treatment of acne if you had difficulty answering this question.

Client needs category: Physiological integrity

Client needs subcategory: Physiological adaptation

Cognitive level: Analyzing

10. The nurse is caring for a 17-year-old male client with Duchenne muscular dystrophy. When assisting the client during a hospitalization for pneumonia, which anticipated nursing interventions would reflect client-specific care? Select all that apply.

☐ **1.** Assisting the client to a Fowler position for a breathing treatment

☐ **2.** Feeding the client a high-calorie breakfast

☐ **3.** Clearing a path to the bathroom for safe and easy access

☐ **4.** Providing directions to the client's educational level

☐ **5.** Completing a bed bath to conserve energy

☐ **6.** Crushing pills for morning medication administration

Ⓓ Rationale: Duchenne muscular dystrophy typically occurs in males with symptoms appearing in the preschool years. The course of the disease is fairly predictable with weakness occurring in the voluntary muscles of the legs and trunk. By the teens, the heart and respiratory muscles can also be affected. Nursing interventions anticipated include assisting the client to an upright position for breathing treatments as the client has difficulty sitting up. Clearing a path to the bathroom is important as the client has an unsteady gait with possible braces and is unable to safely step over and around medical equipment. If wheelchair bound, a clear path is important for navigating to the bathroom. Some clients have intellectual challenges and will need instructions at his appropriate level. A well-balanced diet is best. Clients are encouraged to exercise and complete all activities of daily living as tolerated. Crushing pills may be needed in the later stages of the disease but is not anticipated for a teenager.

Test-taking strategy: Analyze to determine what information the question asks for, which is nursing interventions that are anticipated for a client with Duchenne muscular dystrophy who is admitted for pneumonia. Recall that "muscular dystrophy" involves the dysfunction of the muscles. Consider strength and coordination. Identify options which focus on these. Review the effects of Duchenne muscular dystrophy if you had difficulty answering this question.

Client needs category: Physiological integrity

Client needs subcategory: Physiological adaptation

Cognitive level: Analyzing

PART SIX

Psychiatric and mental health nursing

Foundations of psychiatric nursing

1. A hospitalized client becomes angry and belligerent toward a nurse after speaking on the phone with his mother. The nurse learns that the mother cannot visit as expected. Which interventions will the nurse use to help the client deal with the displaced anger? Select all that apply.

- ☐ **1.** Explore the client's unmet needs.
- ☐ **2.** Acknowledge the client's behavior as inappropriate.
- ☐ **3.** Suggest that the client direct the anger at his mother.
- ☐ **4.** Invite the client to a quiet place to talk after he has settled down.
- ☐ **5.** Assist the client in identifying alternate ways of approaching the problem.

Answer: 1, 2, 4, 5

Ⓔ **Rationale:** Feelings of displacement or directing his anger toward the nurse need to be identified as inappropriate and understood by the client before the nurse can help guide him to choose appropriate actions. Having the client direct anger at another person is inappropriate. Approaching the client in a calm manner and offering to assist in the problem-solving process allow the client to identify needs that are not being met and explore constructive ways of dealing with his anger.

Test-taking strategy: Analyze to determine what information the question asks for, which is nursing interventions to deal with displaced anger. "Select all that apply" questions require considering each option to decide its merit. Recall therapeutic behaviors to have the client explore his feelings and be able to verbalize thoughts. This strategy is helpful in clarifying thoughts and defusing anger. Focus on the optimal therapeutic approach and effective anger management techniques if you had difficulty answering this question.

Client needs category: Psychosocial integrity

Client needs subcategory: None

Cognitive level: Applying

---

2. The nurse is caring for a client with severe depression. In which conditions would the nurse anticipate the use of electroconvulsive therapy (ECT)? Select all that apply.

- ☐ **1.** The client also has dementia.
- ☐ **2.** The client cannot tolerate monoamine oxidase inhibitors (MAOIs).
- ☐ **3.** The client has not responded to conventional therapy.
- ☐ **4.** The client is undergoing a stressful life change.
- ☐ **5.** The client is having acute suicidal thoughts.

Answer: 2, 3, 5

Ⓜ **Rationale:** ECT is used to treat acute depressive illnesses in an attempt to rapidly reverse a life-threatening situation, such as disturbing delusions, agitation, and attempted suicide or when conventional therapies have been unsuccessful. It is also used when the client cannot tolerate antidepressants, since other medication regimens for depression can take weeks to become fully effective. ECT is usually not indicated for situational depression caused by intense stress. Clients with dementia are not given ECT because ECT may further exacerbate cognitive impairment. The decision to use ECT is not based on where the client lives.

Test-taking strategy: Analyze to determine what information the question asks for, which is when to support the use of ECT. "Select all that apply" questions require considering each option to decide its merit. Recall that the use of ECT is anticipated when the client is experiencing severe mental health problems and traditional therapy is ineffective. Using that rationale leads to the correct answers. Recall the major symptoms of depression and treatment options for depression if you had difficulty answering this question.

Client needs category: Psychosocial integrity

Client needs subcategory: None

Cognitive level: Applying

3. A nurse is working in the emergency room when a police officer walks in with a rape victim to be examined. If the nursing goal is to reduce client anxiety, which interventions would be appropriate? Select all that apply.

☐ **1.** Admit the client to the treatment area right away.

☐ **2.** Encourage the client to undergo an examination immediately in order to get it behind her.

☐ **3.** Assure the client of safety in the examination room.

☐ **4.** Touch the client early on demonstrating the nurse is supportive.

☐ **5.** Allow a third party to be present if the client requests it.

☐ **6.** Ask factual questions to determine the type of assault.

Answer: 1, 3, 5, 6

Ⓜ Rationale: Immediately admitting a rape victim to the treatment area may help the client feel cared for and safe. Allowing a third party to remain if requested also increases feeling of safety. Factual questions help to clarify events in a nonjudgmental way. At a time of great distress, the nurse would pace the interview and examination according to the client's level of comfort. Touching a client who has recently been assaulted may increase anxiety. The nurse would wait for the client to initiate contact or ask permission prior to initiating physical contact.

Test-taking strategy: Analyze to determine what information the question asks for, which is interventions to decrease a rape victim's anxiety. "Select all that apply" questions require considering each option to decide its merit. Consider that victims of violent crimes often feel violated and build trust slowly. Offering of oneself in a nonjudgmental way reduces anxiety and allows the client to express feelings. Review the client's physical and emotional needs after experiencing rape if you had difficulty answering this question.

Client needs category: Psychosocial integrity

Client needs subcategory: None

Cognitive level: Applying

---

4. The nurse is meeting a client on the mental health unit. When beginning a therapeutic relationship, which nursing actions are appropriate? Select all that apply.

☐ **1.** Meet the needs and specific desires of the client.

☐ **2.** Help the client explore different problem-solving techniques.

☐ **3.** Encourage the practice of new coping skills.

☐ **4.** Give health advice to the client.

☐ **5.** Exchange personal information with the client.

☐ **6.** Discuss the client's feelings with family members.

Answer: 2, 3

Ⓒ Rationale: The goal of a therapeutic relationship is to enhance the personal growth of the client. This is achieved by helping clients explore problem-solving techniques and develop coping skills. Giving advice, exchanging personal information, and striving to meet the personal needs and special desires of the client are characteristic of social relationships. Discussing the client's feelings with family members is a breach of confidentiality, unless previously approved by the client.

Test-taking strategy: Analyze to determine what information the question asks for, which is actions within a therapeutic relationship. "Select all that apply" questions require considering each option to decide its merit. The key words are "therapeutic relationship," meaning that it benefits the client in some way to meet specific goals. Review how the nurse assists the client to meet basic needs and review therapeutic communication if you had difficulty answering this question.

Client needs category: Psychosocial integrity

Client needs subcategory: None

Cognitive level: Applying

---

5. A nurse is explaining client rights for psychiatric patients to a client who has voluntarily sought admission to an inpatient psychiatric facility. Which rights would the nurse include in the discussion? Select all that apply.

☐ **1.** Right to select health care team members

☐ **2.** Right to refuse treatment

☐ **3.** Right to a written treatment plan

☐ **4.** Right to obtain disability benefits

☐ **5.** Right to confidentiality

☐ **6.** Right to personal mail

Answer: 2, 3, 5, 6

Ⓜ **Rationale:** An inpatient client usually receives a copy of client rights, which may include the Bill of Rights for psychiatric patients in the United States, province-specific Charter of Rights and Freedoms, or the British Columbia Mental Health Act. These documents include the right to refuse treatment, to have a written treatment plan, to have all medical information kept confidential, and to receive mail. A client in an inpatient setting does not have the right to select health care team members. Although the client may apply for disability benefits as a result of a chronic or incapacitating illness, obtaining disability compensation is not a client right and members of a psychiatric institution do not decide who would receive it.

Test-taking strategy: Analyze to determine what information the question asks for, which is components within client right documents for psychiatric patients. "Select all that apply" questions require considering each option to decide its merit. Recall that these documents provide guarantees of essential rights such as the right to information, autonomy, and fair treatment. Review the rights of clients in hospitalized settings and the responsibilities of health care providers if you had difficulty answering this question.

Client needs category: Psychosocial integrity

Client needs subcategory: None

Cognitive level: Applying

---

6. A client is brought to the emergency department dead on arrival (DOA) from a gunshot wound. The client's family arrives and is escorted to a private area. A multidisciplinary team composed of a physician, nurse, and social worker interacts with the family. All members work together to complete the following tasks. Which are the **priority** nursing responsibilities? Select all that apply.

☐ **1.** Explaining the cause of the client's death

☐ **2.** Providing therapeutic touch and support as needed

☐ **3.** Arranging disposition of the client's personal belongings

☐ **4.** Caring for body organs that are appropriate for transplantation

☐ **5.** Escorting the client's family for viewing of the body

Answer: 2, 4, 5

Ⓒ **Rationale:** The death of a loved one in a violent nature is extremely painful and unanticipated for families. Nursing responsibilities include care of the family and maintenance of organs that may be used for transplantation. The physician would explain the client's status and cause of death to the family. Since the social worker is involved, coordination with the funeral director and disposition of personal belongings are efficiently completed. All members offer support as needed.

Test-taking strategy: Analyze to determine what information the question asks for, which is nursing responsibilities when working on a multidisciplinary team. Consider each member of the team identified and determine which member would complete which action. Review the priority nursing responsibilities when working on a multidisciplinary team if you had difficulty answering this question.

Client needs category: Psychosocial integrity

Client needs subcategory: None

Cognitive level: Analyzing

---

7. In the emergency department, a client reveals to the nurse a lethal plan for committing suicide and agrees to a voluntary admission to the psychiatric unit. Which information would the nurse discuss with the client to answer the question "How long do I have to stay here?" Select all that apply.

☐ **1.** "You may leave the hospital at any time unless you're suicidal or homicidal or unable to meet your basic needs."

☐ **2.** "Let's talk more after the health care team has assessed you."

☐ **3.** "Once you've signed the papers, you have no say."

☐ **4.** "Because you have stated that you want to hurt yourself, you must be safe before being discharged."

☐ **5.** "You need a lawyer to help you make that decision."

☐ **6.** "All clients need a court hearing before leaving the hospital."

Answer: 1, 2, 4

ⓒ Rationale: A person who is admitted to a psychiatric hospital may voluntarily sign out of the hospital unless the health care team determines that the person is harmful to self or others. The health care team evaluates the client's condition before discharge. If there is reason to believe that the client may be harmful to self or others, a hearing can be held to determine if the admission status should be changed from voluntary to involuntary. Not all discharges require a hearing. The client still has rights after committing himself or herself to a psychiatric unit. The client does not need a lawyer to leave the hospital. A court hearing is held only if the client may pose a threat to self or others and requires further treatment.

Test-taking strategy: Analyze to determine what information the question asks for, which is answering a client's question of "how long do I have to stay here?" "Select all that apply" questions require considering each option to decide its merit. Recall guidelines for voluntary commitment and subsequent release. Consider safety issues, especially in light of suicide concerns. Review factors that determine length of stay and patient rights if you had difficulty answering this question.

Client needs category: Psychosocial integrity

Client needs subcategory: None

Cognitive level: Applying

8. A nurse has developed a therapeutic relationship with a client who has an addiction problem. Which client behaviors would indicate that the therapeutic interaction is in the working phase? Select all that apply.

☐ **1.** The client discusses how the addiction has contributed to family distress.

☐ **2.** The client reluctantly shares the family history of addiction.

☐ **3.** The client verbalizes difficulty identifying personal strengths.

☐ **4.** The client discusses the financial problems related to the addiction.

☐ **5.** The client expresses uncertainty about what topic to discuss.

☐ **6.** The client acknowledges the addiction's effects on his children.

Answer: 1, 3, 4, 6

Ⓒ Rationale: Acknowledging the addiction's effects on the family and discussing its financial impact will help the client to identify personal strengths in dealing with addiction and strengthen the therapeutic relationship in the process. Discussing the family history of addiction and expressing uncertainty about what topics to address with the nurse typically happen during the introductory phase of a nurse–client relationship.

Test-taking strategy: Analyze to determine what information the question asks for, which is analyzing for a therapeutic interaction. "Select all that apply" questions require considering each option to decide its merit. Note the client statements that suggest open communication with the nurse. Also, analyze each option for characteristics that the client is open to working on goals and displaying personal introspection. Review the dynamics occurring in the introductory phase of a therapeutic relationship if you had difficulty answering this question.

Client needs category: Psychosocial integrity
Client needs subcategory: None
Cognitive level: Evaluating

---

9. A nurse is caring for a client who exhibits behaviors that test the nurse–client relationship. When discussing this behavior at a multidisciplinary team conference, which behaviors would the nurse provide as examples of this behavior? Select all that apply.

☐ **1.** Placing the nurse in the role of parent

☐ **2.** Dressing in a flamboyant or seductive manner

☐ **3.** Requesting personal information from the nurse

☐ **4.** Following the contract established between the nurse and client

☐ **5.** Stating information to try to shock the nurse

☐ **6.** Violating the nurse's personal space

Answer: 1, 3, 5, 6

Ⓒ Rationale: A client will test the nurse–client relationship by acting in ways to control the relationship or to elicit an emotional response from the nurse. Examples of the testing behavior include speaking about things that will shock the nurse, violating personal space, requesting personal information, and placing the nurse in the role of parent. Dressing in a flamboyant or seductive manner demonstrates a lack of rules or expected behaviors; this is a violation of boundary setting. A contract is used to develop or negotiate an agreement between the nurse and the client to achieve a mutual goal.

Test-taking strategy: Analyze to determine what information the question asks for, which is examples of client testing behaviors. "Select all that apply" questions require considering each option to decide its merit. Recall that client testing behaviors test a nurse's response/behavior and deal with controlling the situation by catching the nurse off guard or creating an uncomfortable situation. Review what behaviors test the nurse's professional demeanor if you had difficulty answering this question.

Client needs category: Psychosocial integrity
Client needs subcategory: None
Cognitive level: Analyzing

---

10. A male client states feelings of sadness and is seeking suggestions for strategies to keep active after the loss of his spouse. Which activities might the nurse suggest to the client? Select all that apply.

☐ **1.** A golf league at a club

☐ **2.** Attending regular spiritual/church services

☐ **3.** Walking at sunrise at the local track

☐ **4.** Attending a midday movie at the theater

☐ **5.** Participate in a community charity event

Answer: 1, 2, 5

Ⓜ **Rationale:** It is common after the loss of a spouse to experience sadness related to the grieving process and have difficulty socializing independently. Participating with other individuals in team-related sports or religious activity and having a common goal at a charity event are client-directed activities, which connect the client to others. Independent activities include walking and attending a movie.

Test-taking strategy: Analyze to determine what information the question asks for, which is suggested activities to assist the client with sadness and loneliness. "Select all that apply" questions require considering each option to decide its merit. Compare each option to accomplishing the nursing goal. Ask yourself, "What would increase a client's mood and provide social interaction, thus decreasing loneliness?" Review activities to decrease sadness and increase client participation in activities if you had difficulty answering this question.

Client needs category: Psychosocial integrity

Client needs subcategory: None

Cognitive level: Applying

Anxiety disorders

1. A nurse is caring for a client with agoraphobia. Which signs and symptoms would the nurse anticipate? Select all that apply.

☐ **1.** Hallucinations

☐ **2.** Panic attacks

☐ **3.** Inability to leave home

☐ **4.** Eating disorders

☐ **5.** Alcohol consumption

☐ **6.** Tobacco use

Answer: 2, 3

Ⓜ **Rationale:** Agoraphobia is characterized by extreme anxiety and a fear of being in open places. Panic attacks and an inability to leave home are symptoms associated with the disorder. No correlation exists between fear of open spaces and hallucinations, eating disorders, alcohol consumption, or tobacco use.

Test-taking strategy: Analyze to determine what information the question asks for, which is signs and symptoms anticipated with the diagnosis of agoraphobia. "Select all that apply" questions require considering each option to decide its merit. Use your knowledge of medical terminology to recall the definition of agoraphobia (agora = gathering place; phobia = fear of). Once understood, analyze the options for related symptoms. Review conditions that commonly occur with phobias or unrealistic fears if you had difficulty answering this question.

Client needs category: Psychosocial integrity

Client needs subcategory: None

Cognitive level: Applying

2. A client is being seen in the clinic after returning from military service abroad. The nurse documents restlessness at night with nightmares leaving the veteran irritable and fatigued during the day. When discussing the possibility of post-traumatic stress disorder (PTSD), which statements about PTSD are accurate? Select all that apply.

- ☐ **1.** PTSD is a syndrome that affects only those who have experienced traumatic episodes during war.
- ☐ **2.** PTSD is characterized by nightmares and flashbacks.
- ☐ **3.** Hypervigilance is characteristic of clients with PTSD.
- ☐ **4.** Substance abuse is a common coping mechanism used by clients with PTSD.
- ☐ **5.** Psychotic episodes can occur in clients with PTSD.
- ☐ **6.** Clients with PTSD may complain of feeling empty inside.

Answer: 2, 3, 4, 5, 6

Ⓒ Rationale: PTSD is a serious condition that develops after a person has witnessed a traumatic or terrifying event in which serious physical harm has occurred or is threatened. Although PTSD is commonly associated with combat, it can manifest itself after any kind of trauma. If symptoms occur within 6 months of the traumatic event, the disorder is considered acute. If symptoms occur more than 6 months after the traumatic event, PTSD is considered delayed or chronic. PTSD is characterized by nightmares or flashbacks. Clients are hypervigilant but typically describe themselves as "empty inside." Sometimes, the events can present as a psychotic episode. Substance abuse is a common "symptom" used for coping.

Test-taking strategy: Analyze to determine what information the question asks for, which is accurate statements of PTSD. "Select all that apply" questions require considering each option to decide its merit. If unsure, consider the full name of PTSD and relate symptoms stemming from a trauma or stress. Review the defining characteristics and clinical manifestations of PTSD if you had difficulty answering this question.

Client needs category: Psychosocial integrity
Client needs subcategory: None
Cognitive level: Analyzing

---

3. An 8-year-old child, diagnosed with obsessive–compulsive disorder, is admitted by the nurse to a psychiatric facility. During the admission assessment, which behaviors would be characterized as compulsions? Select all that apply.

- ☐ **1.** Checking and rechecking that the television is turned off before going to school
- ☐ **2.** Repeatedly washing the hands
- ☐ **3.** Brushing teeth three times per day
- ☐ **4.** Routinely climbing up and down a flight of stairs three times before leaving the house
- ☐ **5.** Feeding the dog the same meal every day
- ☐ **6.** Wanting to play the same video game each night

Answer: 1, 2, 4

Ⓔ Rationale: Compulsions involve symbolic rituals that relieve anxiety when they are performed. The disorder is caused by anxiety from obsessive thoughts, and acts are seen as irrational. Examples include repeatedly checking the television set, washing hands, or climbing stairs. An activity such as playing the same video game each night may be indicative of normal development for a school-age child. Frequent brushing of the teeth and feeding the dog a consistent meal are not abnormal.

Test-taking strategy: Analyze to determine what information the question asks for, which is behaviors that indicate a compulsion. "Select all that apply" questions require considering each option to decide its merit. Analyze each option for behaviors that are considered irrational in nature and, many times, repetitive. Review the symptoms of compulsive behavior if you had difficulty answering this question.

Client needs category: Psychosocial integrity
Client needs subcategory: None
Cognitive level: Analyzing

4. A nurse selects a priority nursing diagnosis of *fear related to being embarrassed in the presence of others* for a client who exhibits symptoms of social phobia. Which outcomes, if met, would demonstrate improvement in client's symptoms? Select all that apply.

☐ **1.** The client manages fear in group situations.

☐ **2.** The client develops a plan to avoid situations that may cause stress.

☐ **3.** The client verbalizes feelings that occur in stressful situations.

☐ **4.** The client develops a plan for responding to stressful situations.

☐ **5.** The client denies feelings that may contribute to irrational fears.

☐ **6.** The client uses suppression to deal with underlying fears.

Answer: 1, 3, 4

Ⓒ Rationale: When selecting an outcome for a nursing diagnosis, choose a statement that would demonstrate the progressing toward or achievement of the short-term or long-term goal. Improving stress management skills, verbalizing feelings, and anticipating and planning for stressful situations are adaptive responses to stress. Avoidance, denial, and suppression are maladaptive defense mechanisms.

Test-taking strategy: Analyze to determine what information the question asks for, which is outcomes that demonstrate improvement in social phobia symptoms. "Select all that apply" questions require considering each option to decide its merit. Analyze each option for evidence of positive progress in handling and coping with social phobia. Review client outcomes related to acceptable behaviors in social situations if you had difficulty answering this question.

Client needs category: Psychosocial integrity
Client needs subcategory: None
Cognitive level: Evaluating

---

5. A nurse recognizes improvement in a client with the nursing diagnosis of *ineffective role performance related to the need to perform rituals.* Which behaviors indicate improvement? Select all that apply.

☐ **1.** The client refrains from performing rituals during stress.

☐ **2.** The client verbalizes using "thought stopping" when obsessive thoughts occur.

☐ **3.** The client verbalizes the relationship between stress and ritualistic behaviors.

☐ **4.** The client avoids stressful situations.

☐ **5.** The client rationalizes ritualistic behavior.

☐ **6.** The client performs ritualistic behaviors in private.

Answer: 1, 2, 3

Ⓒ Rationale: Refraining from performing rituals demonstrates that the client manages stress appropriately. Using "thought stopping" demonstrates the client's ability to employ appropriate interventions for obsessive thoughts. Verbalizing the relationship between stress and behaviors indicates that the client understands the disease process. Avoiding stressful situations and rationalizing or hiding ritualistic behaviors are maladaptive methods of managing stress and anxiety.

Test-taking strategy: Analyze to determine what information the question asks for, which is behaviors that demonstrate improvement in the nursing diagnosis of ineffective role performance in relation to ritualistic behavior. "Select all that apply" questions require considering each option to decide its merit. Look for data in the option related to or characteristic of less ritualistic behavior. Review options that promote healthy behaviors if you had difficulty answering this question.

Client needs category: Psychosocial integrity
Client needs subcategory: None
Cognitive level: Analyzing

6. A nurse is caring for a client recently diagnosed with cancer and experiencing situational anxiety. Which interventions would the nurse include in the care plan? Select all that apply.

☐ **1.** Maintain a calm, nonthreatening environment.

☐ **2.** Explain relevant aspects of chemotherapy.

☐ **3.** Encourage the client to verbalize concerns regarding the diagnosis.

☐ **4.** Encourage the client to use deep breathing exercises and other relaxation techniques during periods of increased stress.

☐ **5.** Provide distractions for the client during periods of stress.

☐ **6.** Teach the stages of grieving to the client.

Answer: 1, 3, 4

Ⓒ Rationale: During periods of acute stress, interventions that help the client regain control will help master this new threat. Providing a calm, nonthreatening environment and encouraging verbalization of concerns will help the client face the unknown. Relaxation techniques have a physiologic and psychological effect in calming the client, which in turn allows further exploration of thoughts and feelings as well as problem solving. The ability to learn is limited during extreme stress, so teaching the client about grief and chemotherapy would not be effective at this stage. Providing distractions would be ineffective at this point in the grief process.

Test-taking strategy: Analyze to determine what information the question asks for, which is nursing intervention for a client with extreme stress and anxiety. "Select all that apply" questions require considering each option to decide its merit. Consider anxiety-relieving measures that will assist the client in coping with the diagnosis and regaining control. Review interventions that relieve stress and promote relaxation if you had difficulty answering this question.

Client needs category: Psychosocial integrity

Client needs subcategory: None

Cognitive level: Applying

---

7. The nurse is teaching a client diagnosed with a generalized anxiety disorder how to effectively cope with severe distress. Which interventions would the nurse use to promote effective coping with anxiety? Select all that apply.

☐ **1.** Discuss previous methods that were effective in handling stress.

☐ **2.** Encourage the client to limit to a mutually decided amount of time spent on worrying.

☐ **3.** Help the client to establish a goal and develop a plan to meet the goal.

☐ **4.** Teach the client how to label feelings and how to express them.

☐ **5.** Discuss ways to examine the reality of fears.

☐ **6.** Assist the client to acknowledge the major consequences of blaming others.

Answer: 1, 2, 3, 4

Ⓒ Rationale: To promote effective skills, the nurse would focus on having the client identify successful coping skills used in the past and on building on the client's knowledge of the disorder. Setting a mutually agreed upon limit on the amount of time spent worrying gives the client boundaries and acknowledges the concerns. Establishing a goal and planning to meet the goal allows the client to engage in solving the problem and exercise control over the stressful situation. Labeling and expressing feelings is healthy way to acknowledge feelings. Clients with schizophrenia, not generalized anxiety disorder, require help with focusing on reality-based behaviors. Clients who demonstrate oppositional behavior tend to blame others instead of taking responsibility for their inappropriate behavior.

Test-taking strategy: Analyze to determine what information the question asks for, which is interventions on how to cope with anxiety. "Select all that apply" questions require considering each option to decide its merit. Consider each option for anxiety-reducing strategies and coping skills. Review the defining characteristics and clinical manifestations of generalized anxiety disorder and related coping skills if you had difficulty answering this question.

Client needs category: Psychosocial integrity

Client needs subcategory: None

Cognitive level: Applying

8. The nurse is leading a group session when the nurse notices that a member of the group is tearful and shaking. Which actions would be therapeutic at this time? Select all that apply.

☐ **1.** Ask the client to share the emotions that the client is feeling.

☐ **2.** Allow the client to remain in the group and ignore the behavior.

☐ **3.** Ask the client to leave the group and rejoin once feeling better.

☐ **4.** Apologize to the client and state that you did not mean to cause emotional pain.

☐ **5.** Redirect the group to another topic, which may evoke a less emotional response.

☐ **6.** Direct a staff member to assist the client and continue with the group.

Answer: 1, 6

Ⓓ Rationale: In group therapy, a trained professional leads a small group of people with similar problems to discuss common issues. It is not uncommon for the group to evolve emotions on the topic being discussed. Groups are a safe place to share thoughts and feeling and often must work through negative content before positive outcomes surface. Since groups are a safe place to share emotions, asking the client to share his or her emotions is an appropriate action. A personal interaction with a supportive staff member is also an appropriate action. Ignoring the client or asking the client to leave is discounting the client's feelings.

Test-taking strategy: Analyze to determine what information the question asks for, which is nursing action during group therapy. Consider the goal of group therapy being a supportive, safe environment to discuss and work through common issues. With that in mind, review each option against the benefit of the nursing action. Review nursing actions during group therapy sessions if you had difficulty answering this question.

Client needs category: Psychosocial integrity

Client needs subcategory: None

Cognitive level: Analyzing

Mood, adjustment, and dementia disorders

1. A nurse is conducting a group session for children and adolescents who have been diagnosed with depression. Which behaviors would a nurse anticipate in this group? Select all that apply.

- ☐ **1.** Delusions
- ☐ **2.** Anxiety
- ☐ **3.** Mania
- ☐ **4.** Irritability
- ☐ **5.** Somatic symptoms, such as headache and stomachache
- ☐ **6.** Suicidal thoughts

Answer: 2, 4, 5, 6

Ⓜ **Rationale:** Children and adolescents with depression commonly experience anxiety and irritability as well as somatic symptoms. Suicide is a serious risk in these age groups. These age groups seldom experience psychotic symptoms. If psychotic symptoms do occur, they are more likely to be auditory hallucinations, not delusions. Mania is experienced with bipolar disorder but not depression alone.

Test-taking strategy: Analyze to determine what information the question asks for, which is behaviors of children and adolescents diagnosed with depression. "Select all that apply" questions require considering each option to decide its merit. Consider maturity level, impulsivity, and fluctuating hormones in addition to depressive symptoms. Review the symptoms of children and adolescents with depression if you had difficulty answering this question.

Client needs category: Psychosocial integrity

Client needs subcategory: None

Cognitive level: Applying

2. A rehabilitation nurse is caring for a young client recovering from a motor vehicle accident in which he lost both legs. The client states, "I will never be able to work again or live a normal life." Which responses by the nurse would be considered therapeutic? Select all that apply.

- ☐ **1.** "Losing both legs is hard to accept, how are you feeling now?"
- ☐ **2.** "With a prosthesis, you will be up and walking again soon."
- ☐ **3.** "You must be devastated with your loss. Have you sought legal advice?"
- ☐ **4.** "The occupational therapist will provide you with instructions on potential job opportunities."
- ☐ **5.** "I am here to help you. Let's devise a plan so that you are working toward your goals."

Answer: 1, 5

Ⓓ **Rationale:** Having a life-changing event frequently leaves individuals in a state of shock and overwhelmed with the situation. The client requires a supportive environment to meet his recovery needs. Validating his feelings and having the client express his feelings opens communication. Offering of self is another way to open communication and establish a trusting relationship. Setting mutually established client-centered goals allows the client to feel involved and in control of the rehabilitation process. It is patronizing to state that the client will be up and walking soon. While that may be a true statement, the client has still experienced a significant loss. Asking about legal advice is not the role of the nurse. It is too early to determine job opportunities. The client will determine what opportunities interest him.

Test-taking strategy: Analyze to determine what information the question asks for, which is therapeutic communication with a client who has experienced a significant life-changing event. Recall that client support is necessary at this time. Consider the standards of care beginning with understanding the client perspective. Refer to principles of opening communication and establishing a trusting relationship when analyzing each distracter. Review therapeutic communication techniques if you had difficulty answering this question.

Client needs category: Psychosocial integrity

Client needs subcategory: None

Cognitive level: Applying

---

3. A nurse is caring for a client diagnosed with persistent depressive disorder. Which defining characteristics are associated with this disorder? Select all that apply.

☐ **1.** Insomnia or hypersomnia

☐ **2.** Delusions or hallucinations

☐ **3.** Suicidal thoughts

☐ **4.** Onset of symptoms within a 2-week period

☐ **5.** Symptoms that occur in the winter and resolve in spring

☐ **6.** Appetite disturbance

Answer: 1, 3, 6

ⓒ Rationale: Persistent depressive disorder is a mild, but chronic, form of depression. Sleep and appetite disturbances and suicidal thoughts can appear in clients with this or major depressive disorders. Onset of symptoms is gradual and may appear over weeks or months. Delusions and other psychotic symptoms may occur in major depression but do not occur in persistent depressive disorder. Episodes of depression occurring solely in the winter are indicative of seasonal affective disorder.

Test-taking strategy: Analyze to determine what information the question asks for, which is characteristics of persistent depressive disorder. "Select all that apply" questions require considering each option to decide its merit. Recall that the key point is mild depression; thus, consider options of an altered mood. Review the defining characteristics of persistent depressive disorder if you had difficulty answering this question.

Client needs category: Psychosocial integrity

Client needs subcategory: None

Cognitive level: Applying

4. A nurse is developing a care plan for a client with acute mania. Place the following behaviors according to the order in which they progress in a client with acute mania. All options must be used.

1. Has delusions of grandeur

2. Uses relevant, calm speech patterns

3. Shows high productivity and competitive attitude in work and leisure activities

4. Becomes easily irritated

5. Demonstrates poor judgment and impulse control

Answer: 2, 3, 4, 5, 1

Rationale: Mania is an abnormally elated mental state, typically characterized by feelings of euphoria, lack of inhibition, racing thoughts, risk taking, and irritability. Relevant and calm speech patterns are indicative of normal behavior. An early sign of dysphoria at the beginning of a manic episode is the client's lack of sleep. Since sleep is not a priority, the client soon begins displaying a high level of productivity and competitiveness in work and leisure activities. As the mania increases, the client becomes more easily irritated and requires medication. The client demonstrates poor judgment and impulse control; therefore, client safety becomes a major concern. Lastly, the client becomes psychotic and has grandiose ideas that evolve into delusions of grandeur.

Test-taking strategy: Analyze to determine what information the question asks for, which is progression of symptoms in a client with acute mania. Note that as symptoms progress, they typically progress from minor symptoms to potentially dangerous or debilitating conditions. If unsure, begin with normal behavior and end with the most extreme symptoms. Review the progression of behaviors of mania from mild to major if you had difficulty answering this question.

Client needs category: Psychosocial integrity
Client needs subcategory: None
Cognitive level: Analyzing

5. A nurse is caring for a client displaying extreme mood swings with suicidal tendencies. A physician prescribes lithium and diagnoses the client with bipolar disorder. When teaching the client, which statements, verbalized by the client, indicate a good understanding of the teaching of medication management? Select all that apply.

☐ **1.** "I understand that there is a potential for addiction."

☐ **2.** "I need to watch for signs and symptoms of drug toxicity including blurred vision and ringing in the ears."

☐ **3.** "I will adjust my medication depending upon my symptoms."

☐ **4.** "I will need to be on a low-tyramine diet."

☐ **5.** "I will need to consistently monitor blood levels."

☐ **6.** "The therapeutic effect of the medication takes time to occur."

Answer: 2, 5, 6

Rationale: Client education would cover the signs and symptoms of drug toxicity, which include blurred vision and ringing in the ears. It is important to report toxicity to the health care provider immediately. There is also a need for regular monitoring of drug blood levels. The nurse would also inform the client that mood changes may not be apparent for 7 to 21 days after treatment is initiated. Lithium does not have addictive properties. Birth control should be initiated for sexually active females. There is no need to be on a low-tyramine diet. Tyramine is a potential concern to clients who are also taking monoamine oxidase (MAO) inhibitors.

Test-taking strategy: Analyze to determine what information the question asks for, which is correct statements following client teaching. "Select all that apply" questions require considering each option to decide its merit. Recall that lithium is a potent medication with a narrowed therapeutic index. Review teaching considerations of lithium if you had difficulty answering this question.

Client needs category: Physiological integrity
Client needs subcategory: Pharmacological and parenteral therapies
Cognitive level: Applying

6. After interviewing a client diagnosed with recurrent depression, a nurse determines the client's potential to commit suicide. Which factors listed below might contribute to the client's risk of suicide? Select all that apply.

☐ **1.** Psychomotor retardation

☐ **2.** Impulsive behaviors

☐ **3.** Overwhelming feelings of guilt

☐ **4.** Chronic, debilitating illness

☐ **5.** Decreased physical activity

☐ **6.** Repression of anger

Answer: 2, 3, 4, 6

Ⓒ **Rationale:** Recurrent depression represents a major consideration in suicide prevention because of its high prevalence. Impulsive behavior, overwhelming guilt, chronic illness, and repressed anger are factors that contribute to suicide potential. Psychomotor retardation and decreased physical activity are symptoms of depression, but these do not typically lead to suicide because the client does not have the energy and cognitive abilities to harm self.

Test-taking strategy: Analyze to determine what information the question asks for, which is factors that contribute to client suicide. Consider that the nurse must be aware of the client's feelings, thoughts, and behaviors as they may indicate the likelihood of suicide. Review the risk factors for suicide if you had difficulty answering this question.

Client needs category: Psychosocial integrity

Client needs subcategory: None

Cognitive level: Analyzing

7. A nurse is assessing a client who talks freely about feeling depressed. During the interaction, the nurse hears the client state, "Things will never change." What other indications of hopelessness would the nurse look for? Select all that apply.

☐ **1.** Bouts of anger

☐ **2.** Periods of irritability

☐ **3.** Preoccupation with delusions

☐ **4.** Feelings of worthlessness

☐ **5.** Self-destructive behaviors

☐ **6.** Auditory hallucinations

Answer: 1, 2, 4, 5

Ⓒ **Rationale:** Clients who are depressed and feeling hopeless are often irritable and express inappropriate anger, feelings of worthlessness, and suicidal thoughts. In addition, they may demonstrate self-destructive behaviors. Preoccupation with delusions and auditory hallucinations is generally seen in clients with schizophrenia or other psychotic disorders rather than in those expressing hopelessness.

Test-taking strategy: Analyze to determine what information the question asks for, which is indications of hopelessness. "Select all that apply" questions require considering each option to decide its merit. Recall that many people consider suicide but most people decide to live as they realize that the crisis is temporary and death is permanent. Hopelessness, unfortunately, makes the clients feel that their situation is permanent and they act out feeling angry, irritable, worthless, etc. Review behaviors associated with hopelessness and depression if you had difficulty answering this question.

Client needs category: Psychosocial integrity

Client needs subcategory: None

Cognitive level: Analyzing

8. A nurse interviews the family of a client hospitalized with severe depression and suicidal ideation. What family assessment information is essential to know when formulating an effective plan of care? Select all that apply.

☐ **1.** Physical pain

☐ **2.** Personal responsibilities

☐ **3.** Employment skills

☐ **4.** Communication patterns

☐ **5.** Role expectations

☐ **6.** Current family stressors

Answer: 4, 5, 6

Ⓒ Rationale: When working with the family of a depressed client, it is helpful for the nurse to be aware of the family's communication style, role expectations, and current family stressors. This information can help identify family difficulties and teaching points that could benefit the client and the family. Information concerning physical pain, personal responsibilities, and employment skills would not be helpful because these areas are not directly related to their experience of having a depressed family member.

Test-taking strategy: Analyze to determine what information the question asks for, which is family assessment information essential to planning care. "Select all that apply" questions require considering each option to decide its merit. The key words are "family assessment," meaning that it is information about family relations. It is important to answer the question that is asked. Review the family assessment, not assessment of the client, if you had difficulty answering this question.

Client needs category: Psychosocial integrity

Client needs subcategory: None

Cognitive level: Analyzing

---

9. A client is prescribed sertraline, a selective serotonin reuptake inhibitor. Which adverse effects would the nurse review when creating a medication teaching plan? Select all that apply.

☐ **1.** Agitation

☐ **2.** Agranulocytosis

☐ **3.** Sleep disturbance

☐ **4.** Persistent cough

☐ **5.** Dry mouth

☐ **6.** Seizures

Answer: 1, 3, 5

Ⓒ Rationale: Sertraline is used to treat depression, obsessive–compulsive disorder, and panic and anxiety disorders. Common adverse effects of sertraline are agitation, sleep disturbance, and dry mouth. Agranulocytosis and seizures are adverse effects of clozapine. A persistent cough can be a side effect of antihypertensive medications.

Test-taking strategy: Analyze to determine what information the question asks for, which is the adverse effects of sertraline. "Select all that apply" questions require considering each option to decide its merit. Recall that many select serotonin reuptake inhibitors affect the rapid eye movement sleep causing insomnia. Also, adverse effects may have an opposite effect than the therapeutic effect anticipated. Review the side effects of serotonin reuptake inhibitors if you had difficulty answering this question.

Client needs category: Physiological integrity

Client needs subcategory: Pharmacological and parenteral therapies

Cognitive level: Applying

---

10. A nurse is assessing a client for dementia. What history findings would the nurse anticipate while talking with the client and family? Select all that apply.

☐ **1.** The progression of symptoms has been slow.

☐ **2.** The client admits to feelings of sadness.

☐ **3.** The client acts apathetic and pessimistic.

☐ **4.** The family cannot determine when the symptoms first appeared.

☐ **5.** The client has been exhibiting basic personality changes.

☐ **6.** The client has great difficulty paying attention to others.

Answer: 1, 4, 5, 6

Ⓓ Rationale: Dementia is the loss of brain function. It can affect memory, thinking, language, judgment, and behavior. Dementia is characterized by a slow onset of symptoms, which makes it difficult to determine when symptoms first occurred. It progresses to noticeable changes in the individual's personality and impaired ability to pay attention to other people. Sadness, apathy, and pessimism are symptoms of depression.

Test-taking strategy: Analyze to determine what information the question asks for, which is past history of symptoms of dementia. "Select all that apply" questions require considering each option to decide its merit. Recall clinical manifestations of dementia and relate to the options. Consider the insidious nature of the disease and the symptoms that appear over time. Review the signs and symptoms of dementia if you had difficulty answering this question.

Client needs category: Health promotion and maintenance

Client needs subcategory: None

Cognitive level: Analyzing

---

11. The nurse is caring for a client experiencing panic post fireworks display over the holiday weekend. The client routinely takes a prescribed dose of alprazolam 1.5 mg p.o. t.i.d. A p.r.n. dosage is also prescribed as 1.5 mg p.o. every 4 hours. The maximum daily dose is 8 mg. How many doses of the p.r.n. medication might the client take safely?

_____ doses

Answer: 2

Ⓜ Rationale: The client would have a regularly prescribed dose of 1.5 mg × 3 (t.i.d.) = 4.5 mg. The client only has 2 doses or 3 mg possible to remain under the maximum dosage cap.

Test-taking strategy: Analyze to determine what information the question asks for, which is maximum dose of as-needed medication. Begin with the maximum prescribe dosage and then assess how many potential as-needed doses are possible to remain under the maximum. Review the math or any errors. Review medication abbreviations and subsequent calculations if you had difficulty answering this question.

Client needs category: Physiological integrity

Client needs subcategory: Pharmacological and parenteral therapies

Cognitive level: Applying

12. A client on a mental health unit becomes increasingly agitated and barricades himself in a corner room holding another client hostage. Verbal exchanges indicate an escalation in client desperation. Which nursing actions would be taken at this time? Select all that apply.

☐ **1.** Identify one nurse to interact with the client.

☐ **2.** Pull the fire alarm to obtain help quickly.

☐ **3.** Direct other clients away from the area.

☐ **4.** Speak to the client in an authoritarian manner.

☐ **5.** Discreetly notify security to assist.

☐ **6.** Identify with the client's position and reason for agitation.

Answer: 1, 3, 5, 6

Ⓒ **Rationale:** The goal of the interaction is to defuse client anxiety and maintain the safety of all on the unit. To complete this goal, the nurse must calmly work with the client while obtaining assistance from security in case the situation deteriorates. Identifying one nurse (one with a good client rapport) to work with the client decreases client anxiety as well as a calming voice tone (not authoritarian) and relaxed posture. Identifying with the client allows the client to feel understood. Security precautions include removing the others from the area and notifying security. Pulling the fire alarm would elevate client anxiety.

Test-taking strategy: Analyze to determine what information the question asks for, which is nursing actions in an escalating hostage situation. Recall the phrase, "Calmness is catchy." All actions are focused on reducing the client anxiety. Compare each option to efforts ultimately resolving the situation. Review therapeutic techniques to decrease client anxiety and maintain unit safety if you had difficulty answering this question.

Client needs category: Psychosocial integrity

Client needs subcategory: None

Cognitive level: Analyzing

---

13. A client has been diagnosed with an adjustment disorder with mixed anxiety and depression. What are the primary nursing diagnoses the nurse would associate with this type of adjustment disorder? Select all that apply.

☐ **1.** Activity intolerance

☐ **2.** Impaired social interaction

☐ **3.** Risk for situational low self-esteem

☐ **4.** Disturbed personal identity

☐ **5.** Acute confusion

☐ **6.** Impaired memory

Answer: 2, 3

Ⓒ **Rationale:** Adjustment disorder occurs when an individual is unable to adjust or cope with a particular stressor such as a major life event. A client with an adjustment disorder is likely to exhibit *impaired social interaction* and *risk for situational low self-esteem*. Primary nursing diagnosis would not include the others as the client is able to participate in activities, if desired, and has no deficits in cognition or personal identity.

Test-taking strategy: Analyze to determine what information the question asks for, which is selecting primary nursing diagnoses for a client with adjustment disorder. "Select all that apply" questions require considering each option to decide its merit. The one key is understanding that adjustment disorder occurs from a major life event, not a disease process. Also, to select a "primary" nursing diagnosis, look to the cause and effect of the relationship of major events to psychosocial diagnoses. Review the defining characteristics of adjustment disorder, if you had difficulty answering this question.

Client needs category: Psychosocial integrity

Client needs subcategory: None

Cognitive level: Analyzing

14. A nurse is preparing discharge instructions for a client with resistant depression who was prescribed a new medication regimen that includes phenelzine, a monoamine oxidase inhibitor (MAO inhibitor). If the teaching was successful, what foods would the client state that he/she needs to avoid? Select all that apply.

- ☐ **1.** Aged cheese
- ☐ **2.** Cottage cheese
- ☐ **3.** Milk
- ☐ **4.** Wine
- ☐ **5.** Salami
- ☐ **6.** Fruit

Answer: 1, 4, 5

Ⓜ Rationale: Phenelzine is a medication in the class of MAO inhibitor. MAO is an enzyme responsible for metabolizing neurotransmitters, serotonin and norepinephrine. This drug requires being on a tyramine-free diet to avoid hypertensive crisis. Aged cheese, salami, and wine will cause vasoconstriction and a rise in blood pressure. Cottage cheese, milk, and fruit are allowed on a tyramine-free diet.

Test-taking strategy: Analyze to determine what information the question asks for, which is food selections that a client should avoid when prescribed phenelzine. "Select all that apply" questions require considering each option to decide its merit. First, it is essential to identify that phenelzine is an MAO inhibitor. Once completed, select options that contain tyramine such as are noted above. Review the pharmacologic effects of MAO inhibitors if you had difficulty answering this question.

Client needs category: Physiological integrity

Client needs subcategory: Pharmacological and parenteral therapies

Cognitive level: Applying

---

15. A client, diagnosed with Alzheimer's disease, is a new resident in a long-term care facility. The client has difficulty finding his/her room and is seen wandering into the room of others. When discussing the situation at a multidisciplinary conference, which client-centered actions would the nurse suggest? Select all that apply.

- ☐ **1.** Restrict the client to the client's room and hallway until he/she can recognize that area.
- ☐ **2.** Ensure that the client has prescribed hearing aids and glasses on throughout the day.
- ☐ **3.** Place a box with familiar personal items outside the client's door for visual recognition.
- ☐ **4.** Assign the client to a room close to the nursing station for closer monitoring.
- ☐ **5.** Provide verbal cueing as to where the client's room is located.
- ☐ **6.** Provide a sedative medication to decrease the client's ability to wander.

Answer: 2, 3, 4, 5

Ⓜ Rationale: Alzheimer's disease is a chronic, organic mental disorder that involves a progressive, irreversible loss of memory. Disorientation, especially when brought to an unfamiliar environment, is a common occurrence. Safety of the individual is a priority. Client-centered actions would focus on interventions to promote the identification of the client room and reduce the instances of wandering. Visual recognition via memory boxes, ensuring the client has glasses and hearing aids to facilitate orientation, and verbal cueing are helpful in assisting the client. Placing the client in a location where the nursing staff can interact with the new resident is also helpful. Restricting the client's movement to a small area and medically sedating the client is not a standard of care.

Test-taking strategy: Analyze to determine what information the question asks for, which is nursing suggestions to improve client room recognition. "Select all that apply" questions require considering each option to decide its merit. Analyze each option against standards of care for a client with mental decline. Though the suggestions may be unsuccessful, consider all that reorient the client and limit wandering. Review nursing actions for the client with Alzheimer's disease if you had difficulty answering this question.

Client needs category: Psychosocial integrity

Client needs subcategory: None

Cognitive level: Applying

Psychotic disorders

1. A nurse is assessing a new client and notices clang associations in the speech pattern. From this assessment finding, the nurse begins to evaluate for the potential of which psychiatric conditions? Select all that apply.

☐ **1.** Dissociative identity disorder

☐ **2.** Schizophrenia

☐ **3.** Narcolepsy

☐ **4.** Mania

☐ **5.** Organic disorders

☐ **6.** Intermittent explosive disorder

Answer: 2, 4, 5

Ⓒ Rationale: This speech pattern, characterized by meaningless rhymes, is found most commonly in clients with schizophrenia but may also be present in those with bipolar disorder (during the manic phase) and organic disorders. It is not characteristic of dissociative identity disorders, narcolepsy, or explosive disorders.

Test-taking strategy: Analyze to determine what information the question asks for, which is psychiatric conditions that contain clang associations. "Select all that apply" questions require considering each option to decide its merit. Recall that clang associations are a component of disorganized thinking and even psychosis. Choose options that are characterized by periods of disorganized thinking. Review clang associations related to disease processes if you had difficulty answering this question.

Client needs category: Psychosocial integrity

Client needs subcategory: None

Cognitive level: Analyzing

---

2. A nurse is monitoring a client who appears to be hallucinating. The client is gesturing at a figure on the television and appears agitated with speech containing paranoid content. Which nursing interventions are appropriate at this time? Select all that apply.

☐ **1.** In a firm voice, instruct the client to stop the behavior.

☐ **2.** Reassure the client that there is no danger.

☐ **3.** Acknowledge the presence of the hallucinations.

☐ **4.** Instruct other team members to ignore the client's behavior.

☐ **5.** Immediately implement physical restraints.

☐ **6.** Give simple commands in a calm voice.

Answer: 2, 3, 6

Ⓜ Rationale: Hallucinations are false or distorted sensory perceptions that appear to be real. Using a calm voice and giving simple commands, the nurse would reassure the client of safety. The nurse would not challenge the client; rather, the nurse would acknowledge the hallucinatory experience. It is not appropriate to ask the client to stop the behavior. Ignoring behavior will not reduce the client's agitation. Implementing restraints is not warranted at this time. Although the client is agitated, he/she does not appear to be at risk for harm.

Test-taking strategy: Analyze to determine what information the question asks for, which is nursing interventions when a client is experiencing hallucinations. "Select all that apply" questions require considering each option to decide its merit. Recall that the nurse must use standards of care, which include to facilitate conversation, validate that hallucinations are occurring, and calmly reassure. Review nursing interventions when a client is experiencing hallucinations if you had difficulty answering this question.

Client needs category: Psychosocial integrity

Client needs subcategory: None

Cognitive level: Applying

---

3. The nurse is monitoring a client with schizophrenia who is prescribed clozapine. During a multidisciplinary mental health team meeting, which signs and symptoms would be brought to the psychiatrist's attention? Select all that apply.

☐ **1.** Sore throat

☐ **2.** Pill-rolling movements

☐ **3.** Polyuria

☐ **4.** Fever

☐ **5.** Polydipsia

☐ **6.** Orthostatic hypotension

Answer: 1, 4, 6

ⓓ Rationale: Sore throat, fever, and the sudden onset of other flulike symptoms are signs of agranulocytosis, an adverse effect of clozapine that would be brought to the psychiatrists' attention. The condition is caused by a deficiency of granulocytes (a type of white blood cell), which causes the individual to be susceptible to infection. The client's white blood cell count would be monitored at least weekly during clozapine treatment. Orthostatic hypotension may occur with initial use of the drug. Dizziness upon standing with or without fainting can also occur during clozapine treatment. Extrapyramidal effects (such as pill-rolling) either do not occur or occur at a much lesser rate with the atypical antipsychotic medications. Polydipsia (excessive thirst) and polyuria (increased urination) are common adverse effects of lithium.

Test-taking strategy: Analyze to determine what information the question asks for, which is adverse effects of clozapine. "Select all that apply" questions require considering each option to decide its merit. Recall that, although unknown, clozapine is thought to use an immune mechanism that causes the agranulocytosis with subsequent symptoms. Review the adverse effects of antipsychotic medications, especially clozapine, if you had difficulty answering this question.

Client needs category: Physiological integrity

Client needs subcategory: Pharmacological and parenteral therapies

Cognitive level: Applying

---

4. A delusional client says to a nurse, "I am the Easter bunny," and insists that the nurse refer to him/her as such. The belief appears to be fixed and unchanging. Which nursing interventions would the nurse implement when working with this client? Select all that apply.

☐ **1.** Consistently use the client's name in interactions.

☐ **2.** Smile at the humor of the situation.

☐ **3.** Agree that the client is the Easter bunny.

☐ **4.** Logically point out why the client could not be the Easter bunny.

☐ **5.** Provide an as-needed medication.

☐ **6.** Provide the client with structured activities.

Answer: 1, 6

ⓒ Rationale: This client needs continuous reality-based orientation, so the nurse would use the client's name in all interactions. Structured activities can help the client refocus and resolve this delusion. The nurse would not contribute to the delusion by smiling at the comment or agreeing with the client. Logical arguments and an as-needed medication are not likely to change the client's beliefs.

Test-taking strategy: Analyze to determine what information the question asks for, which is nursing interventions appropriate in working with a delusional client. "Select all that apply" questions require considering each option to decide its merit. Recall that clients with delusions require similar interventions as those with hallucinations. Among those, include a need for safety and security, divert focus back to reality, and teach cognitive recognition strategies. Review nursing interventions when caring for a client with delusion if you had difficulty answering this question.

Client needs category: Psychosocial integrity

Client needs subcategory: None

Cognitive level: Applying

5. A health care provider prescribes haloperidol p.o. 1 mg t.i.d. When assessing the client for extrapyramidal adverse effects, which nursing measures would be initiated? Select all that apply.

☐ **1.** Review subcutaneous injection technique.

☐ **2.** Closely monitor vital signs, especially temperature.

☐ **3.** Observe for increased pacing and restlessness.

☐ **4.** Monitor blood glucose levels.

☐ **5.** Provide the client with sugar-free hard candy.

☐ **6.** Monitor for signs and symptoms of urticaria.

Answer: 2, 3, 5

Ⓒ Rationale: Neuroleptic malignant syndrome is a life-threatening extrapyramidal adverse effect of antipsychotic medications such as haloperidol. It is associated with a rapid increase in temperature. The most common extrapyramidal adverse effect, akathisia, is a form of psychomotor restlessness that is often exhibited as pacing. Haloperidol and the anticholinergic medications that are provided to alleviate its extrapyramidal effects can result in dry mouth. Providing the client with sugar-free hard candy to suck on can help alleviate this problem. Haloperidol is not given subcutaneously and does not affect blood glucose levels. Urticaria is not usually associated with haloperidol administration.

Test-taking strategy: Analyze to determine what information the question asks for, which is nursing measures for assessment of extrapyramidal adverse effects when taking haloperidol. "Select all that apply" questions require considering each option to decide its merit. Choose the options that foreshadow the beginning of extrapyramidal symptoms. Consider the data of which each nursing measure could provide. Review haloperidol administration and extrapyramidal adverse effects if you had difficulty answering this question.

Client needs category: Physiological integrity

Client needs subcategory: Pharmacological and parenteral therapies

Cognitive level: Analyzing

6. When teaching a group of nursing students about the use of antipsychotic medications, the nurse advises them that certain symptoms can occur within the first few weeks of treatment. Which symptoms are likely to occur? Select all that apply.

☐ **1.** Acute dystonic reactions

☐ **2.** Akathisia

☐ **3.** Tardive dyskinesia

☐ **4.** Neuroleptic malignant syndrome

☐ **5.** Hearing loss

☐ **6.** Orthostatic hypotension

Answer: 1, 2, 4, 6

Ⓒ Rationale: Acute dystonia, akathisia, neuroleptic malignant syndrome, and orthostatic hypotension can occur during the first few weeks of treatment with antipsychotic drugs. Tardive dyskinesia does not typically occur until at least 6 months after starting treatment. Hearing loss is not an adverse effect of antipsychotic drugs.

Test-taking strategy: Analyze to determine what information the question asks for, which is early-onset side effects of antipsychotic medications. "Select all that apply" questions require considering each option to decide its merit. The key words are "first few weeks of treatment," indicating a more minor side effect than those with later side effects. Note that an early effect includes motor disturbances because of medication effects in the motor control center of the brain. Review the adverse effects of the different classes of antipsychotic medications if you had difficulty answering this question.

Client needs category: Psychosocial integrity

Client needs subcategory: None

Cognitive level: Analyzing

7. A nurse is working with a schizophrenic client who suddenly begins experiencing auditory hallucinations. Which interactions are appropriate at this time? Select all that apply.

- ☐ **1.** Ask the client, "What are you experiencing right now?"

- ☐ **2.** Encourage the client to relate the history of the hallucinations.

- ☐ **3.** Tell the client, "I'd like to spend time with you to discuss your hallucinations. Is that okay with you?"

- ☐ **4.** Ask the client if he/she has recently taken any drugs or alcohol.

- ☐ **5.** State, "Do you understand the side effects of your medication?"

- ☐ **6.** Question if the client is faking the symptoms for attention.

Answer: 1, 2, 3, 4

ⓒ Rationale: Asking the client about discussing the hallucinations promotes trust, an essential first step in communicating with hallucinating clients. When the client relates the hallucinations, the nurse would observe for nonverbal cues, such as the client's eyes looking around the room. Asking the client about these observations will help promote understanding of the symptoms, increase trust, and decrease the client's perception that the nurse can read his/her mind. Asking the client of recent drug or alcohol activity helps determine the source of the current experience. Once trust is established, the client will be more comfortable discussing the history of the hallucinations, such as when the voices started. This step will be beneficial in helping him/her manage in the present. At this time, discussing medication side effects is inappropriate. Questioning if the client is faking does not promote a trusting relationship.

Test-taking strategy: Analyze to determine what information the question asks for, which is interactions during auditory hallucinations. "Select all that apply" questions require considering each option to decide its merit. Identify the initial interaction as asking for permission, which is essential for communication/trust and decreases anxiety. Once established, assess the history and experience of the client. Review options for interactions with a client experiencing auditory hallucinations if you had difficulty answering this question.

Client needs category: Psychosocial integrity

Client needs subcategory: None

Cognitive level: Applying

8. A client who is taking medication to control schizophrenia asks the nurse to explain the causes of the disorder. The nurse knows that an overactive dopamine system in the brain is one of the leading causes of schizophrenia and tells the client that excessive dopamine activity is responsible for symptoms. Which symptoms is the nurse referring to? Select all that apply.

- ☐ **1.** Hallucinations
- ☐ **2.** Withdrawn behavior
- ☐ **3.** Grandiosity
- ☐ **4.** Delusional thinking
- ☐ **5.** Excessive tearfulness
- ☐ **6.** Hypotension

Answer: 1, 3, 4

Ⓒ Rationale: Hallucinations, grandiosity, and delusional thinking are attributable to the effects of excessive dopamine activity. Withdrawn behavior is not associated with dopamine. Excessive tearfulness and hypotension are not commonly associated with schizophrenia or dopamine activity.

Test-taking strategy: Analyze to determine what information the question asks for, which is symptoms of schizophrenia related to dopamine activity. "Select all that apply" questions require considering each option to decide its merit. Consider that dopamine, a neurotransmitter, is excitable in the structurally changed schizophrenic brain. Recall that when drugs block the dopamine receptors, the symptoms of schizophrenia are reduced. Review the effects of dopamine on the brain and signs and symptoms of schizophrenia if you had difficulty answering this question.

Client needs category: Psychosocial integrity

Client needs subcategory: None

Cognitive level: Analyzing

9. A client with a diagnosis of undifferentiated schizophrenia is admitted to the inpatient unit after developing water intoxication. Which nursing interventions are appropriate? Select all that apply.

- ☐ **1.** Medicate the client at night.
- ☐ **2.** Provide gum for the client.
- ☐ **3.** Lock the unit's kitchen and bathroom.
- ☐ **4.** Weigh the client every day.
- ☐ **5.** Monitor the client's intake and output.
- ☐ **6.** Maintain a structured environment.

Answer: 2, 4, 5, 6

Ⓒ Rationale: Water intoxication is a potentially fatal disturbance in brain functions that results when the normal balance of electrolytes is outside of safe limits by overhydration. It is appropriate for the nurse to monitor intake and output, weigh the client daily, and encourage the client to chew gum rather than drink water. The nurse also provides a structured environment as a way to distract and divert the client away from obtaining fluids. Medicating the client at night and locking the unit's kitchen and bathroom would not be necessary.

Test-taking strategy: Analyze to determine what information the question asks for, which is nursing interventions for a schizophrenic client who has developed water intoxication. "Select all that apply" questions require considering each option to decide its merit. Consider options that monitor the electrolyte status and fluid volume and provide structure for the schizophrenic client. Review water intoxication for a schizophrenic client if you had difficulty answering this question.

Client needs category: Physiological integrity

Client needs subcategory: Reduction of risk potential

Cognitive level: Applying

Substance abuse, eating disorders, and impulse control disorders

1. During the nurse's assessment of a client who has been diagnosed with bulimia nervosa, the nurse evaluates certain assessment findings that accompany binge eating. Which are **most** applicable? Select all that apply.

☐ **1.** Guilt

☐ **2.** Dental caries

☐ **3.** Self-induced vomiting

☐ **4.** Weight loss

☐ **5.** Normal weight

☐ **6.** Introverted behavior

Answer: 1, 2, 3, 5

© Rationale: Bulimia nervosa is an eating disorder in which individuals binge on food and then begin to make up for it by purging, taking laxatives, and starving themselves. Guilt, dental caries, self-induced vomiting, and normal weight are associated with bulimia nervosa. Weight loss and introverted behavior are associated with anorexia nervosa.

Test-taking strategy: Analyze to determine what information the question asks for, which is characteristics of a client with bulimia nervosa and binge eating. "Select all that apply" questions require considering each option to decide its merit. Recall consequences from ingesting and then eliminating food from the body. Consider each option to the effects of gastric contents being eliminated. Review bulimia nervosa, binge eating, and the client's bodily effects if you had difficulty answering this question.

Client needs category: Psychosocial integrity

Client needs subcategory: None

Cognitive level: Analyzing

2. A client, brought to the emergency department by the police, is found wandering the streets of town and appears to be disoriented. When approached by the nurse, the client begins to laugh inappropriately and states feeling dizzy. Which client behaviors suggest the client is symptomatic for huffing aerosols? Select all that apply.

☐ **1.** An unsteady gait

☐ **2.** An elevated temperature

☐ **3.** Multiple bruises on the skin

☐ **4.** Impaired memory of where he/she had been

☐ **5.** A slurred speech during conversation

☐ **6.** Hallucinations of spiders crawling on the bed

Answer: 1, 4, 5, 6

© Rationale: Huffing inhalants includes common household products such as hair spray, paints, and lighter fluids. Signs of abuse are similar to being under the influence of alcohol. These symptoms include slurred speech, an unsteady gait, euphoria, dizziness, confusion, hallucinations, and delusions. An elevated temperature is common in cocaine use and bruising is common with intravenous drug users.

Test-taking strategy: Analyze to determine what information the question asks for, which is symptoms commonly associated with huffing aerosols. Consider the huffing "high" on the central nervous system and relate to stated symptoms. Review the symptoms caused by huffing aerosols if you had difficulty answering this question.

Client needs category: Psychosocial integrity

Client needs subcategory: None

Cognitive level: Applying

3. A nurse is employed at an outpatient rehabilitation facility caring for the client with opioid addiction who is in withdrawal. When assessing clients who present for their counseling session, which findings would be commonly observed? Select all that apply.

☐ **1.** Abdominal cramps

☐ **2.** Dry, warm skin

☐ **3.** Rhinorrhea

☐ **4.** Dilated pupils

☐ **5.** Hypersomnia

☐ **6.** Feelings of hunger

Answer: 1, 3, 4

🄲 **Rationale:** Opioid withdrawal refers to the wide range of symptoms that occur stopping or dramatically reducing opiate drugs. Opioid withdrawal commonly manifests as abdominal cramps, rhinorrhea, dilated pupils, and anorexia (not hunger). Insomnia (not hypersomnia) and diaphoresis (not dry, warm skin) are also common.

Test-taking strategy: Analyze to determine what information the question asks for, which is common signs of opioid withdrawal. "Select all that apply" questions require considering each option to decide its merit. Recall that when withdrawing from opioids, the body needs time to recover from the physical dependence. Many times the client will experience flulike symptoms. Review the withdrawal effects of opioids on the various body systems if you had difficulty answering this question.

Client needs category: Physiological integrity

Client needs subcategory: Pharmacological and parenteral therapies

Cognitive level: Analyzing

---

4. During the nurse's shift in the emergency department, a nurse assesses a client who is suspected of being under the influence of amphetamines. Which symptoms are indicative of amphetamine use? Select all that apply.

☐ **1.** Depressed affect

☐ **2.** Diaphoresis

☐ **3.** Shallow respirations

☐ **4.** Hypotension

☐ **5.** Tremors

☐ **6.** Dilated pupils

Answer: 2, 3, 5, 6

🄲 **Rationale:** A client under the influence of amphetamines may present with euphoria, diaphoresis, shallow respirations, dilated pupils, dry mouth, anorexia, tachycardia, hypertension, hyperthermia, tremors, seizures, and altered mental status. Depressed affect and hypotension are not associated with amphetamine use.

Test-taking strategy: Analyze to determine what information the question asks for, which is symptoms of amphetamine use. "Select all that apply" questions require considering each option to decide its merit. Recall the overall effect of amphetamines as body stimulant. Note the exaggerated effect on the body. Review amphetamine administration and abuse if you had difficulty answering this question.

Client needs category: Physiological integrity

Client needs subcategory: Pharmacological and parenteral therapies

Cognitive level: Applying

5. A nurse is caring for an anorexic client with a nursing diagnosis of *imbalanced nutrition: less than body requirements related to dysfunctional eating patterns*. Which interventions would be supportive for this client? Select all that apply.

☐ **1.** Provide small, frequent meals.

☐ **2.** Monitor weight gain.

☐ **3.** Allow the client to skip meals until the anti-depressant levels are therapeutic.

☐ **4.** Encourage the client to keep a journal.

☐ **5.** Monitor the client during meals and for 1 hour afterward.

☐ **6.** Encourage the client to eat three substantial meals per day.

Answer: 1, 2, 4, 5

C Rationale: Anorexia nervosa is an eating disorder characterized by excessive food restriction and irrational fear of gaining weight. Because the clients are engaged in self-starvation, clients with anorexia rarely can tolerate large meals three times per day. Small, frequent meals may be tolerated better, and they provide a way to gradually increase daily caloric intake. The nurse would monitor the client's weight carefully because a client with anorexia may try to hide the weight loss. The nurse would also monitor the client during meals and for 1 hour afterward to ensure that the client consumes all of the food and does not attempt to purge. The client may be afraid to express feelings; keeping a journal can serve as an outlet for these feelings, which can assist recovery. A client with anorexia is already underweight and should not be permitted to skip meals.

Test-taking strategy: Analyze to determine what information the question asks for, which is nursing interventions for an anorexic client with a nursing diagnosis of imbalanced nutrition. "Select all that apply" questions require considering each option to decide its merit. Focus on the key words of anorexia and nursing diagnosis of imbalanced nutrition and eating patterns. Always answer what the question is asking. Note the relation between the correct answers and the nursing diagnosis. Review nursing interventions for the anorexic client if you had difficulty answering this question.

Client needs category: Psychosocial integrity

Client needs subcategory: None

Cognitive level: Analyzing

6. When assessing a client diagnosed with impulse control disorder, the nurse observes violent, aggressive, and assaultive behavior. Which history and assessment findings is the nurse also likely to find? Select all that apply.

☐ **1.** The client functions well in other areas of life.

☐ **2.** The degree of aggressiveness is out of proportion to the stressor.

☐ **3.** The violent behavior is usually justified by a stressor.

☐ **4.** The client has a history of parental alcoholism and a chaotic, abusive family life.

☐ **5.** The client has no remorse about the inability to control behavior.

Answer: 1, 2, 4

Ⓓ Rationale: A client with an impulse control disorder who displays violent, aggressive, and assaultive behavior generally functions well in other areas of life. The degree of aggressiveness is out of proportion to the stressor, and there is frequently a history of parental alcoholism and a chaotic family life. The client often verbalizes sincere remorse and guilt for the aggressive behavior.

Test-taking strategy: Analyze to determine what information the question asks for, which is findings typically found when assessing a client with impulse control disorder. "Select all that apply" questions require considering each option to decide its merit. Recall that individuals with impulse control disorders cannot resist the urge to do something harmful to themselves or others. Consider that psychological factors are associated with this disorder and remorse is frequently seen. Review the clinical manifestations of impulse control disorder if you had difficulty answering this question.

Client needs category: Psychosocial integrity

Client needs subcategory: None

Cognitive level: Applying

---

7. A nurse is caring for a client with borderline personality disorder. Which interventions are appropriate for clients with this disorder? Select all that apply.

☐ **1.** Providing antianxiety medications

☐ **2.** Providing emotional consistency

☐ **3.** Exploring anger in appropriate ways

☐ **4.** Encouraging independence as soon as possible

☐ **5.** Promoting gradual separation and individuation

☐ **6.** Ensuring the client's safety

Answer: 2, 3, 5, 6

Ⓓ Rationale: In clients with borderline personalities, the primary goal is to ensure a safe environment. As the client begins to learn how to manage his/her behavior, suicide still remains a risk. A key intervention includes providing emotional support that is consistent. The client needs to learn how to manage anger effectively and typically begins needing less support as he/she separates and develops individual coping behaviors. Antianxiety drugs are reserved for clinical emergencies.

Test-taking strategy: Analyze to determine what information the question asks for, which is nursing interventions for a client with borderline personality disorder. "Select all that apply" questions require considering each option to decide its merit. Recall that with borderline personality disorder, how the client views himself/herself is distorted, making the client feel worthless and emotional instability leading to anger, stress, and other problems. Consider each option in relation to clinical manifestations. Review the nursing interventions necessary when caring for a client with borderline personality disorder if you had difficulty answering this question.

Client needs category: Psychosocial integrity

Client needs subcategory: None

Cognitive level: Applying

---

8. A client is prescribed chlordiazepoxide as needed to control the symptoms of alcohol withdrawal. Which symptoms may indicate the need for an additional dose of this medication? Select all that apply.

☐ **1.** Tachycardia

☐ **2.** Mood swings

☐ **3.** Elevated blood pressure and temperature

☐ **4.** Piloerection

☐ **5.** Tremors

☐ **6.** Increasing anxiety

Ⓒ Rationale: Benzodiazepines such as chlordiazepoxide are usually administered based on elevations in heart rate, blood pressure, and temperature, as well as on the presence of tremors and increasing anxiety. Mood swings are expected during the withdrawal period and are not an indication for further medication administration. Piloerection (goosebumps, or a feeling of hair of the skin standing on end) is not a symptom of alcohol withdrawal.

Test-taking strategy: Analyze to determine what information the question asks for, which is symptoms of uncontrolled alcohol withdrawal. "Select all that apply" questions require considering each option to decide its merit. Consider symptom management of alcohol withdrawal and therapeutic chlordiazepoxide effects. Recall that chlordiazepoxide is used to relieve anxiety and control agitation. Review the clinical manifestations of alcohol withdrawal and chlordiazepoxide use if you had difficulty answering this question.

Client needs category: Physiological integrity

Client needs subcategory: Pharmacological and parenteral therapies

Cognitive level: Analysis

9. The nurse is assessing a client who is a polysubstance abuser, with cocaine being one of the drugs most frequently used. Which physiological symptom is suggestive of early (phase 1) cocaine intoxication? Select all that apply.

☐ **1.** Respiratory depression

☐ **2.** Psychomotor agitation

☐ **3.** Cardiac arrhythmias

☐ **4.** Dilated pupils

☐ **5.** Flaccid paralysis

☐ **6.** Slurred speech

Ⓒ Rationale: A polysubstance abuser is an individual who abuses at least three substances. Caffeine and nicotine are not included substances. When assessing for initial cocaine intoxication, the most common physiological symptoms observed are respiratory depression, cardiac arrhythmias, psychomotor agitation, and dilated pupils. Slurred speech is not associated with cocaine intoxication. Flaccid paralysis is characteristic of the last phase (phase III) of cocaine intoxication, typically occurring before death.

Test-taking strategy: Analyze to determine what information the question asks for, which is suggestive symptoms of initial (phase 1) cocaine intoxication. "Select all that apply" questions require considering each option to decide its merit. Recall that cocaine tends to affect the central nervous system immediately. An exaggerated effect would be noted with intoxication. Review the clinical manifestations of initial cocaine intoxication and the effects on body systems if you had difficulty answering this question.

Client needs category: Physiological integrity

Client needs subcategory: Physiological adaptation

Cognitive level: Analyzing

10. The nurse is caring for a mental health client who exhibits passive–aggressive behavior when interacting with the nursing staff. When reporting client behaviors to the next shift, which actions are consistent with this assessment? Select all that apply.

☐ **1.** The client states that problems are not his/her fault.

☐ **2.** The client agrees with the staff but then complains to others.

☐ **3.** The client pouts when he/she does not get his/her way.

☐ **4.** The client feels angry about the group session so he/she scatters papers in the lunchroom.

☐ **5.** The client attacks the nurse and later cries feeling remorse.

Answer: 2, 4

Ⓓ Rationale: The client experiencing passive–aggressive behavior does not confront a situation directly but does something negative and potentially not even related to the situation in which he or she was upset. At times, the client may verbalize one thing and act in a different manner. A client who states that problems are not his/her fault may be refusing to accept responsibility for actions. Pouting reflects immature behavior. Attacking a nurse and then feeling remorse reflects aggressive behavior.

Test-taking strategy: Analyze to determine what information the question asks for, which is client example of passive–aggressive behavior. Use your knowledge of medical terminology (passive = not responding to an action; aggressive = showing a readiness for action) and understanding of opposites to select the correct examples. Review the definition of passive–aggressive behavior if you had difficulty answering this question.

Client needs category: Psychosocial integrity
Client needs subcategory: None
Cognitive level: Applying

---

11. A nurse is caring for a client who has experienced frontal lobe damage in a car accident. Which psychosocial behaviors are indications of this damage? Select all that apply.

☐ **1.** A change in personality

☐ **2.** Overt sexual behavior

☐ **3.** Difficulty controlling temper

☐ **4.** Fewer facial expressions

☐ **5.** Inability to go out in public settings

☐ **6.** A disinterest in family relationships

Answer: 1, 2, 3, 4

Ⓒ Rationale: The frontal lobes are considered our emotional control center and home to our personality. They are involved in motor function, problem solving, spontaneity, memory, language, initiation, judgment, impulse control, and social and sexual behavior. Also, those with frontal damage display fewer spontaneous facial movements, speak fewer words, or the opposite, speak excessively. A client may not be interested in social situations but has the ability to go out in public settings if desired. While there may be personality changes, there is nothing to state a disinterest in family relationships.

Test-taking strategy: Analyze to determine what information the question asks for, which is psychosocial impact of frontal lobe damage. When considering the frontal lobe, think personality and judgment. Review the effect of damage to the frontal lobe of the brain if you had difficulty answering this question.

Client needs category: Physiological integrity
Client needs subcategory: Physiological adaptation
Cognitive level: Applying

Comprehensive tests

Comprehensive test 1

1. The nurse is caring for a client with blood pressure of 210/94 mm Hg. The health care provider prescribes Vasotec 20 mg b.i.d. Which nursing action is **best** when administering a new blood pressure medication to a client?

☐ **1.** Administer the medication to the client explaining that there is a new medication.

☐ **2.** Inform the client about the new medication and provide a handout.

☐ **3.** Inform the client about the new medication, including its name, use, and the reason for the change in medication.

☐ **4.** Administer the medication, and inform the client that the health care provider will later explain the medication.

Answer: 3

Rationale: Medication administration and teaching is in the nurse's scope of practice and a common nursing action. It is important for the nurse to inform the client about the medication, including its name, use, and the reason for the medication change, because teaching the client about treatment regimen promotes compliance. The other responses are not as specific and inclusive.

Test-taking strategy: Analyze to determine what information the question asks for, which is nursing action when administering a new medication. Consider that providing complete and accurate information to a client places the client in the best position to be compliant with the medication regimen. Review nursing actions when a client is prescribed a new medication if you had difficulty answering this question.

Client needs category: Safe and effective care environment

Client needs subcategory: Management of care

Cognitive level: Applying

---

2. The nurse is caring for a client immediately after receiving electroconvulsive therapy for the treatment of severe depression. What is a **priority** intervention for this client?

☐ **1.** Orient the client to the surroundings.

☐ **2.** Educate the client about depression.

☐ **3.** Offer sips of clear liquids orally.

☐ **4.** Administer an opioid analgesic for a headache.

Answer: 1

Rationale: Electroconvulsive therapy uses an electrical current to treat depression and other mental illnesses. After electroconvulsive therapy, the client may be mildly confused or briefly disoriented and requires reorienting to the surroundings. The symptoms after ECT are generally the same as those a client experiences after a seizure. A headache may be present but would not necessitate the administration of an opioid analgesic. Fluids would not be offered until the return of the gag reflex.

Test-taking strategy: Analyze to determine what information the question asks for, which is priority nursing intervention following electroconvulsive therapy. The key words are "immediately after." Consider each option to be completed at this certain time. Eliminate option 2 as not an appropriate time for teaching and option 3 as not offering fluids until the client is fully recovered from procedure. Discriminate between the last two options eliminating the need for an opioid for a headache. Review electroconvulsive therapy if you had difficulty answering this question.

Client needs category: Psychosocial integrity

Client needs subcategory: None

Cognitive level: Analyzing

---

3. A client arrives at the emergency department with chest and stomach pain and a report of black, tarry stools for several months. Which order would the nurse anticipate?

☐ **1.** Cardiac monitoring, oxygen, creatine kinase, and lactate dehydrogenase (LD) levels

☐ **2.** Prothrombin time (PT), partial thromboplastin time (PTT), fibrinogen, and fibrin split product values

☐ **3.** ECG (electrocardiogram), complete blood count, testing for occult blood, and comprehensive serum metabolic panel

☐ **4.** EEG (electroencephalogram), alkaline phosphatase and aspartate aminotransferase levels, and basic serum metabolic panel

Answer: 3

🅔 **Rationale:** An ECG evaluates the report of chest pain, laboratory tests determine anemia, and the test for occult blood determines blood in the stool. Cardiac monitoring, oxygen, and creatine kinase and LD levels are appropriate for a primary cardiac problem. A basic metabolic panel and alkaline phosphatase and aspartate aminotransferase levels assess liver function. PT, PTT, fibrinogen, and fibrin split products are measured to verify bleeding dyscrasias. An EEG evaluates brain electrical activity.

Test-taking strategy: Analyze to determine what information the question asks for, which is anticipated laboratory testing for a client who reports chest and stomach pain. Select the option that reflects laboratory/diagnostic testing that would address client symptoms. Review cardiac and gastrointestinal (GI) diagnostic testing if you had difficulty answering this question.

Client needs category: Physiological integrity

Client needs subcategory: Reduction of risk potential

Cognitive level: Analyzing

---

4. The nurse places the following catheter at the client's bedside for use at which time?

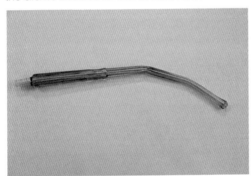

☐ **1.** When the tracheostomy becomes obstructed

☐ **2.** During an ostomy irrigation

☐ **3.** When the oral cavity has thick secretions

☐ **4.** Following nasal surgery

Answer: 3

🅔 **Rationale:** The catheter is a Yankauer suction catheter, which removes oral secretions. It is unable to fit down the tracheostomy tube. It is not used for irrigation. A catheter is not introduced into the airway following nasal surgery.

Test-taking strategy: Analyze to determine what information the question asks for, which is use for the pictured catheter. Note the characteristics of the catheter including size and shape. Consider each use against those characteristics. Eliminate option 4 as nothing would be utilized following nasal surgery. Eliminate option 1 as the characteristics of the catheter do not match with the tracheostomy tube. Review the characteristics and use of a Yankauer catheter if you had difficulty answering this question.

Client needs category: Physiological integrity

Client needs subcategory: Basic care and comfort

Cognitive level: Applying

5. The family of a client, stung by a bee, has rushed the client to the emergency room. The client is experiencing hives and redness at the site. Upon arrival, the client states, "I feel a lump in my throat and I am sweating. I can't breathe! I think I am going to die!" The nurse anticipates which emergency treatment next?

☐ **1.** Administer oxygen 4 L via nasal cannula.

☐ **2.** Administer albuterol 2 puffs stat.

☐ **3.** Administer an injection of epinephrine stat.

☐ **4.** Have the client in high Fowler's position in the bed.

Answer: 3

Ⓔ Rationale: Symptoms of hives and redness at the bee sting site coupled with a progression of symptoms including respiratory difficulty and an impending feeling of doom indicate anaphylaxis. Emergency treatment of anaphylaxis is an injection of epinephrine. Bronchodilators may help but are not the primary treatment. β-Adrenergic blockers are not indicated in the management of anaphylaxis because they may cause bronchospasm. Having the client in high Fowler's position is appropriate but not emergency treatment.

Test-taking strategy: Analyze to determine what information the question asks for, which is emergency treatment for a client in respiratory distress. Analyze the symptoms to conclude that the client is having an anaphylactic reaction. Remember the ABCs (airway, breathing, and circulation) of emergency care, and recall that epinephrine (adrenaline) reduces the body's allergic response. If unsure, consider that an injection enters the blood stream rapidly. Review emergency treatment of anaphylaxis if you had difficulty answering this question.

Client needs category: Physiological integrity

Client needs subcategory: Physiological adaptation

Cognitive level: Analyzing

---

6. A client has a cast applied to the left leg after sustaining a femur fracture during a skiing accident. Which interventions would the nurse provide to avoid complications from the cast application? Select all that apply.

☐ **1.** Apply warm compresses to the casted leg.

☐ **2.** Bivalve the cast on both sides.

☐ **3.** Monitor distal pulses of the affected extremity.

☐ **4.** Maintain the leg elevated above the level of the heart.

☐ **5.** Administer anticoagulation per health care provider's order.

Answer: 3, 4, 5

Ⓜ Rationale: The nurse would monitor the tightness of the cast by assessing the distal pulses and tightness of the cast. Edema can cause the cast to become tight and lead to compartment syndrome. Unless contraindicated, the leg would be elevated above the heart in order to increase venous return and decrease edema. Prophylactic anticoagulation will decrease the risk of clot formation. The nurse would apply cool compresses, not warm. It is not within the nurse's scope of practice to cut the cast or bivalve the cast.

Test-taking strategy: Analyze to determine what information the question asks for, which is actions to prevent complications following cast application. Recall nursing care, which includes monitoring circulatory status. Review complications of cast application if you had difficulty answering this question.

Client needs category: Physiological integrity

Client needs subcategory: Reduction of risk potential

Cognitive level: Analyzing

7. A 9-year-old client with a mild concussion is discharged following a magnetic resonance imaging (MRI) of the brain. Before discharge, the client reports a headache. The mother questions pain medication for home. Which response by the nurse is **most** appropriate?

☐ **1.** "Your child has a mild concussion; acetaminophen can be given."

☐ **2.** "Maybe the health care provider will prescribe aspirin for the head pain."

☐ **3.** "Pain medication is avoided after a head injury to avoid hiding a worsening condition."

☐ **4.** "Opioid medications may lead to vomiting, which increases the intracranial pressure (ICP)."

Answer: 1

Ⓜ **Rationale:** Following MRI of the brain, it is confirmed that there is no bleeding on the brain; thus, pain medication may be administered. The mother asks for medication for a headache. The most appropriate response is that acetaminophen may be given. Opioids may mask changes in the level of consciousness (LOC) that indicate increased intracranial pressure (ICP); therefore, it would not be given. Aspirin is contraindicated in conditions that may involve bleeding, such as traumatic injuries, and for children or young adults with viral illnesses because of the danger of Reye's syndrome.

Test-taking strategy: Analyze to determine what information the question asks for, which is pain medication for a mild concussion once the risk of intracranial bleeding is cleared. Eliminate option 3 following MRI results. Eliminate option 2 related to Reye's syndrome and the client's age. Option 4 is correct, but option 1 answers the mother's question and is the best choice. Review postconcussion care if you had difficulty answering this question.

Client needs category: Physiological integrity

Client needs subcategory: Reduction of risk potential

Cognitive level: Applying

---

8. The nurse is caring for a 15-year-old client with anorexia nervosa and a body mass index (BMI) of 17. Which statement made by the client would indicate to the nurse that the North America Nursing Diagnosis Association (NANDA) diagnosis or patient priority of *Body image altered* is appropriate?

☐ **1.** "Skinny is the best body type."

☐ **2.** "I'm too ugly and fat."

☐ **3.** "I like being a small size."

☐ **4.** "I do not want to gain weight."

Answer: 2

Ⓔ **Rationale:** The NANDA diagnosis of *Body image altered* is defined as the confusion in the mental picture of one's physical self. This is consistent with the patient priority linking body image with the client diagnosis. The client with a BMI of 17 is underweight, but the client sees herself as fat and ugly. The other three responses do not fit the NANDA diagnosis/patient priority because they project a positive image.

Test-taking strategy: Analyze to determine what information the question asks for, which is statement indicating an altered body image. Identify the negative statement in the group. Anytime there is one odd option in a group, always give that option extra consideration. Review client attitudes toward body image when diagnosed with anorexia nervosa if you had difficulty answering this question.

Client needs category: Health promotion and maintenance

Client needs subcategory: None

Cognitive level: Analyzing

9. The nurse is caring for an elderly client with a fractured hip who is on bed rest. Which nursing interventions would be included on the plan of care?

☐ **1.** Encourage coughing and deep breathing, and limit fluid intake.

☐ **2.** Provide only passive range of motion (ROM), and decrease stimulation.

☐ **3.** Have the client lie as still as possible, and give adequate pain medication.

☐ **4.** Turn the client every 2 hours, and encourage coughing and deep breathing.

Answer: 4

Ⓔ Rationale: Appropriate interventions for a bedridden client include turning every 2 hours, providing adequate nutrition, and encouraging coughing and deep breathing. Hydration, active and passive ROM, and adequate pain medication are also appropriate nursing measures. To prevent contractures, the client would not limit fluid intake or lie as still as possible.

Test-taking strategy: Analyze to determine what information the question asks for, which is nursing interventions for a client on bed rest. Discriminate through each option reading carefully as one part of the option may be correct while the other is incorrect. Consider maintaining skin integrity and preventing complications. Review nursing intervention for a client on bed rest if you had difficulty answering this question.

Client needs category: Safe and effective care environment

Client needs subcategory: Management of care

Cognitive level: Applying

---

10. A nurse is providing nutritional teaching for a client with a family history of colon cancer. Which food choice by the client demonstrates an understanding of the correct diet to follow?

☐ **1.** Vegetarian chili

☐ **2.** Hot dogs and sauerkraut

☐ **3.** Egg salad on rye bread

☐ **4.** Spaghetti and meat sauce

Answer: 1

Ⓒ Rationale: A high-fiber, low-fat food, such as vegetarian chili, increases gastric motility and decreases the chance of constipation, helping to reduce the risk of colon cancer. The other choices are not representative of a high-fiber, low-fat diet.

Test-taking strategy: Analyze to determine what information the question asks for, which is nutritional choice for a client with a family history of colon cancer. Recall that most studies state that a plant-based diet rich in fruits, vegetables, legumes, and whole grains is associated with a lower risk of a number of common cancers. Recall dietary guidelines for preventing colon cancer if you had difficulty answering this question.

Client needs category: Health promotion and maintenance

Client needs subcategory: None

Cognitive level: Applying

11. A nurse has a four-patient assignment in the medical step-down unit. When planning care for the clients, which client would have the following treatment goals: fluid replacement, vasopressin replacement, and correction of underlying intracranial pathology?

☐ **1.** The client with diabetes mellitus

☐ **2.** The client with diabetes insipidus

☐ **3.** The client with diabetic ketoacidosis

☐ **4.** The client with syndrome of inappropriate antidiuretic hormone (SIADH) secretion

Answer: 2

Ⓒ Rationale: Maintaining adequate fluid, replacing vasopressin, and correcting underlying intracranial problems (typically lesions, tumors, or trauma affecting the hypothalamus or pituitary gland) are the main objectives in treating diabetes insipidus. Diabetes mellitus does not involve vasopressin deficiencies or an intracranial disorder, but rather a disturbance in the production or use of insulin. Diabetic ketoacidosis results from severe insulin insufficiency. An excess of vasopressin leads to SIADH, causing the client to retain fluid.

Test-taking strategy: Analyze to determine what information the question asks for, which is selecting the client with a specific treatment plan. Discriminate through the options to select the disease process, which includes a disruption in fluid status, lack of vasopressin which is normally secreted by the pituitary gland, and having an intracranial disorder. Review endocrine disorders and their treatment plans if you had difficulty answering this question.

Client needs category: Physiological integrity

Client needs subcategory: Physiological adaptation

Cognitive level: Analyzing

---

12. The nurse states on shift handoff that the client has an elevated uric acid level of 8.2 mg/dl (487.8 mmol/L). Which inflammatory process would the nurse assess for during client assessment?

☐ **1.** Rheumatoid arthritis

☐ **2.** Lupus erythematosus

☐ **3.** Osteoporosis

☐ **4.** Gout

Answer: 4

Ⓔ Rationale: Normal gout levels are 4 to 8 mg/dl (237.9 to 475.9 mmol/L). Uric acid levels that exceed 6 mg/dl (356.9 mmol/L) provide an elevated risk for gout. Gout is a medical condition with symptoms of acute inflammatory arthritis that is caused by high levels of uric acid in the blood. The client can develop uric acid crystal deposits in the joint. The nurse would assess joint areas for pain, redness, and swelling. Rheumatoid arthritis is a chronic disease of joint inflammation and pain. Lupus erythematosus is a chronic tissue disorder of the connective tissue and is known to have an elevated antinuclear antibody level. Osteoporosis has a deficiency in the serum calcium level.

Test-taking strategy: Analyze to determine what information the question asks for, which is inflammatory process associated with an elevated uric acid. Recall that gout is commonly associated with uric acid blood levels. Review the signs and symptoms of gout if you had difficulty answering this question.

Client needs category: Physiological integrity

Client needs subcategory: Reduction of risk potential

Cognitive level: Applying

13. The nurse is working at the local family planning clinic completing family education. When devising a teaching plan, in which client group would the nurse stress the importance of an annual Papanicolaou test?

☐ **1.** Clients with a history of recurrent candidiasis

☐ **2.** Clients who were pregnant before age 20

☐ **3.** Clients infected with the human papillomavirus (HPV)

☐ **4.** Clients with a long history of oral contraceptive use

Answer: 3

Ⓔ Rationale: Annual Papanicolaou testing is a screening to detect potential precancerous and cancerous cells in the endocervical canal of the female reproductive system. HPV causes genital warts, which are associated with an increased incidence of cervical cancer. Recurrent candidiasis, pregnancy before age 20, and use of oral contraceptives do not increase the risk of cervical cancer.

Test-taking strategy: Analyze to determine what information the question asks for, which is client group that would most benefit from annual Papanicolaou testing. Recall the diagnostic findings associated with a Papanicolaou test, and relate these to the risk factors noted in each option. Review the benefits associated with annual Papanicolaou testing if you had difficulty answering this question.

Client needs category: Health promotion and maintenance

Client needs subcategory: None

Cognitive level: Analyzing

---

14. The nurse is caring for an infant diagnosed with thrush. Which instruction would the nurse give to a client's mother who will be administering nystatin oral solution?

☐ **1.** Administer the drug right after meals by swabbing the mouth.

☐ **2.** Administer the drug right before meals by using a gauze pad.

☐ **3.** Mix the drug with small amounts of formula in bottle.

☐ **4.** Administer half the dose before and half after a feeding.

Answer: 1

Ⓜ Rationale: Nystatin oral solution is an antifungal medication used to treat fungal or yeast infections. Nystatin oral solution should be swished around the mouth after eating for the best contact with mucous membranes. Taking the drug before or with meals does not allow for optimal contact with mucous membranes.

Test-taking strategy: Analyze to determine what information the question asks for, which is instructions for a mother administering nystatin oral solution. Recall that the action of the medication needs contact with the mucous membranes. Options 2 and 4 are eliminated as eating after administration removes the medication, and splitting the dosage before provides an incorrect dosage. Option 3 violates the standard of not putting medication in a bottle. Review nystatin administration if you had difficulty answering this question.

Client needs category: Physiological integrity

Client needs subcategory: Pharmacological and parenteral therapies

Cognitive level: Applying

15. A newly admitted client is extremely hostile toward a staff member without apparent reason. According to Freudian theory, the nurse would suspect that the client is exhibiting which phenomenon?

☐ **1.** Intellectualization

☐ **2.** Transference

☐ **3.** Triangulation

☐ **4.** Splitting

Answer: 2

ⓔ Rationale: Transference is the unconscious assignment of negative or positive feelings evoked by a significant person in the client's past to another person. Intellectualization is a defense mechanism in which the client avoids dealing with emotions by focusing on facts. Triangulation refers to conflicts involving three family members. Splitting is a defense mechanism commonly seen in clients with personality disorders in which the world is perceived as all good or all bad.

Test-taking strategy: Analyze to determine what information the question asks for, which is freudian theory demonstrated by hostility toward staff. If unsure, consider possible meaning of each option that will lead directly to the answer (transference = transferring to another person). Review the characteristics of defense mechanisms if you had difficulty answering this question.

Client needs category: Psychosocial integrity

Client needs subcategory: None

Cognitive level: Applying

---

16. A client has a chest tube inserted for the treatment of a pneumothorax. While turning in the bed, the client dislodges the tube and it is found in the bed. As the registered nurse is directing the health care team, place the actions of the registered nurse in the correct order. All options must be used.

1. Assess vital signs and await further medical orders.

2. Tape the dressing on three sides.

3. Apply an occlusive dressing over the puncture site.

4. Direct the licensed practical/vocational nurse to notify the health care provider.

5. Assess the client's respiratory status.

Answer: 3, 2, 4, 5, 1

ⓓ Rationale: A chest tube is a flexible, hollow tube placed through the chest wall and into the pleural space. The chest tube is able to relieve trapped air and fluid. If a chest tube is dislodged and comes out, the nurse would immediately apply an occlusive dressing such as Vaseline gauze (many times kept in the client's room). The dressing is taped on three sides. The first action always focuses on the client. The nurse would direct another licensed nurse to immediately notify the health care provider. The nurse would then assess the respiratory status. The nurse would obtain vital signs and await further orders.

Test-taking strategy: Analyze to determine what information the question asks for, which is priority actions when a chest tube falls out. Always look to the care of the client first. If unsure of the order, look for the first actions and the last or least important action. Narrowing the middle actions allows for careful discrimination and proper ordering. Review nursing actions in the care of a chest tube if you had difficulty answering this question.

Client needs category: Safe and effective care environment

Client needs subcategory: Management of care

Cognitive level: Analyzing

17. A client at 42 weeks of gestation is 3 cm dilated and 30% effaced, with membranes intact and the fetus at 12 station. Fetal heart rate (FHR) is 140 beats/minute. After 2 hours, the nurse notes that, for the past 10 minutes, the external fetal monitor has been displaying an FHR of 190 beats/minute. The client states that her baby has been extremely active. Uterine contractions are strong, occurring every 3 to 4 minutes and lasting 40 to 60 seconds. Which finding would indicate fetal hypoxia?

☐ **1.** Abnormally long uterine contractions

☐ **2.** Abnormally strong uterine intensity

☐ **3.** Excessively frequent contractions, with rapid fetal movement

☐ **4.** Excessive fetal activity and fetal tachycardia

Answer: 4

Ⓔ Rationale: Fetal tachycardia and excessive fetal activity are the first signs of fetal hypoxia. The duration of uterine contractions is within normal limits. Uterine intensity can be mild to strong yet still within normal limits. The frequency of contractions is within normal limits for the active phase of labor.

Test-taking strategy: Analyze to determine what information the question asks for, which is signs of fetal hypoxia. Sift through the data to interpret abnormalities and then relate to a correlation with fetal hypoxia. Recall that restlessness and agitation are key features in hypoxia, which would lead to the correct answer. Review the signs of fetal hypoxia and relate them to FHR if you had difficulty answering this question.

Client needs category: Physiological integrity
Client needs subcategory: Reduction of risk potential
Cognitive level: Analyzing

---

18. The nurse is caring for a 3-day-old neonate born to an opioid-dependent mother. When attempting to interact with the neonate experiencing drug withdrawal, the nurse recognizes which behavior as a sign of the neonate's willingness to interact?

☐ **1.** Gaze aversion

☐ **2.** Hiccups

☐ **3.** Quiet, alert state

☐ **4.** Yawning

Answer: 3

Ⓔ Rationale: When caring for a neonate experiencing drug withdrawal, the nurse needs to be alert for signs of distress from the neonate. Stimuli would be introduced one at a time when the neonate is in a quiet, alert state. Gaze aversion, yawning, sneezing, hiccups, and body arching are distress signals that the neonate cannot handle stimuli at that time.

Test-taking strategy: Analyze to determine what information the question asks for, which is signs of willingness to interact. Recall that "willingness to interact" includes behaviors of a more relaxed state without agitation. In this state, the neonate is able to accept stimuli, including positive stimuli of touch, soothing vocalization, and eye contact. Review characteristics of drug withdrawal in the neonate if you had difficulty answering this question.

Client needs category: Psychosocial integrity
Client needs subcategory: None
Cognitive level: Analyzing

19. A nurse in the telemetry unit is caring for a client with diagnosis of postoperative coronary artery bypass graft (CABG) surgery from 2 days ago. On assessment, the nurse notes a paradoxical pulse of 88. Which surgical complication would the nurse suspect?

☐ **1.** Left-sided heart failure

☐ **2.** Aortic regurgitation

☐ **3.** Complete heart block

☐ **4.** Pericardial tamponade

Ⓜ **Rationale:** A paradoxical pulse (a palpable decrease in pulse amplitude on quiet inspiration) signals pericardial tamponade, a complication of CABG surgery. Left-sided heart failure can cause pulsus alternans (a pulse amplitude alteration from beat to beat, with a regular rhythm). Aortic regurgitation may cause a bisferious pulse (an increased arterial pulse with a double systolic peak). Complete heart block may cause a bounding pulse (a strong pulse with increased pulse pressure).

Test-taking strategy: Analyze to determine what information the question asks for, which is complication from CABG surgery with signs of a paradoxical pulse. Knowledge of the term *paradoxical* pulse is essential in interpreting the type of pulse changes and correlating with correct answer. Recall that pericardial tamponade compresses and constricts the function of the heart because of fluid around the pericardial sac resulting in the stated pulse changes. Review signs and symptoms of a paradoxical pulse and complication from CABG if you had difficulty answering this question.

Client needs category: Physiological integrity

Client needs subcategory: Physiological adaptation

Cognitive level: Applying

20. A nurse is caring for a client recovering from cardiac revascularization surgery of 3 days ago. Upon analysis of lab reports, the nurse notes the client's platelet count decreased from 230,000 to 5,000 ml (5,000 mmol/L). Which condition is suspected?

☐ **1.** Pancytopenia

☐ **2.** Idiopathic thrombocytopenic purpura (ITP)

☐ **3.** Disseminated intravascular coagulation (DIC)

☐ **4.** Heparin-associated thrombosis and thrombocytopenia (HATT)

Ⓜ **Rationale:** HATT may occur after cardiac revascularization surgery because of heparin use during surgery. Pancytopenia is a reduction in all blood cells. Although ITP and DIC cause platelet aggregation and bleeding, neither is common in a client after revascularization surgery.

Test-taking strategy: Analyze to determine what information the question asks for, which is conditions causing a noted drop in platelet count. Recall that HATT is an immune system complication of using heparin therapy, resulting in devastating thromboembolic outcomes. Review complication of cardiac revascularization surgery and heparin use if you had difficulty answering this question.

Client needs category: Physiological integrity

Client needs subcategory: Physiological adaptation

Cognitive level: Applying

21. The nurse is suctioning a client's tracheostomy. For what reason during the procedure does the nurse complete the following action?

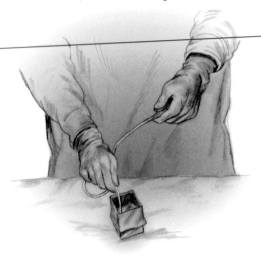

☐ **1.** To loosen the client's thick, tracheal secretions

☐ **2.** To regulate the suction pressure

☐ **3.** To clear secretions from the tubing

☐ **4.** To lubricate the outside of the suction catheter

Answer: 3

Ⓜ **Rationale:** The picture shows a nurse inserting the suction catheter in a container of water. The hole on the catheter is then occluded creating suction. The water is used to clear the catheter and tubing of secretions. The tubing does not need to be primed or lubricated. The catheter removes the secretions but does not loosen them.

Test-taking strategy: Analyze to determine what information the question asks for, which is rationale for nursing action. Consider all of the steps required in the procedure. Ask yourself, "What is the nurse doing and then why?" Gain clues from the picture. Review the standard procedure of suctioning a tracheostomy if you had difficulty answering this question.

Client needs category: Physiological integrity

Client needs subcategory: Basic care and comfort

Cognitive level: Analyzing

22. The nurse is caring for a comatose client who needs a nasopharyngeal airway for suctioning. After the airway is inserted, the client gags and coughs. Which action would the nurse take?

☐ **1.** Remove the airway and insert a shorter one.

☐ **2.** Reposition the airway.

☐ **3.** Leave the airway in place until the client gets used to it.

☐ **4.** Remove the airway and attempt suctioning without it.

Answer: 1

Ⓒ **Rationale:** If the client gags or coughs after nasopharyngeal airway placement, the tube may be too long. The nurse would remove it and insert a shorter one. Simply repositioning the airway will not solve the problem. The client will not get used to the tube because it is the wrong size. Suctioning without a nasopharyngeal airway causes trauma to the natural airway.

Test-taking strategy: Analyze to determine what information the question asks for, which is correct procedure for placing a nasopharyngeal airway. Recall the symptoms in relation to the anatomy of the respiratory system indicating a problem. Eliminate options 2 and 3 as not correcting the problem. Eliminate option 4 as inappropriate nursing care. Review the procedure for nasopharyngeal airway placement and suctioning if you had difficulty answering this question.

Client needs category: Physiological integrity

Client needs subcategory: Reduction of risk potential

Cognitive level: Applying

23. The nurse is caring for a client with a head injury. Which client goal is **most** appropriate for the acute phase of a neurological injury?

☐ **1.** The client will use the adaptive devices to assist with feeding.

☐ **2.** The client's vital signs will stabilize, returning to normal range.

☐ **3.** The client's skin will remain clean, dry, and intact.

☐ **4.** The client will return to optimal level of functioning.

Answer: 2

Ⓔ Rationale: During the acute phase of a neurological injury, the goal of nursing management is to stabilize the client to prevent further neurological damage. A client goal would be to have the vital signs stabilize, indicating an improvement in status, and also returning to normal range. Using adaptive devices would occur in the recovery or chronic phase of a neurological deficit. The client's skin and returning to optimal level of functioning is a goal for later in the recovery process.

Test-taking strategy: Analyze to determine what information the question asks for, which is a goal for an acute head injury. There are several key words in the stem that impact how to answer this question. They are "client goal" and "acute phase." Assess each option for an immediate client goal for care. Review nursing goals in the acute phase of a neurological injury if you had difficulty answering this question.

Client needs category: Physiological integrity

Client needs subcategory: Physiological adaptation

Cognitive level: Analyzing

24. A nurse is caring for a client following a hypophysectomy. Included in the postoperative orders is vasopressin intramuscularly. Which rationale is **most** correct for the administration of this medication?

☐ **1.** To treat growth failure

☐ **2.** To prevent SIADH

☐ **3.** To reduce cerebral edema and lower ICP

☐ **4.** To replace antidiuretic hormone (ADH) normally secreted from the pituitary

Answer: 4

Ⓜ Rationale: After hypophysectomy, or removal of the pituitary gland, the body cannot synthesize ADH. Vasopressin replaces the hormone and acts on the kidney and blood vessels. Somatotropin or growth hormone, not vasopressin, is used to treat growth failure. SIADH results from excessive ADH secretion. Mannitol or corticosteroids are used to reduce cerebral edema.

Test-taking strategy: Analyze to determine what information the question asks for, which is rationale for vasopressin administration. Recall that vasopressin is the man-made form of the ADH. Review nursing care after a hypophysectomy and vasopressin administration if you had difficulty answering this question.

Client needs category: Physiological integrity

Client needs subcategory: Pharmacological and parenteral therapies

Cognitive level: Applying

25. The orthopedic nurse is providing discharge instructions to a surgical client. Which action, by the client, would demonstrate proper touchdown weight bearing?

☐ **1.** Bearing full weight on the affected extremity

☐ **2.** Bearing 30% to 50% of weight on the affected extremity

☐ **3.** Bearing no weight on the extremity but allowing the extremity to touch the floor

☐ **4.** Bearing no weight on the extremity and keeping the extremity elevated at all times

Answer: 3

Ⓜ **Rationale:** Touchdown weight bearing involves bearing no weight on the extremity but allowing the affected extremity to touch the floor. Full weight bearing allows for full weight to be put on the affected extremity. Partial weight bearing allows for 30% to 50% weight bearing on the affected extremity. Non–weight bearing refers to bearing no weight on the affected extremity.

Test-taking strategy: Analyze to determine what information the question asks for, which is the correct procedure for touchdown weight bearing. Use the terminology "touchdown," which suggests very little weight bearing, to provide a clue. Review the term *touchdown* and guidelines for the amount of weight bearing and extremity activity allowed if you had difficulty answering this question.

Client needs category: Safe and effective care environment

Client needs subcategory: Management of care

Cognitive level: Applying

---

26. A client has an indwelling urinary catheter and is prescribed physical therapy. As the client is being placed in a wheelchair, which action by the assistant would need further clarification by the nurse?

☐ **1.** The catheter drainage bag is placed on the lower side of the wheelchair.

☐ **2.** The assistant brings a container to drain the urine from the bag.

☐ **3.** The catheter bag is placed upon the client's lap for safe transport.

☐ **4.** The assistant checks to make sure the tubing is not kinked.

Answer: 3

Ⓔ **Rationale:** The nurse would clarify to the assistant that the catheter bag needs to be placed lower than the client's bladder so as not to have backflow from the catheter tubing to the bladder. Placing the catheter on a lower portion of the wheelchair allows urine to flow through the tubing and does not encourage backflow. It is appropriate to drain the urine from the catheter bag before physical therapy and to make sure that there are no kinks in the tubing preventing urine flow to the drainage bag.

Test-taking strategy: Analyze to determine what information the question asks for, which is incorrect action by the assistant regarding the care of a urinary catheter. Discriminate through each option and compare to standard practices. Consider the impact of each action. Review care of the urinary catheter if you had difficulty answering this question.

Client needs category: Safe and effective care environment

Client needs subcategory: Safety and infection control

Cognitive level: Analyzing

27. A medication nurse is preparing to administer 9 AM medications to a client with liver cancer. Which consideration is the nurse's highest **priority?**

☐ **1.** Frequency of the medication

☐ **2.** Purpose of the medication

☐ **3.** Necessity of the medication

☐ **4.** Metabolism of the medication

Answer: 4

🅔 **Rationale:** The rate and ability of the liver to metabolize medications will be altered in a client with liver cancer. Therefore, it is essential to understand how each medication is metabolized. The other considerations are important but not as vital.

Test-taking strategy: Analyze to determine what information the question asks for, which is nursing priority in administering medications to a client with liver cancer. The key word is "liver" as the liver plays a key role in medication metabolism. If unsure, use the key words in the options of frequency, purpose, necessity, and metabolism to guide your priority selection. Review normal drug metabolism and the pathophysiology of liver cancer as it relates to medication administration if you had difficulty answering this question.

Client needs category: Physiological integrity

Client needs subcategory: Pharmacological and parenteral therapies

Cognitive level: Analyzing

28. A registered nurse (RN) and licensed practical/vocational nurse (LPN/VN) are working together in the emergency department to care for a client who is hemorrhaging. Which actions would be delegated to the LPN/VN? Select all that apply.

☐ **1.** Assessment of the wound

☐ **2.** Reassessment of vital signs

☐ **3.** Initiation of blood products

☐ **4.** Dressing of the wound

☐ **5.** Documentation of vital signs during infusion of blood products

☐ **6.** Repositioning of the client off of the wound site

Answer: 2, 4, 5, 6

🅒 **Rationale:** The RN has the primary responsibility of the client in the acute situation. The RN is able to delegate tasks within the scope of practice of the LPN/VN. Assessment of an acutely ill client falls to the RN. In this situation, that includes the assessment of the wound and initiation of blood products and assessing for a transfusion reaction. Once the client is stable, the nurse may choose to delegate reassessment (not initial) of vital signs and documentation (also obtaining) of vital signs during the blood transfusion. Once the RN has assessed the wound, the dressing procedure can be delegated and the client may be repositioned.

Test-taking strategy: Analyze to determine what information the question asks for, which is delegation of care. Always consider standards of practice and scope of practice when delegating. The National Council of State Boards of Nursing (NCSBN) has a delegation algorithm on its Web site for guidance. Review delegation principles if you had difficulty answering this question.

Client needs category: Safe and effective care environment

Client needs subcategory: Management of care

Cognitive level: Analyzing

29. A nurse is caring for a client diagnosed with Cushing's syndrome. When considering fluid balance, sodium and water retention contribute to which common disorder?

☐ **1.** Hypoglycemia and dehydration

☐ **2.** Hypotension and hyperglycemia

☐ **3.** Pulmonary edema and dehydration

☐ **4.** Hypertension and heart failure

Answer: 4

Ⓜ Rationale: In Cushing's syndrome, increased mineralocorticoid activity results in sodium and water retention, which commonly contributes to hypertension and heart failure. Hypoglycemia and dehydration are uncommon in a client with Cushing's syndrome. Diabetes mellitus and hyperglycemia may develop, but hypotension is not part of the disease process. Pulmonary edema and dehydration also are not complications of Cushing's syndrome.

Test-taking strategy: Analyze to determine what information the question asks for, which is a common disorder effecting sodium and water retention. The key word is "retention." Eliminate options 1, 2, and 3 as each has a component of dehydration and hypotension, common in fluid loss. Review the effects of water and sodium retention on various body systems if you had difficulty answering this question.

Client needs category: Physiological integrity

Client needs subcategory: Physiological adaptation

Cognitive level: Analyzing

---

30. The Women's Clinic nurse is instructing a client on the proper use of an applicator to instill vaginal cream. Which of the following instructions is applicable when teaching a client about vaginal medication insertion?

☐ **1.** Insert the nozzle about 3″ (8 cm) into the vagina.

☐ **2.** Direct the tip of the applicator toward the sacrum.

☐ **3.** Instill the cream slowly over 5 minutes.

☐ **4.** Sterilize the applicator in boiling water to prepare for next use.

Answer: 2

Ⓒ Rationale: The normal position of the vagina slants up and back toward the sacrum. Directing the tip of the applicator toward the sacrum allows it to follow the normal slant of the vagina and minimizes tissue trauma. The applicator would be inserted about 2″ (5 cm). The medication can be administered by placing continuous pressure until the tip of the plunger hits the applicator, taking 10 to 15 seconds. This eliminates the medication from the applicator placing it in the vagina. Should the applicator need to be reused, the applicator may be washed thoroughly and placed on a towel to dry.

Test-taking strategy: Analyze to determine what information the question asks for, which is correct application of vaginal cream. Consider the location and condition of the vagina when discriminating through the options. Review the anatomy of the female reproductive system and clean versus sterile technique if you had difficulty answering this question.

Client needs category: Safe and effective care environment

Client needs subcategory: Safety and infection control

Cognitive level: Applying

31. A nurse is caring for a premenopausal client who had precancerous cells found during a routine Papanicolaou (Pap) test. At which time during the menstrual cycle would the nurse schedule a cervical biopsy?

- ☐ **1.** One week after the end of the menstrual period
- ☐ **2.** Immediately before the menstrual period begins
- ☐ **3.** During ovulation
- ☐ **4.** At the end of the menstrual period

Answer: 1

Ⓜ Rationale: The nurse is most correct to schedule a cervical biopsy 1 week after the end of the menstrual period when the cervix is less vascular. The cervix is most vascular immediately before menstruation and during ovulation. A biopsy would not be scheduled when vaginal discharge remains.

Test-taking strategy: Analyze to determine what information the question asks for, which is timing for a cervical biopsy. Consider the normal menstrual cycle and times of menstrual flow. Because of the nature of the biopsy, timing would be kept away from the time of menstrual flow and increased vascularity. Review the timing of a cervical biopsy with a woman's menstrual cycle if you had difficulty answering this question.

Client needs category: Physiological integrity

Client needs subcategory: Reduction of risk potential

Cognitive level: Applying

---

32. A registered nurse (RN) is to obtain a wound culture from a client's gaping surgical incision. The RN delegates the nursing action to a licensed practical nurse/licensed vocational/registered practical nurse. Which instruction would the RN state to ensure proper culture collection?

- ☐ **1.** Thoroughly irrigate the wound with normal saline before collecting the culture.
- ☐ **2.** Use a sterile swab to wipe the crusty area around the outside of the wound.
- ☐ **3.** Gently roll a sterile swab from the center of the wound outward to collect drainage.
- ☐ **4.** Use one sterile swab to collect drainage from several possible infected sites along the incision.

Answer: 3

Ⓔ Rationale: Rolling a swab from the center outward is the correct way to culture a wound. Irrigating the wound washes away drainage, debris, and many of the microorganisms colonizing or infecting the wound. The outside of the wound may be colonized with microorganisms from this wound or another wound, or from normal microorganisms found on the client's skin. These may grow in culture and confuse the interpretation of results. All of the sources of drainage from an incision or a surgical wound may not be infected, or they may be infected with different microorganisms; consequently, each swab should be used on only one site.

Test-taking strategy: Analyze to determine what information the question asks for, which is the correct procedure to obtain a surgical wound culture. Visualize the procedure and consider ways to obtain drainage from the surgical site. Focus on obtaining draining at the site of any crusting, redness, or drainage. Review the standard procedure for obtaining a surgical wound culture if you had difficulty answering this question.

Client needs category: Safe and effective care environment

Client needs subcategory: Safety and infection control

Cognitive level: Applying

33. A mental health nurse in an outpatient clinic is caring for a client who is newly diagnosed with a phobic disorder. Which individual counseling approach is **best** to assist the client in daily activities?

☐ **1.** Have the client keep a daily journal.

☐ **2.** Help the client identify the source of the anxiety.

☐ **3.** Teach the client effective ways to problem-solve.

☐ **4.** Develop strategies to prevent the client from using substances.

Answer: 2

🄴 **Rationale:** By understanding the source of the anxiety, the client will understand how this anxiety has been displaced as a phobic response. Keeping a journal is an effective method in many situations; however, its use is limited in the treatment of phobias. Problem solving is a more useful technique for clients with obsessive–compulsive disorder than for clients with phobias. People with phobias do not tend to self-medicate like clients with other psychiatric disorders.

Test-taking strategy: Analyze to determine what information the question asks for, which is approach to assist the client in daily activities. Consider that phobias are fears and are a type of anxiety disorder. Review the defining characteristics of phobic disorders, and focus on the optimal therapeutic approach if you had difficulty answering this question.

Client needs category: Psychosocial integrity

Client needs subcategory: None

Cognitive level: Applying

34. A client with antisocial personality disorder is trying to manipulate the health care team. Which strategy is **most** important for the staff to use?

☐ **1.** Focus on how to teach the client more effective behaviors for meeting basic needs.

☐ **2.** Help the client verbalize underlying feelings of hopelessness and learn coping skills.

☐ **3.** Remain calm and do not emotionally respond to the client's manipulative actions.

☐ **4.** Help the client eliminate the intense desire to have everything in life turn out perfectly.

Answer: 3

🄴 **Rationale:** The best strategy to use with a client trying to manipulate staff is to stay calm and refrain from responding emotionally. Negative reinforcement of inappropriate behavior increases the chance it will be repeated. Later, it may be possible to address how to meet the client's basic needs. Clients with antisocial personality disorder do not tend to experience feelings of hopelessness or to desire life events to turn out perfectly. In most cases, these clients negate responsibility for their behavior.

Test-taking strategy: Analyze to determine what information the question asks for, which is a strategy to use with an antisocial personality who is manipulative. Recall that manipulation is a client attempt for control. Focus on the strategy that does not reinforce the client's behavior. Review how to interact with manipulative clients if you had difficulty answering this question.

Client needs category: Psychosocial integrity

Client needs subcategory: None

Cognitive level: Analyzing

35. The nurse is working in the labor and birth unit when a mother with active herpes simplex virus type 2 (HSV-2) appears in active labor. Which adjustment in the plan of care is anticipated?

☐ **1.** Administer an intravenous antibiotic to the mom while in labor.

☐ **2.** Complete a full assessment of the newborn on birth.

☐ **3.** Prepare the mother for a cesarean section.

☐ **4.** Place an antibacterial ointment on the mother's lesions.

Answer: 3

E **Rationale:** The nurse is most accurate to prepare for a cesarean section since the mother has an active lesion and does not want to transmit the virus to the newborn. Antibiotic therapy, at this time, does not prevent the transmission of the infection. A full assessment is always completed on the newborn and is not an adjustment in the plan of care. Antibacterial ointment is not placed on the mother's lesions.

Test-taking strategy: Analyze to determine what information the question asks for, which is adjustment in the plan of care for a laboring woman with HSV-2. Consider that the virus is transmittable and ways to prevent transmission. Review care for a laboring client with HSV-2 if you had difficulty answering this question.

Client needs category: Physiological integrity

Client needs subcategory: Reduction of risk potential

Cognitive level: Analyzing

---

36. A child is admitted to the hospital for an asthma exacerbation. The nursing history reveals this client was exposed to varicella (chickenpox) 1 week ago. When, if at all, would this client require isolation?

☐ **1.** Isolation is not required at this time.

☐ **2.** Immediate isolation is required in a private room.

☐ **3.** Isolation would be required 10 days after exposure.

☐ **4.** Isolation would be required 12 days after exposure.

Answer: 2

M **Rationale:** The incubation period for varicella (chickenpox) is 2 to 3 weeks, usually 13 to 17 days. A client is commonly isolated 1 week after exposure to avoid the risk of an earlier breakout. A person is infectious from 1 day before eruption of lesions to 6 days after the vesicles have formed crusts.

Test-taking strategy: Analyze to determine what information the question asks for, which is when isolation is necessary after chickenpox exposure. Recall the communicable nature and incubation period for chickenpox, and relate this to the timing of isolation. If unsure, also consider the immunocompromised status of hospital clients and the need to protect. Review isolation precautions especially related to communicable diseases if you had difficulty answering this question.

Client needs category: Safe and effective care environment

Client needs subcategory: Safety and infection control

Cognitive level: Applying

37. The school nurse is monitoring the diet of a child with cystic fibrosis. Which type of diet would be stressed to the family?

☐ **1.** Fat restricted

☐ **2.** High calorie

☐ **3.** Low protein

☐ **4.** Sodium restricted

Answer: 2

🅔 **Rationale:** A well-balanced high-calorie, high-protein diet is recommended for a child with cystic fibrosis because of the impaired intestinal absorption. Fat restriction is not required because digestion and absorption of fat in the intestine are impaired. The child usually increases enzyme intake along with the consumption of high-fat foods. Low-sodium foods can lead to hyponatremia; therefore, high-sodium foods are recommended, especially during hot weather or when the child has a fever.

Test-taking strategy: Analyze to determine what information the question asks for, which is dietary recommendation for a client with cystic fibrosis. Recall that clients with cystic fibrosis need to ingest 50% more calories because of malabsorption. Also, clients who are in a good nutritional state are able to fight off infections and viruses. Review the disease process of cystic fibrosis in relation to children's nutritional needs if you had difficulty answering this question.

Client needs category: Safe and effective care environment

Client needs subcategory: Management of care

Cognitive level: Applying

---

38. A child has just returned to the pediatric unit following ventriculoperitoneal shunt placement for hydrocephalus. Which intervention would a nurse perform **first?**

☐ **1.** Assess intake and output.

☐ **2.** Place the child on the side opposite the shunt.

☐ **3.** Offer fluids because the child has a dry mouth.

☐ **4.** Administer pain medication by mouth as ordered.

Answer: 2

🅜 **Rationale:** Following shunt placement surgery, the child would be placed on the side opposite of the surgical site to prevent pressure on the shunt valve. Intake and output will also need to be assessed, but that is not the nurse's priority. The child is usually on nothing-by-mouth status until the nasogastric (NG) tube is removed and bowel sounds return. Pain medication should be administered by an intravenous route initially postoperatively.

Test-taking strategy: Analyze to determine what information the question asks for, which is postoperative priority for a client with shunt placement. Consider safety needs following surgery and immediate nursing care. Review nursing care in the immediate postoperative period if you had difficulty answering this question.

Client needs category: Physiological integrity

Client needs subcategory: Basic care and comfort

Cognitive level: Applying

39. The nurse is caring for a client in the diagnostic studies area of the hospital. Which information would a nurse provide to the parents of a child undergoing testing for muscular dystrophy?

- ☐ **1.** Genitals will be covered by a lead apron.
- ☐ **2.** Local anesthetic will be used for the test.
- ☐ **3.** Electrode wires will be attached to the scalp.
- ☐ **4.** A fiberoptic endoscope will be inserted into a joint.

Answer: 2

Ⓜ Rationale: A muscle biopsy, used to confirm the diagnosis of muscular dystrophy, shows the degeneration of muscle fibers and infiltration of fatty tissue. It is typically performed using a local anesthetic. Genitals are covered by a lead apron during an x-ray examination, which is used to detect osseous, not muscular, problems. Electrode wires are attached to the scalp during an electroencephalography to observe brain wave activity; this test is not used to diagnose muscular dystrophy. Arthroscopy, also not used to test for muscular dystrophy, involves the insertion of a fiberoptic scope into a joint.

Test-taking strategy: Analyze to determine what information the question asks for, which is information to provide parents on diagnostic testing for muscular dystrophy. Recall that muscular dystrophy involves analysis of nerve fibers obtained invasively leading to the answer of local anesthetic. Eliminate options 1, 3, and 4 as these diagnostic testing sites include areas not used in muscle fiber testing. Review definite testing for muscular dystrophy if you had difficulty answering this question.

Client needs category: Physiological integrity

Client needs subcategory: Basic care and comfort

Cognitive level: Applying

---

40. The nurse is completing a sexual history on a client. The client reports a history of having a sexually transmitted infection (STI), which lies dormant in the body and can reoccur, but does not remember the name. Which STI matches the client's description?

- ☐ **1.** Chlamydia
- ☐ **2.** Herpes infection
- ☐ **3.** Gonorrhea
- ☐ **4.** Syphilis

Answer: 2

Ⓔ Rationale: The nurse is most accurate to identify the herpes infection as the virus can remain dormant in the ganglia of the nerves. Symptoms are usually more severe with the initial outbreak. Subsequent episodes are usually shorter and less intense. The other infections do not have the same characteristics and, if identified, will be documented in the history.

Test-taking strategy: Analyze to determine what information the question asks for, which is STI with possible recurrence. Analyze each option against this distinctive characteristic. Review timing and signs and symptoms of infections/exacerbations if you had difficulty answering this question.

Client needs category: Safe and effective care environment

Client needs subcategory: Safety and infection control

Cognitive level: Applying

41. A nurse is caring for a 7-month-old who has just had surgical repair of a cleft palate. Which instruction would be included in the discharge teaching to the parents?

☐ **1.** Continue a normal diet.

☐ **2.** Continue using arm restraints at home.

☐ **3.** Do not allow the child to drink from a cup.

☐ **4.** Establish good mouth care and proper brushing.

Answer: 2

Ⓜ **Rationale:** Cleft palate is a congenital deformity that, if not treated, causes speech problems, feeding difficulty, and maxillofacial growth and dentition deviations. Surgical repair is suggested before the client is 1 year old. Discharge instructions include arm restraints used at home to keep the child's hands away from the mouth until the palate is healed. The hands can interfere with the healing process and also introduce bacteria into the surgical site. A soft diet is recommended; no food harder than mashed potatoes can be eaten. Fluids are best taken from a cup. Proper mouth care is encouraged after the palate is healed.

Test-taking strategy: Analyze to determine what information the question asks for, which is discharge instruction following cleft palate repair. Recall the nature and placement of cleft palate including special care needs for the areas inside and coming in contact with the mouth. Eliminate options 1 and 4 as appropriate for a normal oral cavity. Eliminate option 3 as the cup is acceptable following repair. Review the child's age and immediate home care needs, and recall postoperative interventions following cleft palate repair if you had difficulty answering this question.

Client needs category: Safe and effective care environment

Client needs subcategory: Safety and infection control

Cognitive level: Applying

---

42. A pediatric nurse in a public health clinic is collecting data on an initial visit to the clinic. Which comment made by the mother of a neonate at the 2-week office visit would alert the nurse to suspect congenital hypothyroidism?

☐ **1.** "My baby is unusually quiet and good."

☐ **2.** "My baby seems to be a yellowish color."

☐ **3.** "After feedings, my baby pulls the legs up and cries."

☐ **4.** "My baby seems to really look at my face during feeding time."

Answer: 1

Ⓓ **Rationale:** Parental remarks about an unusually "quiet and good" neonate together with any of the early physical manifestations would lead to a suspicion of hypothyroidism, which requires a referral for specific tests. If a neonate begins to look yellow in color, hyperbilirubinemia may be the cause. If the neonate is pulling the legs up and crying after feedings, it might be showing signs of colic. Neonates like looking at the human face and would show interest in this when 2 weeks old.

Test-taking strategy: Analyze to determine what information the question asks for, which is maternal statements indicating potential hypothyroidism. Consider that hypothyroidism causes a decrease in metabolism; thus, select a statement indicating a decrease in energy or activity. Review the pathophysiology of congenital hypothyroidism if you had difficulty answering this question.

Client needs category: Health promotion and maintenance

Client needs subcategory: None

Cognitive level: Applying

43. In teaching a group of parents about monitoring for urinary tract infection (UTI) in preschoolers, the nurse would mention which finding as **most** indicative of the need to have a child evaluated?

☐ **1.** The child voids only twice in any 6-hour period.

☐ **2.** The child exhibits incontinence after being toilet trained.

☐ **3.** The child has difficulty sitting still for more than a 30-minute period.

☐ **4.** The child's urine smells strongly of ammonia after it stands for more than 2 hours.

Answer: 2

Ⓔ Rationale: A child who exhibits incontinence after being toilet trained would be evaluated for UTI. Most urine smells strongly of ammonia after standing for more than 2 hours, so this does not necessarily indicate UTI. The other options are not reasons for parents to suspect problems with their child's urinary system.

Test-taking strategy: Analyze to determine what information the question asks for, which is indications of a UTI in preschoolers. Consider the common signs and symptoms of UTI and relate to a preschool-age child. Recall that in the adult, UTI symptoms include urinary frequency and relate to incontinence to the preschooler. Review signs of UTI in pediatrics if you had difficulty answering this question.

Client needs category: Safe and effective care environment

Client needs subcategory: Management of care

Cognitive level: Applying

---

44. A nurse is evaluating essential nutrition for a pediatric burn client. Which statement **best** describes the nutritional needs?

☐ **1.** A child needs 100 cal/kg during hospitalization.

☐ **2.** The hypermetabolic state after a burn injury leads to poor healing.

☐ **3.** Caloric needs can be lowered by maintaining a neutral environmental temperature.

☐ **4.** Maintaining a hypermetabolic rate will lower the child's risk of infection.

Answer: 2

Ⓓ Rationale: A burn injury causes a hypermetabolic state that leads to protein and lipid catabolism, which affects wound healing. Caloric intake would be 1½ to 2 times the basal metabolic rate, with a minimum of 1.5 to 2 g/kg of body weight of protein daily. Keeping the temperature within a normal range lets the body function efficiently and use calories for healing and normal physiological processes. If the temperature is too warm or cold, energy must be used for warming or cooling, taking energy away from tissue repair. High metabolic rates increase the risk of infection.

Test-taking strategy: Analyze to determine what information the question asks for, which is the nutritional needs of a burn client. Consider the increased nutritional needs related to metabolism and wound healing. Without the essential nutrients in the diet, healing and growth and development may be compromised. Review the nutritional needs of the pediatric burn client if you had difficulty answering this question.

Client needs category: Physiological integrity

Client needs subcategory: Basic care and comfort

Cognitive level: Analyzing

45. A charge nurse is preparing client care assignments for the next shift. A client who underwent femoral–popliteal bypass surgery is scheduled to return from the postanesthesia care unit. Which staff member would receive this client?

☐ **1.** Registered nurse (RN) with 1 year of experience

☐ **2.** Registered practical nurse/licensed practical or vocational nurse with 5 years of experience

☐ **3.** Nursing assistant/unregulated health care worker with 15 years of experience

☐ **4.** Charge nurse with 10 years of experience

Answer: 1

Ⓒ Rationale: Because this client requires frequent neurovascular assessments, an RN would receive the client. A registered practical nurse/licensed practical or vocational nurse, although experienced and capable of collecting data, would not be receiving the client and report from the operating room as skilled assessments are necessary. The nursing assistant/unregulated health care worker lacks the necessary assessment skills. The charge nurse needs to be available to direct the care of other clients and management of unit.

Test-taking strategy: Analyze to determine what information the question asks for, which is nurse assignment for receiving a postoperative client. Recall that the client has changing hemodynamics and care needs following surgical procedures. In general, assignment needs to be made to an RN who is skilled in assessment. Review the postoperative needs of the client to determine staff assignments if you had difficulty answering this question.

Client needs category: Safe and effective care environment

Client needs subcategory: Management of care

Cognitive level: Analyzing

46. A scrub nurse is assigned to the operating room for an appendectomy case. Which action by the scrub nurse violates the standards of sterility during the operation?

☐ **1.** Crossing arms while waiting for the surgery to begin

☐ **2.** Removing a blood sponge from the body cavity

☐ **3.** Tying the back of another nurse's gown

☐ **4.** Passing a sterile gauze pad to the surgeon

Answer: 3

Ⓒ Rationale: Scrub nurses, also called perioperative nurses, are registered nurses who assist in surgical procedures by setting up the room before the operation, working with the doctor during surgery, and preparing the patient for the move to the recovery room. The scrub nurse must remain sterile during the operation as a primary responsibility is assisting the surgeon with surgical equipment. Touching the back of a nonsterile gown breaks sterility. All of the other measures maintain sterility.

Test-taking strategy: Analyze to determine what information the question asks for, which is an error by the scrub nurse breaking sterility. Begin by understanding the role of the scrub nurse being to assist the surgeon during the surgical procedure. Eliminate options 2 and 4 as proper and necessary during the surgery. Discriminate between the remaining options. Review sterile procedures if you had difficulty answering this question.

Client needs category: Safe and effective care environment

Client needs subcategory: Safety and infection control

Cognitive level: Analyzing

47. A nurse is employed on a medical unit specializing in blood cancers. According to a standard staging classification of Hodgkin's lymphoma, which criterion reflects stage II?

☐ **1.** Involvement of extralymphatic organs or tissues

☐ **2.** Involvement of a single lymph node region or structure

☐ **3.** Involvement of two or more lymph node regions or structures

☐ **4.** Involvement of lymph node regions or structures on both sides of the diaphragm

Ⓔ Rationale: Hodgkin's lymphoma is a cancer originating from the white blood cells (WBCs). Hodgkin's lymphoma is characterized by the orderly spread of disease from one lymph node group/region to another. Stage II involves two or more lymph node regions. Stage I involves only one lymph node region, stage III involves nodes on both sides of the diaphragm, and stage IV involves extralymphatic organs or tissues (metastasis).

Test-taking strategy: Analyze to determine what information the question asks for, which is criteria for stage II Hodgkin's lymphoma. Recall that cancer involvement rises with numerical value typically ending with stage IV indicating metastasis. Consider stage II coordinating with at least two lymph node regions. Review the criteria for staging of Hodgkin's lymphoma if you had difficulty answering this question.

Client needs category: Physiological integrity

Client needs subcategory: Physiological adaptation

Cognitive level: Applying

---

48. Which nursing action **best** addresses the outcome: *The client will be free from falls*?

☐ **1.** Use large muscle group when transferring client from bed to chair.

☐ **2.** Encourage use of grab bars and railings in the bathroom and halls.

☐ **3.** Place emergency contact's telephone number in a prominent place.

☐ **4.** Install a monitoring system to help the client in an emergency situation.

Ⓔ Rationale: To address the client outcome of being free from falls, it is best to place assistive devices of grab bars especially in the bathroom and railings in the halls to promote balance. It is a nursing-focused action to use large muscle groups when transferring a client. It is important to place an emergency contact number close by and have an emergency monitoring system; however, they will not prevent falls.

Test-taking strategy: Analyze to determine what information the question asks for, which is addressing the client outcome of safety. First, ensure that the client is the focus of the action; thus, eliminate option 1. Next, make sure that the action directly results in meeting the outcome. Eliminate options 3 and 4. Note that the options can be all correct actions, but choose the one that answers the question. Review client safety for fall prevention if you had difficulty answering this question.

Client needs category: Safe and effective care environment

Client needs subcategory: Safety and infection control

Cognitive level: Analyzing

49. A healthy client comes to the clinic for a routine examination. When auscultating lower lung lobes, the nurse anticipates which type of breath sound?

☐ **1.** Bronchial

☐ **2.** Tracheal

☐ **3.** Vesicular

☐ **4.** Bronchovesicular

Answer: 3

Ⓜ **Rationale:** Vesicular breath sounds are soft, low-pitched sounds normally heard over the lower lobes of the lung. They are prolonged on inhalation and shortened on exhalation. Bronchial breath sounds are loud, high-pitched sounds normally heard next to the trachea; they are discontinuous and loudest during exhalation. Tracheal breath sounds are harsh, discontinuous sounds heard over the trachea during inhalation or exhalation. Bronchovesicular breath sounds are medium-pitched, continuous sounds that occur during inhalation or exhalation and are best heard over the upper third of the sternum and between the scapulae.

Test-taking strategy: Analyze to determine what information the question asks for, which is anticipated breath sounds in a healthy client. Memorization and recognition of normal breath sounds are essential to answer this question. Review the anatomy of the lungs and breath sound characteristics if you had difficulty answering this question.

Client needs category: Health promotion and maintenance

Client needs subcategory: None

Cognitive level: Applying

---

50. The nurse is preparing to do a 12-lead ECG on a client. Indicate the correct area where the V_2 electrode would be placed on the figure below.

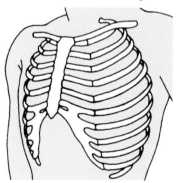

Answer:

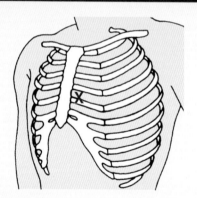

Ⓓ **Rationale:** The V_2 electrode would be placed over the fourth intercostal space, at the left sternal border.

Test-taking strategy: Analyze to determine what information the question asks for, which is placement of the V_2 electrode during ECG monitoring. Recall that V_2 is one of the six precordial leads. Review the anatomy of chest and correct placement of electrodes for a 12-lead ECG if you had difficulty answering this question.

Client needs category: Safe and effective care environment

Client needs subcategory: Management of care

Cognitive level: Applying

51. A client arrives at a public health clinic worried that she has breast cancer after finding a lump in her breast. When assessing the breast, which assessment finding provides an indication that the lump is more typical of fibrocystic breast disease?

- ☐ **1.** One breast is larger than the other.
- ☐ **2.** The lump is firm and nonmovable.
- ☐ **3.** The lump is round and movable.
- ☐ **4.** Nipple retractions are noted.

Answer: 3

ⓔ Rationale: When assessing a breast with fibrocystic disease, the lumps typically are different from cancerous lumps. The characteristic breast mass of fibrocystic disease is soft to firm, circular, movable, and unlikely to cause nipple retraction. A cancerous mass is typically irregular in shape, firm, and nonmovable. Lumps typically do not make one breast larger than the other. Nipple retractions are suggestive of cancerous masses.

Test-taking strategy: Analyze to determine what information the question asks for, which is signs and symptoms differentiating fibrocystic breast disease and a cancerous breast mass. Consider that the cell makeup of a cancerous lump is a group of disorganized cells that reproduce at a high rate and also need a blood supply. Because of this fact, the mass is often firm and nonmovable. Fibrocystic breast disease thus is round and movable.

Client needs category: Physiological integrity
Client needs subcategory: Physiological adaptation
Cognitive level: Applying

---

52. A client is ready to be discharged after arthroscopic knee surgery. Which information would the nurse expect the health care provider to write on the discharge instructions?

- ☐ **1.** "Ice and elevate the extremity for 12 hours after discharge."
- ☐ **2.** "Infection would not be a problem because of the small incision size."
- ☐ **3.** "Swelling and coolness of the joint and limb are normal right after surgery."
- ☐ **4.** "Take ibuprofen every 6 hours as necessary for pain relief."

Answer: 4

ⓒ Rationale: Mild to moderate pain is normal after this type of surgery and can be relieved by oral nonsteroidal anti-inflammatory drugs (NSAIDs). To minimize swelling, the client would ice and elevate the extremity for at least 24 hours after surgery. Infection is a potential problem after an invasive procedure, regardless of the incision size. Swelling and coolness of the joint and limb may indicate complications from tourniquet use during surgery.

Test-taking strategy: Analyze to determine what information the question asks for, which is anticipated discharge instructions. Consider that pain is a priority concern after a surgical procedure. Review postoperative management and the potential complications of arthroscopy if you had difficulty answering this question.

Client needs category: Physiological integrity
Client needs subcategory: Basic care and comfort
Cognitive level: Applying

53. The nurse is caring for a client with possible Cushing's syndrome undergoing diagnostic testing. The health care provider orders lab work and a dexamethasone suppression test. Which parameter would the nurse assess on the dexamethasone suppression test?

☐ **1.** The amount of dexamethasone in the system

☐ **2.** Cortisol levels after the system is challenged

☐ **3.** Changes in certain body chemicals, which are altered in depression

☐ **4.** Cortisol levels before and after the system is challenged with a synthetic steroid

Answer: 4

Ⓜ **Rationale:** The dexamethasone suppression test measures cortisol levels before and after the system is challenged with a synthetic steroid. The dexamethasone suppression test does not measure dexamethasone or body chemicals altered in depression. Dexamethasone is used to challenge the cortisol level.

Test-taking strategy: Analyze to determine what information the question asks for, which is the parameter measured in a dexamethasone suppression test. The key word is "suppression," indicating a reduction. Recall that dexamethasone is an exogenous steroid that provides negative feedback to the pituitary to suppress the secretion of adrenocorticotropic hormone. A normal result in the decrease is cortisol level. Review the dexamethasone suppression test if you had difficulty answering this question.

Client needs category: Health promotion and maintenance

Client needs subcategory: None

Cognitive level: Applying

54. During a routine physical examination, a firm mass is palpated in the right breast of a 35-year-old female client. Which assessment finding in the client's history would suggest breast cancer rather than fibrocystic disease?

☐ **1.** History of early menarche

☐ **2.** Cyclic change in mass size

☐ **3.** History of anovulatory cycles

☐ **4.** Dimpling of the skin on the breast

Answer: 4

Ⓜ **Rationale:** Dimpling of the breast is consistent with breast cancer. A dimpling is a pulling of the skin, which may occur when the arm is raised or the client leans forward. Early menarche as well as late menopause or a history of anovulatory cycles is associated with fibrocystic disease. Masses associated with fibrocystic disease of the breast are firm and increase in size prior to menstruation. They may be bilateral in a mirror image and are typically well demarcated and freely movable.

Test-taking strategy: Analyze to determine what information the question asks for, which is assessment finding in the client's history associated with breast cancer. Consider that a dimpling of the breast may be seen in breast cancer. Recall that any irregularities of the breast must be brought to the health care provider's attention. Review the pathophysiology and clinical manifestations of breast cancer and fibrocystic disease if you had difficulty answering this question.

Client needs category: Health promotion and maintenance

Client needs subcategory: None

Cognitive level: Applying

55. A client with disseminated herpes zoster is ordered intravenous hydrocortisone, 40 mg b.i.d. Which laboratory value would the nurse expect to be elevated as a result of this therapy?

☐ **1.** Calcium

☐ **2.** Glucose

☐ **3.** Magnesium

☐ **4.** Potassium

Answer: 2

E **Rationale:** Hydrocortisone is used in the treatment of a variety of disease processes mainly for the medication's anti-inflammatory immunosuppressant activity. Corticosteroids increase blood sugar and tend to lower serum potassium and calcium levels. Their effect on magnesium is not substantial.

Test-taking strategy: Analyze to determine what information the question asks for, which is anticipated lab value elevation following hydrocortisone administration. Consider the action of corticosteroids within the body and also that illness affects blood glucose levels. Review the action of corticosteroids in the body and laboratory values if you had difficulty answering this question.

Client needs category: Physiological integrity

Client needs subcategory: Pharmacological and parenteral therapies

Cognitive level: Analyzing

---

56. When caring for a client on the medical unit, which precaution, unique to phenytoin, must be taken when administering via a nasogastric (NG) tube?

☐ **1.** Check the phenytoin level after giving the drug to monitor for toxicity.

☐ **2.** Elevate the head of the bed before giving phenytoin through the NG tube.

☐ **3.** Give phenytoin 1 hour before or 2 hours after NG tube feedings to ensure absorption.

☐ **4.** Verify proper placement of the NG tube by placing the end of the tube in a glass of water and observing for bubbles.

Answer: 3

M **Rationale:** Nutritional supplements and milk interfere with the absorption of phenytoin, decreasing its effectiveness. Phenytoin levels are typically checked before giving the drug, and the drug is withheld for elevated levels to avoid compounding toxicity. The head of the bed would be elevated when giving any drug or solution, so this is not specific to phenytoin administration. The nurse verifies NG tube placement by checking for stomach contents before giving drugs and feedings.

Test-taking strategy: Analyze to determine what information the question asks for, which is precautions when administering phenytoin via an NG tube. Consider both (1) precautions when giving the medication through the NG tube and (2) normal considerations of the medication use. Notice that only one option noted the NG tube and is incorrect. Recall phenytoin considerations the same as oral administration. Review safety precautions specific to NG tubes and phenytoin administration if you had difficulty answering this question.

Client needs category: Physiological integrity

Client needs subcategory: Pharmacological and parenteral therapies

Cognitive level: Applying

57. The nurse is educating a client who insists that the newly prescribed imipramine is not working for her feelings of depression. When evaluating the client's statement, which question is most important to ask **first?**

☐ **1.** "Do you feel worse since taking the medication?"

☐ **2.** "How long have you been taking the medication?"

☐ **3.** "What time of day are you taking the medication?"

☐ **4.** "What is the dosage of medication that you are prescribed?"

Answer: 2

Ⓔ Rationale: Clients are often hopeful of positive results when a new medication is prescribed. It is frustrating to the client when symptom relief does not occur in a time frame which the client feels is acceptable. Understanding that symptom relief takes time, the nurse's next question is to ask how long she has been taking the medication. The nurse is correct to realize that one disadvantage of cyclic antidepressants is the lag time between initiation of drug therapy and relief of depressive symptoms. Nursing instruction includes maintaining the medication for at least a month before medication adjustments are made. Confirming the other questions is appropriate.

Test-taking strategy: Analyze to determine what information the question asks for, which is priority questions when assessing a client's cyclic antidepressant medication concern. Recall that it takes 4 to 6 weeks for symptom improvement for many individuals; thus, knowing when the client began taking the medication is a priority. Review imipramine use and side effects if you had difficulty answering this question.

Client needs category: Physiological integrity

Client needs subcategory: Pharmacological and parenteral therapies

Cognitive level: Evaluating

---

58. A client is undergoing peritoneal dialysis. The dialysate dwell time is completed, and the clamp is opened to allow the dialysate to drain. The nurse notes that drainage has stopped and that only 500 ml has drained; the amount of dialysate instilled was 1,500 ml. Which intervention would be done **first?**

☐ **1.** Change the client's position.

☐ **2.** Call the physician.

☐ **3.** Check the catheter for kinks or obstruction.

☐ **4.** Clamp the catheter and instill more dialysate at the next exchange time.

Answer: 3

Ⓔ Rationale: The first intervention would be to check for kinks and obstructions because that could be preventing drainage. After checking for kinks, have the client change position to promote drainage. Do not give the next scheduled exchange until the dialysate is drained because abdominal distention will occur, unless the output is within the parameters set by the health care provider. If unable to get more output despite checking for kinks and changing the client's position, the nurse would then call the health care provider to determine the proper intervention.

Test-taking strategy: Analyze to determine what information the question asks for, which is nursing action when peritoneal dialysate drainage has stopped. Note the key word as "first" intervention, indicating that other choices could be correct but completed at a later time. Focus on the most obvious causes of lack of dialysate drainage, and use the process of elimination to select the answer. Review care for peritoneal dialysis if you had difficulty answering this question.

Client needs category: Physiological integrity

Client needs subcategory: Physiological adaptation

Cognitive level: Analyzing

---

59. A client has been hospitalized with a diagnosis of conversion disorder blindness. Which statement **best** explains this manifestation?

- [ ] **1.** The client is suppressing true feelings.
- [ ] **2.** The client's anxiety has been relieved through physical symptoms.
- [ ] **3.** The client is acting indifferent because he/she does not want to show actual fear.
- [ ] **4.** The client's needs are being met, so he/she does not need to be anxious.

Ⓜ **Rationale:** Conversion accomplishes anxiety reduction through the production of a physical symptom symbolically linked to an underlying conflict. The client is not aware of the internal conflict. Hospitalization does not remove the source of the conflict.

Test-taking strategy: Analyze to determine what information the question asks for, which is explanation of conversion disorder. Recall that conversion disorder is an anxiety disorder. Also, note that conversion means changing in form or function. Discriminate between options 2 and 4 as they are the only options dealing with anxiety. Eliminate option 4 as client needs are not being met. Review conversion disorders if you had difficulty answering this question.

Client needs category: Psychosocial integrity

Client needs subcategory: None

Cognitive level: Analyzing

60. A pediatric nurse is providing discharge instructions for the family of a school-aged child with idiopathic thrombocytopenia. Which activity would be restricted until further notice?

- [ ] **1.** Swimming
- [ ] **2.** Bicycle riding
- [ ] **3.** Computer games
- [ ] **4.** Exposure to large crowds

Ⓔ **Rationale:** When routine blood counts reveal the platelet level is 100,000/mm³ (100,000 × 10⁹/L) or less, the child would not engage in contact sports, bicycle or scooter riding, climbing, or other activities that could lead to injury (especially to the head). Swimming releases energy, builds muscle, and allows the child to compete without risking injury, as long as the child follows normal safety precautions. Computer games do not cause physical injury. It is not necessary for this child to avoid large crowds because idiopathic thrombocytopenia does not suppress the immune system.

Test-taking strategy: Analyze to determine what information the question asks for, which is activity restriction for a pediatric client with idiopathic thrombocytopenia. Recall the definition of thrombocytopenia as an abnormal drop in platelet count. Select the option that could include possible bruising or bleeding. Review idiopathic thrombocytopenia if you had difficulty answering this question.

Client needs category: Safe and effective care environment

Client needs subcategory: Safety and infection control

Cognitive level: Applying

61. A toddler in respiratory distress is admitted to the pediatric intensive care unit. When the toddler refuses to keep the oxygen face mask on, the mother tries to help. Which action by the nurse is **most** appropriate?

☐ **1.** Giving the child a puzzle to play with

☐ **2.** Asking the mother to read the child's favorite book

☐ **3.** Administering a strong sedative so the child will sleep

☐ **4.** Telling the child that the face mask will help with breathing

Answer: 2

ⓒ Rationale: Having the mother read the child's favorite book will ease anxiety and provide comfort to the child. The child needs the mother's comfort because the face mask is frightening. A puzzle must be very basic to be developmentally appropriate. When a child is in respiratory distress, the child's focus would not be on putting a puzzle together. Sedation is contraindicated because it can mask signs of respiratory distress. A toddler is too young to understand that something will make him/her feel better.

Test-taking strategy: Analyze to determine what information the question asks for, which is nursing action most appropriate when attempting to get a toddler to wear a face mask. Recall that toddlers are fearful of strange surroundings and strangers. Consider that the mother might be most successful in getting the toddler to comply. Review the child's age and the circumstances surrounding hospitalization, with ways to obtain cooperation if you had difficulty answering this question.

Client needs category: Safe and effective care environment

Client needs subcategory: Management of care

Cognitive level: Applying

---

62. Which assignment made by a charge nurse would be appropriate?

☐ **1.** An RN assigned to an infant newly diagnosed with bacterial meningitis

☐ **2.** A senior level student nurse assigned to an adolescent with cystic fibrosis who is receiving several medications

☐ **3.** A registered practical nurse/licensed practical or vocational nurse assigned to a newly admitted child with acute leukemia who is receiving a blood transfusion

☐ **4.** A nursing assistant assigned to a transferred client with a head injury and frequent seizures

Answer: 1

ⓔ Rationale: An RN would be appropriately assigned to care for an infant with meningitis. The RN would make frequent assessments and provide a high level of care. Student nurses, even at the senior level, may not be allowed to give medications without supervision, and it may be easier for the RN or registered practical nurse/licensed practical or vocational nurse to provide care to this client. In many states, registered practical nurses/licensed practical or vocational nurses are not allowed to initiate blood or blood products. A client transferred to the unit with a head injury would need frequent assessments that only a licensed nurse would be able to provide.

Test-taking strategy: Analyze to determine what information the question asks for, which is staff assignments appropriate to various clients. Recall the scope of practice and nursing's career ladder. Consider the client's needs, and relate them to the skill level of the staff members. Review nursing's career ladder if you had difficulty answering this question.

Client needs category: Safe and effective care environment

Client needs subcategory: Management of care

Cognitive level: Evaluating

63. A 6-year-old boy is admitted to a pediatric unit for the treatment of osteomyelitis. Which essential medication classification would the nurse anticipate as documented on the medication report?

☐ **1.** Anti-inflammatory

☐ **2.** Analgesic

☐ **3.** Antibiotic

☐ **4.** Antipyretic

Answer: 3

Ⓜ **Rationale:** *Staphylococcus aureus* is the most common causative pathogen of osteomyelitis; the usual source of the infection is an upper respiratory infection (URI) or skin lesion. The nurse anticipates an intravenous antibiotic as the essential medication. The nurse may have an anti-inflammatory medication as adjunct therapy. By decreasing the infection, the client may decrease his or her pain, thus not needing an analgesic. The nurse would administer an antipyretic if the child was febrile.

Test-taking strategy: Analyze to determine what information the question asks for, which is medication classification essential for osteomyelitis. Recall that osteo means bone and myelitis means infection, and consider possible medication classifications to treat a bone infection. Eliminate options 1, 2, and 3 as either causative organisms for other disorders or normal to healthy individuals. Review osteomyelitis sources if you had difficulty answering this question.

Client needs category: Physiological integrity

Client needs subcategory: Pharmacology and parenteral therapies

Cognitive level: Applying

---

64. The nurse is preparing to teach a client about the prescribed spironolactone and to monitor for adverse effects of the drug. The nurse would instruct the client about which adverse effects? Select all that apply.

☐ **1.** Confusion

☐ **2.** Fatigue

☐ **3.** Hypertension

☐ **4.** Leg cramps

☐ **5.** Weakness

☐ **6.** Urinary retention

Answer: 1, 2, 5

Ⓒ **Rationale:** Spironolactone is used to treat hypertension and edema by removing excess fluid. Spironolactone is known as a potassium-sparing diuretic. Confusion, fatigue, and weakness are signs of hyperkalemia, an adverse effect of spironolactone. Spironolactone is used to treat hypertension, so it would not produce this effect. Leg cramps are an adverse effect of hypokalemia. Urinary retention is a side effect of anticholinergics.

Test-taking strategy: Analyze to determine what information the question asks for, which is adverse effects of spironolactone. Consider the action of the medication and its potassium-sparing quality. Recall that adverse effects can be an extension of a therapeutic effect. Review spironolactone actions and adverse effects if you had difficulty answering this question.

Client needs category: Physiological integrity

Client needs subcategory: Pharmacological and parenteral therapies

Cognitive level: Analyzing

65. The nurse is managing the care of a client diagnosed with Alzheimer's disease, who is being cared for at home. During a conference with the client's family and multidisciplinary team members, the nurse structures care around which **priority** nursing diagnosis or patient **priority**?

☐ **1.** Chronic confusion

☐ **2.** Impaired memory

☐ **3.** Impaired verbal communication

☐ **4.** Impaired swallowing

Answer: 4

Ⓜ Rationale: When working with the client's family and multidisciplinary team, it is most important to select priority nursing diagnosis/patient priority that, many times, includes safety concerns. The nurse is most correct to select impaired swallowing as the highest priority. Impaired swallowing can affect fluid and electrolytes status and nutrition and potentially cause pneumonia. Impaired memory and chronic confusion alone is manageable with appropriate supervision. Impaired verbal communication is an obstacle in expressing thoughts and feelings.

Test-taking strategy: When identifying a priority, select the diagnosis/patient priority that could be the most harmful. Eliminate option 3 as not a safety issue. Also, note that options 1 and 2 are very similar, canceling them as options. Review nursing diagnosis/patient priority and interventions for Alzheimer's disease if you had difficulty answering this question.

Client needs category: Safe and effective care environment

Client needs subcategory: Management of care

Cognitive level: Evaluating

---

66. A client presents to the emergency room with abdominal pain and upper gastrointestinal bleeding. The client is sweating and appears to be in moderate distress. Which nursing action would be a **priority** at this time?

☐ **1.** Obtain vital signs.

☐ **2.** Document history of the symptoms.

☐ **3.** Assess bowel sounds and abdominal tenderness.

☐ **4.** Insert an NG tube and connect to suction.

Answer: 1

Ⓔ Rationale: The priority nursing action is vital signs. Vital signs provide valuable information on the internal body system. Symptoms of shock, such as low blood pressure, a rapid weak pulse, cold clammy skin, and restlessness, can be monitored. Assessing bowel sounds and abdominal tenderness can provide useful data but is not a priority. Documentation is a lower priority, and a health care provider's order is needed for a nasogastric tube placement.

Test-taking strategy: Analyze to determine what information the question asks for, which is a priority action for a client with abdominal pain and an upper gastrointestinal bleed. The key word is "priority," which indicates that one action occurs before another. Use the ABCs to determine priority with vital sign focus. Review symptoms of upper gastrointestinal bleeding and priority nursing actions if you had difficulty answering this question.

Client needs category: Physiological integrity

Client needs subcategory: Physiological adaptation

Cognitive level: Analyzing

67. A client has received dietary instructions as part of the treatment plan for diabetes type 1. Which statement by the client would alert the nurse of needing additional instructions?

☐ **1.** "I'll need a bedtime snack because I take an evening dose of NPH insulin."

☐ **2.** "I can eat whatever I want as long as I cover the calories with sufficient insulin."

☐ **3.** "I can have an occasional low-calorie drink as long as I include it in my meal plan."

☐ **4.** "I should eat meals as scheduled, even if I'm not hungry, to prevent hypoglycemia."

E **Rationale:** Diabetes mellitus is a chronic condition associated with abnormally high glucose in the blood. The goal of dietary therapy in diabetes mellitus is to attain and maintain ideal body weight. Each client is prescribed a specific caloric intake and insulin regimen to help accomplish this goal. The other statements are correct.

Test-taking strategy: Analyze to determine what information the question asks for, which is nursing statement alerting the nurse that additional client teaching on dietary therapy is needed. The key words are "additional teaching," indicating that the statement is incorrect. Recall that dietary management of diabetes mellitus requires regular monitoring of diet along with blood sugar readings. Review the goals of dietary therapy for type 1 diabetes mellitus if you had difficulty answering this question.

Client needs category: Physiological integrity

Client needs subcategory: Basic care and comfort

Cognitive level: Analyzing

68. The nurse is caring for a 3-year-old diagnosed with a Wilms' tumor. If both kidneys are affected, the nurse would understand that treatment prior to surgery might include which of the following?

☐ **1.** Peritoneal dialysis

☐ **2.** Abdominal gavage

☐ **3.** Radiation and chemotherapy

☐ **4.** Antibiotics and intravenous fluid therapy

M **Rationale:** If both kidneys are involved, the child may be treated with radiation therapy or chemotherapy preoperatively to shrink the tumor, allowing more conservative therapy. Peritoneal dialysis would be needed only if the kidneys are not functioning. Abdominal gavage would not be indicated. Antibiotics are not needed because Wilms' tumor is not an infection.

Test-taking strategy: Analyze to determine what information the question asks for, which is treatment when a Wilms' tumor involves both kidneys. Recall that a Wilms' tumor is the most common cause of kidney cancer in children. Option 3 is the only option dealing with cancer treatment. Review Wilms' tumor nursing care and treatment if you had difficulty answering this question.

Client needs category: Safe and effective care environment

Client needs subcategory: Management of care

Cognitive level: Applying

69. Topical treatment with 2.5% hydrocortisone is prescribed for a 6-month-old infant with eczema. The mother is instructed to use the cream for no longer than 1 week. Why is this time limit appropriate?

☐ **1.** The drug loses its efficacy after prolonged use.

☐ **2.** This reduces adverse effects, such as skin atrophy and fragility.

☐ **3.** If no improvement is seen after 1 week, a stronger concentration will be prescribed.

☐ **4.** If no improvement is seen after 1 week, an antibiotic will be prescribed.

Ⓜ **Rationale:** Eczema is a chronic skin disorder that involves scaly and itchy rashes. Hydrocortisone cream helps to soothe dry, itchy, or healing patches but would be used for brief periods to decrease such adverse effects as atrophy of the skin. The drug does not lose efficacy after prolonged use. A stronger concentration may not be prescribed if no improvement is seen, and an antibiotic would be inappropriate in this instance.

Test-taking strategy: Analyze to determine what information the question asks for, which is treatment protocol of hydrocortisone cream for eczema. Recall that hydrocortisone is a synthetic steroid with adverse effects in which benefits can outweigh risks. Review the use of hydrocortisone cream for eczema and the effects on various body systems if you had difficulty answering this question.

Client needs category: Physiological integrity

Client needs subcategory: Pharmacological and parenteral therapies

Cognitive level: Applying

---

70. The registered nurse (RN) is referred to a client's home when a husband and wife have been confirmed to have scabies. The family asks, "How will we get rid of this?" When instructing on the proper procedure to wash contaminated clothing and sheets, which nursing instruction is a **priority?**

☐ **1.** Use commercial grade laundry detergent.

☐ **2.** Pretreat clothing where scabies contact existed.

☐ **3.** Wash clothes through 2 laundry cycles.

☐ **4.** Use hot water throughout wash cycle.

Ⓔ **Rationale:** The nurse instructs to use hot water throughout the wash cycle. Using hot water kills scabies and infectious agents on the laundry. If using the correct wash settings, the client does not need to use commercial grade laundry detergent and the clothing does not need to be pretreated or washed through 2 cycles. The family would also be instructed to dry the articles in a dryer. The family would clean all belongings thoroughly because of the ease of transmission.

Test-taking strategy: Analyze to determine what information the question asks for, which is priority teaching to rid a household of scabies. Consider that hot water and heat kill. The other option may be helpful but not as effective.

Client needs category: Physiological integrity

Client needs subcategory: Basic care and comfort

Cognitive level: Applying

71. A 23-year-old client develops cardiac tamponade when his/her car hits a telephone pole; the client was not wearing a seat belt. The nurse helps the health care provider perform a pericardiocentesis. Which outcome would indicate that pericardiocentesis has been effective?

- ☐ **1.** Neck vein distention
- ☐ **2.** Pulsus paradoxus
- ☐ **3.** Increased blood pressure
- ☐ **4.** Muffled heart sounds

Ⓔ Rationale: Cardiac tamponade is associated with decreased cardiac output, which in turn reduces blood pressure. By removing a small amount of blood, pericardiocentesis increases blood pressure. Neck vein distention, pulsus paradoxus, and muffled heart sounds indicate persistent cardiac tamponade, meaning pericardiocentesis has not been effective.

Test-taking strategy: Analyze to determine what information the question asks for, which is signs that pericardiocentesis has been effective. Consider options that would include improved cardiac output, improved vital signs, and normalization of heart sounds. Review the disease process of cardiac tamponade with treatment results if you had difficulty answering this question.

Client needs category: Physiological integrity

Client needs subcategory: Physiological adaptation

Cognitive level: Analyzing

72. A client arrives at the emergency department with a heart rate of 210 beats/minute and the following pattern on the cardiac monitor. The nurse is correct to alert the health care provider to the presence of which disorder?

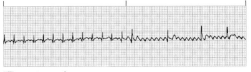

- ☐ **1.** Asystole
- ☐ **2.** Premature ventricular contraction
- ☐ **3.** Atrial flutter
- ☐ **4.** Ventricular fibrillation

Ⓔ Rationale: Atrial flutter (a sawtooth pattern on the monitor) is a disorder in which a single atrial impulse outside the SA node causes the atria to contract at an exceedingly rapid rate. The atrioventricular (AV) node conducts only some impulses to the ventricle, resulting in a ventricular rate slower than the atrial rate, thus forming a sawtooth pattern on the heart monitor. Asystole is the absence of cardiac function (a flat line) and can indicate death. Premature ventricular contraction indicates an early electric impulse and does not necessarily produce an exceedingly rapid heart rate. Ventricular fibrillation is the inefficient quivering of the ventricles and indicative of a dying heart.

Test-taking strategy: Analyze to determine what information the question asks for, which is cardiac monitor rhythm. Note the distinctive pattern on the monitor strip. Identify the pattern using the term "sawtooth" pattern. Review cardiac rhythms if you had difficulty answering this question.

Client needs category: Physiological integrity

Client needs subcategory: Physiological adaptation

Cognitive level: Analyzing

73. The nurse is caring for a child with a history of strep throat. Upon current assessment, the child states abdominal pain and joint achiness. Which laboratory data would the nurse communicate to the health care provider immediately?

☐ **1.** Leukocytosis

☐ **2.** Anemia

☐ **3.** Low hemoglobin level

☐ **4.** Marginal erythrocyte sedimentation rate

Answer: 1

🅴 **Rationale:** Leukocytosis can be seen as an immune response triggered by colonization of the pharynx with group A streptococci. This finding is expected in a client with rheumatic fever. Laboratory data indicating anemia or a low hemoglobin level will need to be addressed but are not critical and associated with the current disease process. A marginal erythrocyte sedimentation rate would be communicated on the laboratory report.

Test-taking strategy: Analyze to determine what information the question asks for, which are laboratory data that need to be brought to the health care provider's attention. Recall that a history of strep throat can lead to serious complications. Analyze current symptoms and which lab data could confirm a new diagnosis, such as rheumatic fever. Review complications of strep throat and associated laboratory data if you had difficulty answering this question.

Client needs category: Physiological integrity

Client needs subcategory: Reduction of risk

Cognitive level: Analyzing

---

74. A nurse is caring for a client newly diagnosed with multiple myeloma. Which blood cells are associated with abnormal values early in the disease process?

☐ **1.** Immunoglobulins

☐ **2.** Platelets

☐ **3.** Red blood cells (RBCs)

☐ **4.** WBCs

Answer: 1

🅲 **Rationale:** Multiple myeloma is characterized by malignant plasma cells that produce an increased amount of immunoglobulin that is not functional. As more malignant plasma cells are produced, there is less space in the bone marrow for RBC production. In late stages, platelets and WBCs are reduced as the bone marrow is infiltrated by malignant plasma cells.

Test-taking strategy: Analyze to determine what information the question asks for, which is abnormal blood characteristics early in the disease process. The key word is "early," indicating a change from the later stages of the disease. Review the pathophysiology of multiple myeloma and the effect on various cells of the body if you had difficulty answering this question.

Client needs category: Health promotion and maintenance

Client needs subcategory: None

Cognitive level: Analyzing

---

75. A 20-year-old client with cystic fibrosis is being discharged with a high-frequency chest wall oscillating vest. Which statement by the client indicates an understanding of how to use the vest?

- ☐ **1.** "I'll wear the vest for 5 minutes each time a treatment is due."
- ☐ **2.** "I'll lie down to use the vest."
- ☐ **3.** "I'll require help in applying the vest."
- ☐ **4.** "I can be in any position to use the vest."

Ⓜ **Rationale:** The high-frequency chest wall oscillating vest offers airway clearance treatment for individuals with cystic fibrosis. The vest system does not require special positioning or breathing to be effective. In most cases, treatments last 15 to 20 minutes and clients can manage therapy without any assistance.

Test-taking strategy: Analyze to determine what information the question asks for, which is correct statement indicating understanding of vest usage. Consider the meaning of the word oscillating, meaning to move to or from and relate to the benefits in a client with cystic fibrosis. Analyze each option for a correct statement. Review the purpose and correct use of the vest if you had difficulty answering this question.

Client needs category: Physiological integrity
Client needs subcategory: Basic care and comfort
Cognitive level: Analyzing

76. The nurse is evaluating the therapeutic goal of a client with history of cardiac dysrhythmias and newly completed radiofrequency catheter ablation. Which client-centered goal is **most** appropriate?

- ☐ **1.** The client will experience reprofusion of ischemic heart tissue.
- ☐ **2.** The client will have a lowered blood pressure from the dilation of arterial vessels.
- ☐ **3.** The client will have a regular heart rhythm from destruction of errant tissue of the heart.
- ☐ **4.** The client will have no fainting from over-stimulation of the heart.

Ⓜ **Rationale:** The therapeutic goal of radiofrequency catheter ablation is to destroy errant tissue in hopes of allowing impulse conduction to travel over appropriate pathways. The goal does not include dilation of blood vessels or reprofusion of heart tissue. There is no stimulation of the heart.

Test-taking strategy: Analyze to determine what information the question asks for, which is goal of radiofrequency catheter ablation. Use your knowledge of medical terminology (ablation = to destroy). Review the goals of cardiac ablation if you had difficulty answering this question.

Client needs category: Physiological integrity
Client needs subcategory: Physiological adaptation
Cognitive level: Evaluating

77. The nurse in a rehabilitation center is caring for a client injured in a swimming accident. Which intervention is **most** appropriate to include in a bladder program for a client in rehabilitation for a spinal cord injury?

☐ **1.** Insert an indwelling urinary catheter.

☐ **2.** Schedule intermittent catheterization every 2 to 4 hours.

☐ **3.** Perform a straight catheterization every 8 hours while the client is awake.

☐ **4.** Perform Credé's maneuver to the lower abdomen before the client voids.

Answer: 2

Ⓜ **Rationale:** Intermittent catheterization would begin every 2 to 4 hours early in treatment. When residual volume is less than 400 ml, the schedule may advance to every 4 to 6 hours. Indwelling catheters may predispose the client to infection and are removed as soon as possible. Credé's maneuver is applied after voiding to enhance bladder emptying.

Test-taking strategy: Analyze to determine what information the question asks for, which is nursing interventions to include in a bladder program. Analyze each option for the best possible method for urinary elimination. Eliminate option 4 as not relating to urinary elimination. Discriminate between the remaining three options as to which best meets the goal. Review the bladder programs if you had difficulty answering this question.

Client needs category: Physiological integrity

Client needs subcategory: Basic care and comfort

Cognitive level: Applying

---

78. The nurse is caring for a client on the urinary unit. When providing report to the next shift, it is noted that the client has osteopenia and history of renal calculi. Which of the following disorders would the nurse suspect?

☐ **1.** Hyperparathyroidism

☐ **2.** Hypoparathyroidism

☐ **3.** Hypopituitarism

☐ **4.** Hypothyroidism

Answer: 1

Ⓜ **Rationale:** Hyperparathyroidism is characterized by osteopenia and renal calculi secondary to overproduction of parathyroid hormone. The hallmark symptom of hypoparathyroidism is tetany from hypocalcemia. Hypopituitarism presents with extreme weight loss and atrophy of all endocrine glands. Symptoms of hypothyroidism include hair loss, weight gain, and cold intolerance.

Test-taking strategy: Analyze to determine what information the question asks for, which is disorder characterized by osteopenia and renal calculi. Focus on the pathophysiology of the disorders mentioned, and review the clinical manifestations of each. Review the endocrine disorders if you had difficulty answering this question.

Client needs category: Physiological integrity

Client needs subcategory: Physiological adaptation

Cognitive level: Analysis

---

79. A client arrives to the emergency department with suspected appendicitis. The admitting nurse performs an assessment. Order the following steps according to the sequence in which they are performed. All options must be used.

1. Percuss all four abdominal quadrants.

2. Obtain a health history.

3. Inspect the abdomen, noting the shape, contours, and any visible peristalsis or pulsations.

4. Auscultate bowel sounds in all four quadrants.

5. Gently palpate all four quadrants, saving the painful area for last.

Answer: 2, 3, 4, 1, 5

Ⓜ Rationale: The first step in the data collection process is to obtain a health history. Then, the nurse would visually inspect the abdomen. Of the three remaining steps, it is important to auscultate before percussing or palpating the client's abdomen. Touching or palpating the abdomen before listening may actually change the bowel sounds, leading to faulty data.

Test-taking strategy: Analyze to determine what information the question asks for, which is sequence of actions with suspected appendicitis. Always begin with questioning for data collection. Second, begin the abdominal-focused assessment progressing from least contact to most contact. Review basic assessment techniques if you had difficulty answering this question.

Client needs category: Physiological integrity
Client needs subcategory: Reduction of risk potential
Cognitive level: Analyzing

---

80. A mother infected with human immunodeficiency virus (HIV) asks the nurse about the possibility of breast-feeding her neonate. Which response by the nurse would be **most** appropriate?

☐ **1.** "Breast-feeding isn't an option because of risk of virus transmission."

☐ **2.** "Breast-feeding would be best for your baby."

☐ **3.** "Breast-feeding is only an option if the mother is taking zidovudine."

☐ **4.** "Breast-feeding is an option if milk is expressed and fed by a bottle."

Answer: 1

Ⓔ Rationale: Mothers infected with HIV are unable to breast-feed because the virus has been isolated in breast milk and could be transmitted to the infant. Taking zidovudine does not prevent transmission. The risk of breast-feeding is not associated with direct contact with the breast but with the possibility of the HIV contained in the breast milk.

Test-taking strategy: Analyze to determine what information the question asks for, which is correct information regarding HIV transmission in breast milk. Recall how HIV is transmitted and that HIV has been found in breast milk. If unsure, eliminate options 2 and 4 as essentially the same. Eliminate option 3 as medication does not eliminate the virus completely. Review breast-feeding and HIV transmission if you had difficulty answering this question.

Client needs category: Health promotion and maintenance
Client needs subcategory: None
Cognitive level: Applying

81. A child with a diagnosis of meningococcal meningitis develops signs of sepsis and a purpuric rash over both lower extremities. The primary health care provider would be notified immediately because these signs could be indicative of which complication?

☐ **1.** A severe allergic reaction to the antibiotic regimen with impending anaphylaxis

☐ **2.** Onset of the SIADH

☐ **3.** Meningococcemia

☐ **4.** Adhesive arachnoiditis

Answer: 3

Ⓜ **Rationale:** Meningococcemia is a serious complication usually associated with meningococcal infection. A client with a severe allergic reaction and impending anaphylaxis would most likely have signs and symptoms of respiratory distress, GI problems (abdominal pain, cramps, and diarrhea), hypotension, hives, itching, and anxiety. SIADH can be an acute complication, but it would not be accompanied by the purpuric rash. Adhesive arachnoiditis occurs in the chronic phase of the disease and leads to obstructed flow of cerebrospinal fluid.

Test-taking strategy: Analyze to determine what information the question asks for, which is complication of meningococcal meningitis. If unsure, note that the answer is associated with the diagnosis. Review the symptoms in relation to the pathophysiology of meningococcal meningitis if you had difficulty answering this question.

Client needs category: Physiological integrity
Client needs subcategory: Reduction of risk potential
Cognitive level: Applying

---

82. The nurse is working in the intensive care unit with a client in shock. During handoff, the nurse reports the results of which assessment findings that signal early signs of the decompensation stage? Select all that apply.

☐ **1.** Vital signs

☐ **2.** Nutrition

☐ **3.** Skin color

☐ **4.** Gait

☐ **5.** Urine output

☐ **6.** Peripheral pulses

Answer: 1, 3, 5, 6

Ⓜ **Rationale:** Shock is a medical emergency in which the organs and tissues of the body are not receiving adequate blood flow. Although shock can develop and progress quickly, the nurse monitors evidence of early signs that blood volume and circulation is becoming compromised. Vital signs, skin color, urine output related to blood perfusion of the kidneys, and peripheral pulses all provide assessment data relating blood volume and circulation. Nutrition and gait is not related to blood circulation.

Test-taking strategy: Analyze to determine what information the question asks for, which is assessment data related to the decompensation stage of shock. The key word is "decompensation" indicating further deterioration. Recall that a diagnosis of shock means a decreasing blood flow to the tissues. Identify types of assessments that provide data on blood flow. Review shock particularly in the decompensation stage if you had difficulty answering this question.

Client needs category: Physiological integrity
Client needs subcategory: Physiological adaptation
Cognitive level: Applying

83. When a 6-month-old infant is admitted for intestinal obstruction, which assessment finding would alert the nurse to a potential problem?

☐ **1.** Presence of the Moro reflex

☐ **2.** The child's playing with his/her feet

☐ **3.** Eruption of the first tooth

☐ **4.** Rolling from the stomach to back

Answer: 1

Ⓜ Rationale: By 6 months of age, the Moro (startle) reflex would no longer be observed. Playing with the feet, eruption of the first tooth, and rolling from the stomach to back are all normal for a 6-month-old infant.

Test-taking strategy: Analyze to determine what information the question asks for, which is an assessment finding that is inconsistent with 6 months of age. Note that there is no relation to the diagnosis needed. Recall developmental milestones. If unsure, recall that the Moro reflex is assessed at birth. Review the infant's age and developmental milestones if you had difficulty answering this question.

Client needs category: Health promotion and maintenance

Client needs subcategory: None

Cognitive level: Analyzing

---

84. The nurse is administering noon medications. Which assessment finding would alert the nurse to change the intranasal route for medication administration?

☐ **1.** Mucous membrane irritation

☐ **2.** Severe coughing

☐ **3.** Sore throat

☐ **4.** Pneumonia

Answer: 1

Ⓒ Rationale: Mucous membrane irritation caused by a cold or allergy renders the intranasal route unreliable. Severe coughing, pneumonia, or a sore throat would not interfere with the intranasal route.

Test-taking strategy: Analyze to determine what information the question asks for, which is assessment finding requiring a change from intranasal route. Focus on nasal structures that eliminate options 2 and 4. Recall the route of administration, and consider which assessment finding would interfere with the drug's absorption. Review the intranasal route of administration if you had difficulty answering this question.

Client needs category: Physiological integrity

Client needs subcategory: Pharmacological and parenteral therapies

Cognitive level: Applying

85. A nurse is developing a teaching plan for a client who will undergo a stapedectomy for the treatment of otosclerosis. Which instruction would the plan include?

☐ **1.** Ringing in the ears is common after surgery.

☐ **2.** Vertigo and dizziness are common after surgery.

☐ **3.** Hearing should return immediately after surgery.

☐ **4.** Excessive drainage is common after surgery.

Answer: 2

Ⓜ **Rationale:** Vertigo is the most common complication of stapedectomy. The client would move slowly to avoid triggering or worsening vertigo and would ask for assistance with ambulation. Ringing in the ears (tinnitus) rarely follows this surgery and would be reported to the health care provider. Hearing typically decreases after surgery because of ear packing and tissue swelling, but commonly returns over the next 2 to 6 weeks. Usually, postoperative drainage and pain are minimal; excessive drainage would be reported.

Test-taking strategy: Analyze to determine what information the question asks for, which is instruction included in the teaching plan. Recall the physiology and function of the stapes, which is impacted by the surgery. Also, consider that the middle ear is essential in the function of balance. Review complication from a stapedectomy if you had difficulty answering this question.

Client needs category: Physiological integrity

Client needs subcategory: Reduction of risk potential

Cognitive level: Applying

---

86. The nurse is caring for a client of African descent who is having increased respiratory difficulty. When assessing the client's oxygen status, which assessment technique is used to evaluate client cyanosis? Select all that apply.

☐ **1.** Inspecting the nail beds

☐ **2.** Inspecting the conjunctiva

☐ **3.** Noting a dullness in skin color

☐ **4.** Assessing the earlobe

☐ **5.** Assessing the lips and gums

Answer: 1, 2, 5

Ⓒ **Rationale:** The color of a client's skin is determined by the amount of pigment it contains and the blood flowing through it. In clients with highly pigmented skin, cyanosis is accurately detected by inspecting the conjunctiva and nail beds and assessing the oral mucous membranes including the lips and gums. The other options do not provide the assessment for cyanosis.

Test-taking strategy: Analyze to determine what information the question asks for, which is assessment technique when evaluating an African client's cyanosis. Since a client's skin pigment interferes with the ability to note cyanotic status, the nurse must look to other areas that reflect cyanosis. Recall that mucous membranes provide an assessment area. Review assessment techniques for client's with pigmented skin if you had difficulty answering this question.

Client needs category: Physiological integrity

Client needs subcategory: Physiological adaptation

Cognitive level: Applying

---

87. A female client with diabetes has a decreased level of consciousness and a fingerstick glucose level of 39 mg/dl (39 mmol/L). Her family reports that she has been skipping meals in an effort to lose weight. When managing the client's care after discharge, which nursing intervention is **most** appropriate?

- ☐ **1.** Placing a Salem sump tube and providing tube feedings
- ☐ **2.** Administering a 500-ml bolus of normal saline solution
- ☐ **3.** Administering 1 ampule of 50% dextrose solution
- ☐ **4.** Providing a high-protein, high-caloric snack

Ⓔ Rationale: The client will have the blood sugars be normalized in the health care facility, but upon discharge, the client needs to effectively manage her care. Administering 50% dextrose solution helps preserve and restore the client's physiologic integrity. Providing a feeding tube and ingesting a snack is appropriate only in a less urgent situation, Consider that during the time it takes to insert an NG tube, administer a feeding, and wait for digestion to occur, the client may suffer permanent brain damage and seizures from severe hypoglycemia. A blood pressure drop was not mentioned; a bolus of normal saline solution would correct only the client's fluid status, not glucose level.

Test-taking strategy: Analyze to determine what information the question asks for, which is nursing intervention for a client with a critical blood sugar reading of 39 mg/dl (39 mmol/L). Recall that a blood sugar of 39 mg/dl (39 mmol/L) is an emergency situation requiring immediate blood sugar elevation. Instilling dextrose intravenously is the best option. Review hypoglycemic protocol if you had difficulty answering this question.

Client needs category: Safe and effective care environment

Client needs subcategory: Management of care

Cognitive level: Applying

88. The nurse is caring for a client diagnosed with genitourinary tuberculosis (TB). Which statement, made by the client, about genitourinary TB demonstrates an understanding?

- ☐ **1.** "It isn't infectious and I can't pass it from one person to another."
- ☐ **2.** "I can't pass it sexually to my partner."
- ☐ **3.** "It's a late manifestation of respiratory tuberculosis."
- ☐ **4.** "It's an early manifestation of an autoimmune disorder."

Ⓔ Rationale: Genitourinary TB is usually a late manifestation of respiratory TB and can occur if the disease spreads through the bloodstream from the lungs. *Bacillus* in the urine is infectious, and urine would be handled cautiously. A condom would be used during sex to prevent spread of the infection.

Test-taking strategy: Analyze to determine what information the question asks for, which is identifying the correct statement regarding genitourinary TB. Note that the correct answer has the same title as in the question. Review the pathophysiology of TB if you had difficulty answering this question.

Client needs category: Physiological integrity

Client needs subcategory: Physiological adaptation

Cognitive level: Applying

89. A client having an acute asthmatic attack is admitted to the emergency room. The health care provider writes an order for *epinephrine 1:1,000 injection 0.3 ml subcutaneous stat*. The nurse reads in the unit's drug reference that epinephrine 1:1,000 contains 1 mg/ml. Instructions direct the nurse to dilute each milligram of the 1:1,000 concentration with 10 ml of normal saline, resulting in a solution that contains 0.1 mg/1 ml. How many milligrams of epinephrine will be administered to the client after the nurse has added the diluent? Record your answer using three decimal places.

_____ mg

Answer: 0.03

Ⓓ Rationale: Using the ratio-and-proportion method, calculate the correct dosage by using the following formula:

Dose on hand/quantity on hand = X/dose prescribed

0.1 mg/1 ml = X mg/0.3 ml

$$\frac{0.1 \text{ mg}}{1 \text{ ml}} = \frac{X \text{ mg}}{0.3 \text{ ml}}$$

$$X = 0.03$$

Test-taking strategy: Analyze to determine what information the question asks for, which is calculated dosage for medication administration. Use the above formula to enter question data. Proofread the math calculation. Review dosage calculations formulas if you had difficulty answering this question.

Client needs category: Physiological integrity

Client needs subcategory: Pharmacological and parenteral therapies

Cognitive level: Applying

---

90. The nurse is reviewing a pediatric client's plan of care. Which method is considered the definitive treatment for hypopituitarism because of growth hormone deficiency?

☐ **1.** Treatment with desmopressin acetate (DDAVP)

☐ **2.** Replacement of ADH

☐ **3.** Treatment with testosterone or estrogen

☐ **4.** Replacement with biosynthetic growth hormone

Answer: 4

Ⓜ Rationale: The definitive treatment for growth hormone deficiency, replacement with biosynthetic growth hormone, is successful in 80% of affected children. DDAVP is used to treat diabetes insipidus. ADH deficiency causes diabetes insipidus and is not related to hypopituitarism. Testosterone or estrogen may be given during adolescence for normal sexual maturation, but neither is the definitive treatment for hypopituitarism.

Test-taking strategy: Analyze to determine what information the question asks for, which is definitive treatment for hypopituitarism and growth hormone deficiency. Consider the action of the pituitary gland as producing growth hormone. Treatment options would include stimulating the pituitary for more hormones or replacing the hormone, which leads to the correct answer. Review treatment for hypopituitarism if you had difficulty answering this question.

Client needs category: Physiological integrity

Client needs subcategory: Pharmacological and parenteral therapies

Cognitive level: Applying

91. When providing discharge teaching for a client with uric acid calculi, the nurse would include an instruction to avoid which type of diet?

☐ **1.** Low calcium

☐ **2.** Low oxalate

☐ **3.** High oxalate

☐ **4.** High purine

Ⓜ **Rationale:** To control uric acid calculi, the client would follow a low-purine diet, which excludes high-purine foods such as organ meats. The other diets do not control uric acid calculi.

Test-taking strategy: Analyze to determine what information the question asks for, which is dietary instruction for a client with uric acid calculi. Recall the cause of uric acid calculi and dietary guidelines of a low-purine diet as uric acids are the waste product of purines. Review a low-purine diet if you had difficulty answering this question.

Client needs category: Physiological integrity

Client needs subcategory: Basic care and comfort

Cognitive level: Applying

---

92. Parents of a child diagnosed with bacterial meningitis are asking the nurse questions regarding the disease process. Which description about the development of sequelae in infants with bacterial meningitis is **most** accurate?

☐ **1.** They usually occur during the first 2 months of life.

☐ **2.** They only occur in children with meningo-coccal meningitis.

☐ **3.** They primarily involve the fourth ventricle of the brain.

☐ **4.** They tend to affect the ocular nerves, leading to retinal damage.

Ⓜ **Rationale:** In infants with bacterial meningitis who are younger than 2 months old, communicating hydrocephalus and the effects of cerebritis on the immature brain lead to the frequent occurrence of sequelae. Sequelae are least common in children with meningococcal meningitis. Meningitis affects the meninges (the connective tissue layers of the brain), not the ventricles, and it primarily affects the nerves for hearing, not vision.

Test-taking strategy: Analyze to determine what information the question asks for, which is potential sequelae in infants with bacterial meningitis. Consider that the bacteria/infection is located in the sac surrounding the brain. Recall the growth and development of the infant brain if you had difficulty answering this question.

Client needs category: Physiological integrity

Client needs subcategory: Physiological adaptation

Cognitive level: Applying

93. The nurse is caring for a client with chronic hypertension who struggles with medication compliance because of financial issues. When reviewing recent lab work results, which reflects the client's blood pressure issues? Select all that apply.

☐ **1.** Blood urea nitrogen (BUN)

☐ **2.** Complete blood count

☐ **3.** Creatinine

☐ **4.** Cardiac enzymes

☐ **5.** Alanine aminotransferase (ALT)

☐ **6.** Calcium

Answer: 1, 3, 6

Ⓓ Rationale: Financial issues can lead to a client inability to afford medication and, thus, chronic issues with hypertension. Blood urea nitrogen (BUN) and creatinine levels reveal kidney function and, if abnormal, are reflective of chronic hypertension. Calcium levels fluctuate as calcium leaves the bone. Calcification of major blood vessels in the body can occur. Hypertension is not reflective in the complete blood count levels. Cardiac enzymes may indicate a myocardial infarction. Alanine aminotransferase (ALT) is a liver enzyme reflective of liver function.

Test-taking strategy: Analyze to determine what information the question asks for, which is lab work that reflects the effects of chronic hypertension. Recall that chronic hypertension can damage the kidney causing renal perfusion dysfunction (noted in the BUN/creatinine levels). Because of the kidney dysfunction, serum phosphate levels and serum calcium levels have a reciprocal relationship. Review the effects of chronic hypertension if you had difficulty answering this question.

Client needs category: Physiological integrity

Client needs subcategory: Reduction of risk potential

Cognitive level: Analyzing

---

94. The nurse is caring for a client who has a type I second-degree atrioventricular (AV) block. Which ECG rhythm would the nurse expect to see?

☐ **1.**

☐ **2.**

☐ **3.**

☐ **4.**

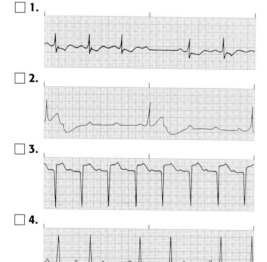

Answer: 4

Ⓜ Rationale: Type I second-degree AV block is characterized by a progressively longer PR interval until a QRS complex is dropped (option 4). Option 1 shows a type II second-degree AV block, which has a PR interval that may be prolonged but stays constant until a QRS complex is dropped. Option 2 shows a third-degree AV block, which has a constant PR interval and a constant interval between the QRS complexes, but there is no apparent relationship between the P waves and the QRS complexes. Option 3 shows a first-degree AV block, which has a consistent prolonged PR interval. No QRS complexes are dropped.

Test-taking strategy: Analyze to determine what information the question asks for, which is identifying a type I second-degree AV block. Focus on the different characteristics of each type of heart block and relate to the pattern shown on the rhythm strip. Review the rationale for definitions and findings on the rhythm strip. Review ECG tracings if you had difficulty answering this question.

Client needs category: Physiological integrity

Client needs subcategory: Physiological adaptation

Cognitive level: Analyzing

95. The nurse is caring for a client who has been placed on phenobarbital 30 mg daily for newly diagnosed seizure activity. Which instruction would be included in client teaching specifically related to anticonvulsant drug efficacy?

☐ **1.** Wear a medical identification bracelet.

☐ **2.** Maintain a seizure frequency chart.

☐ **3.** Avoid potentially hazardous activities.

☐ **4.** Discontinue the drug immediately if adverse effects are suspected.

Answer: 2

Ⓜ **Rationale:** Efficacy means the capacity for beneficial change. Ongoing evaluation of therapeutic effects can be accomplished by maintaining a seizure frequency chart that indicates the date, time, and nature of all seizure activities. These data are helpful in making dosage alterations and specific drug selection. Avoidance of hazardous activities and wearing a medical identification bracelet are ways to minimize dangers related to seizure activity, but these factors do not affect drug efficacy. Anticonvulsant drugs would never be discontinued abruptly because of the risk of developing status epilepticus.

Test-taking strategy: Analyze to determine what information the question asks for, which is instruction specifically related to drug efficacy. The key words are "drug efficacy," which means amount of drug to produce the drug effect. The option reflecting therapeutic effect is to maintain tracking of seizure activity. Review the therapeutic activity of anticonvulsants if you had difficulty answering this question.

Client needs category: Physiological integrity

Client needs subcategory: Pharmacological and parenteral therapies

Cognitive level: Applying

---

96. The nurse is caring for a client on hemodialysis who has an arteriovenous (AV) fistula in the right arm. When managing a client's plan of care, which nursing instructions/actions are appropriate? Select all that apply.

☐ **1.** Maintaining the right arm above the heart

☐ **2.** Utilizing a splint to maintain the right arm in an extended position

☐ **3.** Avoiding all blood pressure readings and trauma to the right arm

☐ **4.** Assessing the shunt by auscultating a bruit

☐ **5.** Completing arm and finger exercises

☐ **6.** Encouraging wearing tight-fitted shirts

Answers: 3, 4, 5

Ⓜ **Rationale:** An AV fistula is a connection between an artery and a vein creating a ready source with a rapid flow of blood. The fistula is located under the skin and is used during dialysis to access the bloodstream. When managing the care of the client, instruction is needed to ensure the patency of the fistula. The client would not have any blood pressure readings, lab work drawn, or trauma to the right arm. To check the fistula for adequate blood flow, the client would feel the thrill of the blood moving through the vessels and auscultate a bruit hearing the swish in the vessels. Arm and finger exercises are encouraged for blood flow. The client would not elevate the right arm above the heart as would be done to decrease swelling or inflammation or split the arm. Tight-fitting clothes are to be avoided.

Test-taking strategy: Analyze to determine what information the question asks for, which is instruction needed to manage care of a client with an AV fistula. Recall that the fistula allows access to the arteriovenous circulation. The primary goal is to maintain the blood flow and patency of the fistula. Consider each option against that goal. Review the care and maintenance of an AV fistula if you had difficulty answering this question.

Client needs category: Safe and effective care environment

Client needs subcategory: Management of care

Cognitive level: Analyzing

97. A float nurse is assigned to a surgical unit. The nurse is receiving 2 clients from the postanesthesia care unit (PACU) at the same time. When delegating tasks to other PACU personnel who are not known to the nurse, which question would be **most** important to ask?

☐ **1.** What is your highest educational level?

☐ **2.** How long have you worked on this floor?

☐ **3.** Are you comfortable in performing the tasks being assigned?

☐ **4.** Who provided you the unit training?

Answer: 3

ⓔ Rationale: Since the float nurse is not familiar with staff, it is important to ask the worker if he/she is comfortable and had instruction in the task assigned. Principles of delegation state that the right task in the right situation by the right personnel is essential to client care. Asking the highest educational level, how long they worked on the floor, and who provided their training is not as important as if they are comfortable with performing the task.

Test-taking strategy: Analyze to determine what information the question asks for, which is question to ask when delegating tasks. The key word is "float," meaning that the assigning nurse is unsure of the skill of the others on the unit. The nurse must ensure the understanding and ability of those they are delegating to. Review delegating guidelines if you had difficulty answering this question.

Client needs category: Safe and effective care environment

Client needs subcategory: Management of care

Cognitive level: Analyzing

---

98. The nurse is triaging phone calls at a local pediatrician's office. Which statement by the parent of a child being treated for pinworms indicates that further teaching is needed?

☐ **1.** "I'll make my child wash his/her hands well before meals."

☐ **2.** "I'll warn my child to avoid sharing hairbrushes and hats to prevent spreading pinworms to others."

☐ **3.** "I'll give my child only one dose of medication."

☐ **4.** "I'll keep my child's nails short."

Answer: 2

ⓒ Rationale: Sharing hairbrushes and hats reduces the spread of lice, not pinworms. Hands would be washed well before food preparation and eating to avoid ingesting eggs that may be under the fingernails from scratching the itchy infested perianal area. Only a single dose of medication, such as mebendazole, is needed to treat pinworms. Keeping the fingernails short reduces the risk of carrying eggs under the nails.

Test-taking strategy: Analyze to determine what information the question asks for, which is parent statements that need further instruction. The key words are "need further instruction" indicating an incorrect statement. Analyze each option for an incorrect statement related to pinworms. Recall the cause and location of pinworms, which will lead to the correct answer. Review nursing instruction of pinworms if you had difficulty answering this question.

Client needs category: Safe and effective care environment

Client needs subcategory: Safety and infection control

Cognitive level: Analyzing

99. The nurse is caring for a homeless client with pneumonia. Laboratory testing reveals the following results: blood urea nitrogen (BUN) 180 mg/dl, creatinine 30 mg/dl (2,652 mmol/L), potassium 6.2 mEq/L (6.2 mmol/L), and hemoglobin 6.2% (62 g/L). Based on the health care provider's order below, which drug order would the nurse question?

Physician Orders	
12/21/15 0900	Gentamicin 180 mg I.V. piggyback every 8 hours
	Erythropoietin 50 units/kg subcutaneously Monday, Wednesday, and Friday
	Aluminum hydroxide gel 500 mg P.O. four times daily
	Ferrous sulfate 325 mg P.O. three times daily ————— Garry Reynolds, MD

☐ **1.** Gentamicin sulfate

☐ **2.** Erythropoietin

☐ **3.** Aluminum hydroxide gel

☐ **4.** Ferrous sulfate

Answer: 1

Ⓜ Rationale: Based on the high BUN, creatinine, and potassium levels, the client is in renal failure. Gentamicin sulfate is nephrotoxic and can exacerbate the renal failure. Ferrous sulfate and erythropoietin would be given to treat the client's anemia. Aluminum hydroxide gel would also be appropriate because it binds with phosphate, which is elevated in renal failure.

Test-taking strategy: Analyze to determine what information the question asks for, which is drug order to be questioned. The key word is "questioned" indicating a problem. Analyze each option for correct drug, adverse effects, etc., in relation to the laboratory information provided in the question. Review the laboratory results and medication contraindications if you had difficulty answering this question.

Client needs category: Physiological integrity

Client needs subcategory: Reduction of risk potential

Cognitive level: Analyzing

---

100. The nurse is caring for a client with a nasogastric tube and in mitt restraints. Which nursing action is required every 1 to 2 hours?

☐ **1.** Assist the client to the bathroom.

☐ **2.** Assess cognitive status.

☐ **3.** Offer the client sips of clear liquids.

☐ **4.** Remove restraints and assess skin and circulation.

Answer: 4

Ⓔ Rationale: Placing a client in any type of restraint is a controversial issue. Strict guidelines exist. The client in restraints must have the skin integrity and circulation assessed every 1 to 2 hours. It is also appropriate to massage the area and provide range-of-motion exercises. On a regular basis, the client would be offered to use a bedpan or ambulate to the bathroom and the nurse would assess the cognitive status. A client with a nasogastric tube would not be offered fluids.

Test-taking strategy: Analyze to determine what information the question asks for, which is nursing action required every 1 to 2 hours for the client in a restraint. First, understand the time frame and ask yourself, "What requires frequent assessment when in a restraint?" Compare each option with that standard. Review nursing care for a client in a restraint.

Client needs category: Safe and effective care environment

Client needs subcategory: Safety and infection control

Cognitive level: Analyzing

1. The nurse is working in an internal medicine office. A daughter brings her elderly mother to the doctor's appointment. Upon reviewing the medication list, the daughter states, "Which medication is prescribed to prevent a stroke?" The nurse is correct to answer which medication?

☐ **1.** Allopurinol

☐ **2.** Claritin

☐ **3.** Ticlopidine

☐ **4.** Methylprednisolone

Answer: 3

E Rationale: Ticlopidine inhibits platelet aggregation by interfering with adenosine diphosphate release in the coagulation cascade and, therefore, is used to prevent thromboembolic stroke. Allopurinol is an antigout medication used to reduce uric acid. Claritin is an over-the-counter allergy medication. Methylprednisolone, a steroid with anticoagulant properties, is not used to treat thromboembolic stroke.

Test-taking strategy: Analyze to determine what information the question asks for, which is medication prescribed to prevent a stroke. Consider each option for the action and property of the medication. Review the indications for the medications listed if you had difficulty answering this question.

Client needs category: Physiological integrity

Client needs subcategory: Pharmacological and parenteral therapies

Cognitive level: Analyzing

2. A telemetry nurse is assessing a client's ECG. The ECG is showing ST elevation in leads V_2, V_3, and V_4. Which artery is most likely occluded?

☐ **1.** Circumflex artery

☐ **2.** Internal mammary artery

☐ **3.** Left anterior descending artery

☐ **4.** Right coronary artery

Answer: 3

C Rationale: The client's ECG changes suggest an anterior wall myocardial infarction (MI). The left anterior descending artery is the primary source of blood for the anterior wall of the heart. The circumflex artery supplies the lateral wall of the heart, the internal mammary artery supplies the anterior chest wall and breasts, and the right coronary artery supplies the inferior wall of the heart.

Test-taking strategy: Analyze to determine what information the question asks for, which is analyzing the ECG and determining the occluded artery. First, consider the location of the electrode transmitting information and interpret ECG tracing. Review the relationship between the heart's electrical conduction system and the specific coronary arteries mentioned if you had difficulty answering this question.

Client needs category: Physiological integrity

Client needs subcategory: Physiological adaptation

Cognitive level: Analyzing

3. The nurse is caring for a client with possible immune deficiency. Which subjective data would be **most** indicative?

☐ **1.** "I get up every morning with a stuffy nose and sore throat."

☐ **2.** "Just as I get over a virus, it seems that I get another."

☐ **3.** "I have had a sore on my leg that just won't heal."

☐ **4.** "I sneeze and have watery eyes throughout the spring and summer."

Answer: 2

© Rationale: Immune deficiencies make it harder for the body to fight infection. With a low resistance, the client is susceptible to obtaining more circulating viruses. Having morning stuffiness and a sore throat is indicative of sinus congestion. Having a leg sore is indicative of cardiovascular insufficiency or diabetes. Sneezing with watery eyes indicates seasonal allergies.

Test-taking strategy: Analyze to determine what information the question asks for, which is a statement indicating immune deficiency. Focus on the word immune indicating a prevention of disease. Option 2 states a frequency in obtaining illness. Review the etiology and symptoms of immune deficiency if you had difficulty answering this question.

Client needs category: Physiological integrity

Client needs subcategory: Physiological adaptation

Cognitive level: Analyzing

---

4. A client with physical deficits related to a recent cerebral vascular accident states with tears in her eyes, "I no longer can take care of myself." Which statement by the nurse is **most** therapeutic?

☐ **1.** "It is hard not to be able to care for yourself."

☐ **2.** "You will get back to normal after you have some physical therapy."

☐ **3.** "Let me help you dress and then we can get some breakfast."

☐ **4.** "Let's focus on the positive things that you can still do."

Answer: 1

© Rationale: Therapeutic communication is client centered in which the client is in control of the topic and expressing feelings of which they are concerned. Providing open-ended questions allows the client an opportunity for that discussion. The nurse would not offer condescending words stating that the client will be back to normal. It is also not appropriate to deflect the client feelings by changing the topic to breakfast or focusing on another topic.

Test-taking strategy: Analyze to determine what information the question asks for, which is a therapeutic response to a client with recent physical deficits. When you think of therapeutic communication, think of allowing the expression of feeling and open-ended questions. Review therapeutic communication techniques if you had difficulty answering this question.

Client needs category: Psychosocial integrity

Client needs subcategory: None

Cognitive level: Analyzing

5. A nurse teaches a group of police officers about the spread of tuberculosis (TB). Which statement by an officer indicates that teaching has been effective?

☐ **1.** "I could get TB by being in close proximity for a brief time with someone who has the disease."

☐ **2.** "I could get TB if I inhale infected droplets when an infected individual coughs."

☐ **3.** "I could get TB if I search the home of someone infected with TB."

☐ **4.** "I could get TB if I come in contact with blood from an infected person."

Answer: 2

Ⓔ Rationale: TB infection typically occurs from inhaling infected droplets after a person with TB coughs. Transmission usually requires close, frequent, and prolonged contact. HIV, not TB, is spread through contact with an infected person's blood.

Test-taking strategy: Analyze to determine what information the question asks for, which is correct statement related to TB transmission. Recall the transmission precautions for TB as airborne requiring inhalation for transmission. Review transmission-based precautions if you had difficulty answering this question.

Client needs category: Safe and effective care environment

Client needs subcategory: Safety and infection control

Cognitive level: Analyzing

---

6. A nurse manager is making morning assignments for the nursing team. Which duties can be assigned to the nursing assistant/unlicensed worker? Select all that apply.

☐ **1.** Changing the linen of a client on a pressure-releasing mattress

☐ **2.** Transferring a client from the bed to the chair using a mechanical lift

☐ **3.** Teaching a client on an anticoagulant about using an electric razor

☐ **4.** Totaling the intake and output for the entire unit

☐ **5.** Obtaining vital signs on a client being admitted to the unit

☐ **6.** Repositioning a client on complete bed rest

Answer: 1, 2, 4, 6

Ⓒ Rationale: The nursing assistant/unlicensed worker can assist the nurse in duties that do not require skilled nursing and nursing judgment. Changing linen, transferring a client using a mechanical lift, totaling the intake and output, and repositioning a client are in the scope of practice of the nursing assistant/unlicensed worker. Skills that require a registered nurse include medication teaching and vital sign assessment on admission.

Test-taking strategy: Analyze to determine what information the question asks for, which is duties that can be assigned to a nursing assistant/unlicensed worker. Consider that this skill of worker has approximately 120 to 150 hours of total training. They are taught very important tasks but not skilled assessment and nursing interventions. Review nursing assistant skills and duties if you had difficulty answering this question.

Client needs category: Safe and effective care environment

Client needs subcategory: Management of care

Cognitive level: Analyzing

7. The emergency room nurse is caring for a client who fell breaking the tibia. The nurse determines that a client understands the risk of compartment syndrome when knowing to report which early symptom following treatment?

☐ **1.** Heat

☐ **2.** Paresthesia

☐ **3.** Skin pallor

☐ **4.** Swelling

Answer: 2

Ⓜ Rationale: Compartment syndrome is the compression of the nerves, blood vessels, and muscle inside a closed space. Paresthesia is the earliest sign of compartment syndrome. Pain, heat, and swelling are also signs but occur after paresthesia. Skin pallor is not a sign of compartment syndrome.

Test-taking strategy: Analyze to determine what information the question asks for, which is an early symptom of compartment syndrome. Consider that compartment = compression. Recall the structures that compartment syndrome effects (nerves), which lead to the correct answer. Review the signs of compartment syndrome if you had difficulty answering this question.

Client needs category: Physiological integrity

Client needs subcategory: Physiological adaptation

Cognitive level: Analyzing

8. The nurse is providing dietary instruction for the client with fibrocystic breast disease. Which of the client's favorite foods are discouraged? Select all that apply.

☐ **1.** Lasagna

☐ **2.** Chocolate pudding

☐ **3.** Organ meat

☐ **4.** Cola products

☐ **5.** Popcorn

☐ **6.** Nuts

Answer: 2, 4

Ⓓ Rationale: When instructing the client on appropriate food choices, the nurse instructs the client to avoid caffeine. Caffeine is in products such as chocolate and cola drinks. Lasagna is discouraged in clients with digestive disorders. Organ meats are discouraged in clients with high cholesterol. Popcorn and nuts are discouraged in clients with disorders such as diverticulitis.

Test-taking strategy: Analyze to determine what information the question asks for, which is dietary instruction for a client with fibrocystic breast disease. The key word is "discourage," meaning it interacts poorly with fibrocystic breast disease. Review dietary concerns in clients with fibrocystic breast disease if you had difficulty answering this question.

Client needs category: Health promotion and maintenance

Client needs subcategory: None

Cognitive level: Applying

9. A client presented to the outpatient center for a gastroscopy, which revealed redness and inflammation of the stomach indicating acute gastritis. Which action would be included in the immediate management?

☐ **1.** Advising the client to reduce work-related stress

☐ **2.** Preparing the client for gastric resection

☐ **3.** Treating the underlying cause of disease

☐ **4.** Administering enteral tube feedings

Answer: 3

Ⓔ Rationale: Discovering and treating the cause of gastritis is the most beneficial approach in the immediate management phase. Reducing the amount of stress and reducing or eliminating oral intake until the symptoms are gone is important in the recovery phase. A gastric resection is considered only when serious erosion has occurred.

Test-taking strategy: Analyze to determine what information the question asks for, which is immediate management for acute gastritis. The key word is *"immediate."* Recall the acute nature of the situation. The goal of treatment and management is to reduce the redness and irritation, which leads to the correct answer. Review the management of acute gastritis if you had difficulty answering this question.

Client needs category: Physiological integrity

Client needs subcategory: Reduction of risk potential

Cognitive level: Analyzing

---

10. A client arrives in the emergency department following an arm injury while playing football. The nurse suspects the diagnosis of a possible fracture of the humerus based on which assessment finding?

☐ **1.** Pain that is radiating to the wrist and unrelated to movement

☐ **2.** Pain that is sharp and related to movement

☐ **3.** Pain that is sharp and unrelated to movement

☐ **4.** Pain that is dull, deep, and related to movement

Answer: 2

Ⓜ Rationale: Fracture pain is sharp, occurring at the site of the fracture and related to movement. Pain that is dull, deep, and unrelated to movement is not typical of a fracture, eliminating a fracture as an option.

Test-taking strategy: Analyze to determine what information the question asks for, which is assessment finding consistent with that of a fracture. Focus on the client's specific symptoms, and review the pathophysiology of a fracture, particularly with respect to type of pain. Recall that this is an acute injury. Review signs and symptoms of a fracture if you had difficulty answering this question.

Client needs category: Physiological integrity

Client needs subcategory: Physiological adaptation

Cognitive level: Analyzing

11. A health care provider and nurse are discussing treatment options with a client diagnosed with severe ulcerative colitis. When providing client teaching during early treatment, the symptoms of which diagnosis would be discussed?

☐ **1.** Gastritis

☐ **2.** Bowel herniation

☐ **3.** Bowel outpouching

☐ **4.** Bowel perforation

Answer: 4

Ⓜ Rationale: Bowel perforation, obstruction, or hemorrhage and toxic megacolon are common complications of ulcerative colitis that may require surgery. Gastritis and herniation are not associated with irritable bowel diseases, and outpouching of the bowel wall is diverticulosis.

Test-taking strategy: Analyze to determine what information the question asks for, which is teaching of disease complications with ulcerative colitis. The key word is "severe," indicating a significant nature to the disease. Recall that ulcerative colitis (colitis = colon) is composed of ulcers and open sores in the colon, which could lead to a perforation. Review complications of ulcerative colitis if you had difficulty answering this question.

Client needs category: Physiological integrity

Client needs subcategory: Physiological adaptation

Cognitive level: Applying

---

12. A nurse is reviewing the medication regimen with a client who was recently discharged from the hospital. The nurse notes that the client was started on metformin and glyburide. Which symptoms does the nurse anticipate that the client had initially prior to treatment?

☐ **1.** Polydipsia, polyuria, and weight loss

☐ **2.** Weight gain, tiredness, and bradycardia

☐ **3.** Irritability, diaphoresis, and tachycardia

☐ **4.** Diarrhea, abdominal pain, and weight loss

Answer: 1

Ⓔ Rationale: Symptoms of hyperglycemia include polydipsia, polyuria, and weight loss. Metformin and glyburide are commonly ordered oral antidiabetic medications. Weight gain, tiredness, and bradycardia are symptoms of hypothyroidism. Irritability, diaphoresis, and tachycardia are symptoms of hypoglycemia. Symptoms of Crohn's disease include diarrhea, abdominal pain, and weight loss.

Test-taking strategy: Analyze to determine what information the question asks for, which is signs indicating the need for oral antidiabetic medication. Recall that metformin and glyburide are used for the management of type 2 diabetes and may be used with diet, insulin, or other sulfonylurea/oral hypoglycemics to control blood sugar. To require these medications, blood sugar readings would need to be elevated. Review the signs of diabetes if you had difficulty answering this question.

Client needs category: Physiological integrity

Client needs subcategory: Pharmacological and parenteral therapies

Cognitive level: Analyzing

13. The client has been prescribed vaginal cream for a yeast infection to be administered via a vaginal applicator. In which position would the nurse instruct the client to take for appropriate administration?

☐ **1.** Supine position

☐ **2.** Low Fowler's position

☐ **3.** Sims' position

☐ **4.** Dorsal recumbent position

Answer: 4

Ⓜ **Rationale:** The dorsal recumbent position (supine with the hips and knees bent) allows easy access to the vaginal orifice and proper placement for the medication. The other positions do not allow access to the vaginal orifice as the legs are closed.

Test-taking strategy: Analyze to determine what information the question asks for, which is correct position to insert vaginal medication. Recall medical terminology to discriminate through the positions. Visualize each position and the ability to access the vaginal. Review vaginal medication administration if you had difficulty answering this question.

Client needs category: Physiological integrity

Client needs subcategory: Pharmacological and parenteral therapies

Cognitive level: Applying

---

14. The nurse is caring for a client diagnosed with cancer of the cervix. When instructing on intracavitary radiation, which explanation **best** explains the importance of emptying the bowel?

☐ **1.** Feces in the bowel increase the risk of ileus.

☐ **2.** An empty bowel allows the applicator to be positioned with little or no discomfort.

☐ **3.** Bowel movements increase the risk of inadvertent contamination of the vagina and urethra.

☐ **4.** Pressure changes in the pelvis associated with bowel movements can alter the position of the applicator and the radiation source.

Answer: 4

Ⓔ **Rationale:** A position change of the radioactive implant could deliver more radiation to healthy tissue and less to the malignant lesion. This increases the risk of injury to healthy tissue and decreases the effectiveness of treatment on the cancer. Feces in the bowel increase the likelihood of a bowel movement, which can change the position of the applicator and radiation source. Feces in the bowel do not increase the risk of ileus or inadvertent contamination of the vagina and urethra from a bowel movement. Applicators are usually inserted under anesthesia in the operating room.

Test-taking strategy: Analyze to determine what information the question asks for, which is best explanation of the importance of emptying the bowel prior to radioactive implant placement. Consider the goal of radioactive implant therapy, which is to insert a radioactive source into a hollow organ to deliver a high radiation dose to the lesion while sparing the surrounding tissue. To accomplish the goal, it is best for there to be limited fecal matter for bowel movements. Review radioactive implants and intracavitary radiation for cervical cancer if you had difficulty answering this question.

Client needs category: Physiological integrity

Client needs subcategory: Reduction of risk potential

Cognitive level: Analyzing

---

15. The assessment of a client on the first day after thoracotomy shows a temperature of 100°F (37.8°C); heart rate, 96 beats/minute; blood pressure, 136/86 mm Hg; and shallow respirations at 24 breaths/minute, with rhonchi at the bases. The client states incisional pain. Which nursing action has **priority?**

☐ **1.** Medicate the client for pain.

☐ **2.** Help the client get out of bed.

☐ **3.** Give ibuprofen as ordered to reduce the fever.

☐ **4.** Encourage the client to cough and deep breathe.

Answer: 1

Ⓒ **Rationale:** Although the interventions are incorporated in the client's care plan, the priority is to relieve the client's pain and make the client comfortable. This would give the client energy and stamina to achieve the other objectives.

Test-taking strategy: Analyze to determine what information the question asks for, which is priority nursing action following a thoracotomy. First, analyze the data given and prioritize actions according to abnormalities. Note shallow breathing, rhonchi, and pain. Recall that pain impedes the client's desire to ambulate and cough and deep breath, which are essential to diminish the presenting symptoms. Review nursing actions that prioritize interventions according to the most beneficial to the client symptoms if you had difficulty answering this question.

Client needs category: Physiological integrity

Client needs subcategory: Basic care and comfort

Cognitive level: Analyzing

---

16. After telling a nurse to "pray for me," a client gives away personal possessions and shows a sudden calmness. The nurse recognizes that this behavior may signal which condition?

☐ **1.** Major depression

☐ **2.** Panic attack

☐ **3.** Suicidal ideation

☐ **4.** Severe anxiety

Answer: 3

Ⓔ **Rationale:** Verbal clues to suicidal ideation include such statements as "Pray for me" and "I won't be here when you get back." Nonverbal clues include giving away personal possessions, a sudden calmness, and risk-taking behaviors. The nurse would recognize the combination of these signs as indicating suicidal ideation—not depression, panic, or anxiety. Clients with major depression generally do not exhibit suicidal behavior until their outlook on their problems begins to improve (an improvement in behavior should raise suspicion, especially if accompanied by sudden calmness).

Test-taking strategy: Analyze to determine what information the question asks for, which is behavior associated with a psychosocial condition. Focus on the client's actions and words, and use the process of elimination to select the answer. Eliminate options 2 and 4 as not consistent with the calmness of the client. Although the client may be depressed, giving away possessions may indicate no use for them leading to suicide. Review behavior consistent with suicide if you had difficulty answering this question.

Client needs category: Psychosocial integrity

Client needs subcategory: None

Cognitive level: Applying

17. The nurse is working in a psychiatric facility on an anxiety disorder unit. The unit is locked, and clients have scheduled group and family therapy sessions. Which other standard is maintained on this unit for a client diagnosed with panic disorder?

☐ **1.** Clients may come and go as they desire.

☐ **2.** Clients may eat anything that is facility prepared.

☐ **3.** Suicide precautions are instituted.

☐ **4.** A security guard is present at the door.

Answer: 3

Ⓜ **Rationale:** Clients with anxiety disorders including panic disorder are at risk for suicide because they can be impulsive. Unit standards include maintaining suicide precautions. Nutritional problems do not typically accompany panic disorder, and family can bring in client requests. Clients, depending on their status, typically remain on the unit; however, while there is facility security, there is no guard at the unit door.

Test-taking strategy: Analyze to determine what information the question asks for, which is unit standards of care for a panic disorder. Consider that every client is individual but there are priority standard precautions for safety and client behavior. Review nursing precautions for a client with panic disorder if you had difficulty answering this question.

Client needs category: Psychosocial integrity

Client needs subcategory: None

Cognitive level: Applying

---

18. A 24-year-old client is admitted with acute schizophrenic reaction. Which method does the nurse anticipate as the **most** appropriate therapy for this type of schizophrenia?

☐ **1.** Counseling to produce insight into behavior

☐ **2.** Biofeedback to reduce agitation associated with schizophrenia

☐ **3.** Drug therapy to reduce symptoms associated with acute schizophrenia

☐ **4.** Electroconvulsive therapy to treat the mood component of schizophrenia

---

Answer: 3

Ⓔ **Rationale:** Schizophrenia is a thought disorder marked by delusions, hallucinations, and disorganized speech and behavior. Drug therapy is usually successful in normalizing behavior and reducing or eliminating hallucinations, delusions, disordered thinking, affect flattening, apathy, and asociality. Counseling would not be appropriate at this time. Electroconvulsive therapy might be considered for schizoaffective disorder, which has a mood component; it is also one of the treatments of choice for clinical depression. Biofeedback reduces anxiety and modifies behavioral responses, but it is not a major component in treating schizophrenia.

Test-taking strategy: Analyze to determine what information the question asks for, which is anticipated therapy for a client with schizophrenic reaction. Consider each option for ability to assist with the symptoms of schizophrenia. Also, consider how each treatment might benefit the client and how that benefit may impact the client's ability to function. Review the treatment plan for schizophrenic reaction if you had difficulty answering this question.

Client needs category: Psychosocial integrity

Client needs subcategory: None

Cognitive level: Applying

---

19. A client recovering from alcohol addiction asks the nurse how he/she should talk to his/her children about the impact of his/her addiction on them. Which response is **most** appropriate?

☐ **1.** "Try to limit references to the addiction, and focus on the present."

☐ **2.** "Talk about all the hardships you've had in working to remain sober."

☐ **3.** "Tell them you're sorry, and emphasize that you're doing so much better now."

☐ **4.** "Talk to them by acknowledging the difficulties and pain your drinking caused."

Answer: 4

Ⓔ Rationale: Part of the healing process for the family is to acknowledge the pain, embarrassment, and overall difficulties the client's drinking problem caused to family members. The first option facilitates the client's ability to deny the problem. The second option prevents the client from acknowledging the difficulties the children endured. The third option might lead the client to believe that only a simple apology is needed. The addiction must be addressed and the children's pain acknowledged.

Test-taking strategy: Analyze to determine what information the question asks for, which is nursing guidance on facilitating therapeutic communication between the parent and the child. Consider therapeutic communication in an open environment and which statement will be most helpful in the healing process of the family. Review therapeutic communication if you had difficulty answering this question.

Client needs category: Psychosocial integrity
Client needs subcategory: None
Cognitive level: Applying

---

20. A 26-year-old man is reported missing after being the victim of a violent crime. Two months later, a family member finds him working in a city 100 miles from his home. The man does not recognize the family member or recall being the victim of a crime. The nurse anticipates diagnosis of which condition?

☐ **1.** Depersonalization disorder

☐ **2.** Dissociative amnesia

☐ **3.** Dissociative fugue

☐ **4.** Dissociative identity disorder

Answer: 3

Ⓒ Rationale: Dissociative fugue is characterized by sudden, unexpected travel from home or usual surroundings after a traumatic event. During the episode, the person may assume a new identity and not recognize people from the past. Depersonalization disorder is the sudden loss of the sense of one's own reality. Dissociative amnesia does not involve flight from work or home. Dissociative identity disorder is the coexistence of two or more personalities in one person.

Test-taking strategy: Analyze to determine what information the question asks for, which is determining the condition that results from a traumatic event. Knowledge of the definitions of the options in this case is essential as terminology is not helpful in discriminating through the options. Consider the client's state of mind and the specifics of the situation, and relate them to the disorders mentioned. Review mental health disorders related to traumatic events if you had difficulty answering this question.

Client needs category: Psychosocial integrity
Client needs subcategory: None
Cognitive level: Applying

21. The nurse is instructing the client at 24 weeks of gestation regarding a glucose tolerance test to screen for gestational diabetes. The client asks, "What will be done if I have this disorder?" The nurse is correct to state that gestational diabetes is managed by which therapy?

☐ **1.** Dietary control of carbohydrates, fats, and proteins

☐ **2.** An oral hypoglycemic agent, metformin

☐ **3.** Ultralente (long-acting) insulin

☐ **4.** Metformin and ultralente (long-acting) insulin

Answer: 1

ⓔ **Rationale:** Clients with gestational diabetes are usually managed by dietary control of carbohydrates, fats, and proteins alone to control their glucose intolerance. Exercise is also suggested. Oral hypoglycemic drugs such as metformin are contraindicated in pregnancy and are considered teratogenic. Long-acting insulin such as ultralente usually is not needed for blood glucose control in the client with gestational diabetes.

Test-taking strategy: Analyze to determine what information the question asks for, which is management of gestational diabetes. Consider the term "gestational" as typically a temporary condition and during pregnancy. Recall that dietary management would be the first step in controlling the high glucose levels. Review the management of gestational diabetes if you had difficulty answering this question.

Client needs category: Health promotion and maintenance

Client needs subcategory: None

Cognitive level: Applying

---

22. During a vaginal examination of a client in labor, the nurse palpates the fetus's larger, diamond-shaped fontanelle positioned toward the anterior portion of the client's pelvis. Considering this assessment finding, the nurse determines nursing care using which rationale?

☐ **1.** The client can expect a brief, intense labor with possible lacerations.

☐ **2.** The client is at risk for uterine rupture and needs constant monitoring.

☐ **3.** The client may need interventions to ease back pain and change the fetal position.

☐ **4.** The fetus will be delivered using forceps or a vacuum extractor.

Answer: 3

ⓜ **Rationale:** The fetal position is occiput posterior, a position that commonly produces intense back pain during labor. Most of the time, the fetus rotates during labor to occiput anterior position. Positioning the client on her side can facilitate this rotation. An occiput posterior position would most likely result in prolonged labor. Occiput posterior alone does not create a risk of uterine rupture. The fetus would be delivered with forceps or vacuum extractor only if its presenting part does not rotate and descend spontaneously.

Test-taking strategy: Analyze to determine what information the question asks for, which is care required when a fetus is presenting in the occiput posterior position. First, use the data presented to make decisions regarding the status/position of the fetus. Next, recall that labor becomes more difficult as the bony part of the fetal head is in contact with the bony part of the mother's pelvis initiating back pain. Review the position of the fetus's fontanelles and relate this to the anatomy of the female reproductive system if you had difficulty answering this question.

Client needs category: Safe and effective care environment

Client needs subcategory: Management of care

Cognitive level: Analyzing

23. The nurse is instructing a prenatal class in the progression of behaviors experienced in the postpartum period. The nurse states that clients can expect to observe which behavior on the fourth postpartum day?

☐ **1.** The client asks many questions about the baby's care.

☐ **2.** The client wants to relate her birth experience.

☐ **3.** The client asks the nurse to select her meals for her.

☐ **4.** The client asks the nurse to help her bathe herself.

Answer: 1

🅔 **Rationale:** The taking-hold phase usually lasts from days 3 to 10 postpartum. During this stage, the mother strives for independence and autonomy; she also becomes curious and interested in the care of the baby and is most ready to learn. During the taking-in phase, which usually lasts 2 to 3 days, the mother is passive and dependent and expresses her own needs. During this taking-in phase, the client may ask the nurse to help her with self-care, wants to talk about the birth experience, and lets others make decisions for her.

Test-taking strategy: Analyze to determine what information the question asks for, which is behaviors by the client on the fourth postpartum day. Consider the mother's behavior of focusing on herself and the birth experience to focusing on the newborn and his/her needs. Review the transition phases of the postpartum period and when each phase occurs if you had difficulty answering this question.

Client needs category: Psychosocial integrity

Client needs subcategory: None

Cognitive level: Applying

---

24. A 29-week gestation client arrives in the labor and birth suite for an emergency cesarean section. The neonate is born, and artificial surfactant is administered. Which action **best** explains the main function and goal of surfactant use?

☐ **1.** Assists with ciliary body maturation in the upper airways eliminating mucus

☐ **2.** Helps maintain a rhythmic breathing pattern reducing tachypnea

☐ **3.** Promotes mucus production lubricating the respiratory tract

☐ **4.** Helps lungs remain expanded after the initiation of breathing improving oxygenation

Answer: 4

🅜 **Rationale:** Surfactant works by reducing surface tension in the lung. It allows the lung to remain slightly expanded, decreasing the amount of work required for inspiration. Improved oxygenation, as determined by arterial blood gases, is noted. Surfactant has not been shown to influence ciliary body maturation, regulate the neonate's breathing pattern, or lubricate the respiratory tract.

Test-taking strategy: Analyze to determine what information the question asks for, which is function and goal of surfactant in a premature neonate. Recall that surfactant is given to promote lung maturity, resulting in more efficient respirations and improving oxygenation. Review complications of prematurity if you had difficulty answering this question.

Client needs category: Health promotion and maintenance

Client needs subcategory: None

Cognitive level: Applying

25. A 6-month-old infant is admitted to the pediatric unit for a 2-week course of antibiotics. The parents can visit only on weekends. Which action indicates that the nurse understands the infant's emotional needs?

☐ **1.** The nurse places the infant in a four-bed pediatric unit near the nurse's station.

☐ **2.** The nurse places the infant in a room away from other children.

☐ **3.** The nurse assigns a float sitter to rock the infant when crying.

☐ **4.** The nurse assigns the infant to the same nurse as often as possible.

Answer: 4

E Rationale: Building a sense of trust is crucial with an infant at this stage of growth and development. Consistent caregivers will promote a sense of trust. Placing the infant in a four-bed unit close to the nurse's station is appropriate for supervision but not the best choice because a 6-month-old child does not play with other children. Placing in a room away from other children would isolate the infant from others, which is neither necessary nor helpful.

Test-taking strategy: Analyze to determine what information the question asks for, which is nursing actions that meet the infant's emotional needs. The key words are "emotional needs," which in infancy are safety, security, and feelings of well-being. Review the child's age, developmental level, and emotional needs if you had difficulty answering this question.

Client needs category: Safe and effective care environment

Client needs subcategory: Management of care

Cognitive level: Applying

---

26. A nurse is caring for a client with symptoms of epigastric pain. When teaching the action of gastric contents related to functioning of the body, which actions occur in the stomach? Select all that apply.

☐ **1.** Vitamin B_{12} absorption

☐ **2.** Emulsifying fats

☐ **3.** Breaking down food fibers

☐ **4.** Killing microorganisms

☐ **5.** Activating the enzyme pepsin

☐ **6.** Vitamin B_6 absorption

Answer: 1, 3, 4, 5

D Rationale: Vitamin B_{12} absorption, dissolving of food fibers, killing microorganisms, and activating the enzyme pepsin all occur in the stomach. Intrinsic factor is secreted in the fundus of the stomach and is essential for vitamin B_{12} absorption, and hydrochloric acid is needed for breaking down food fibers, killing microorganisms, and activating the enzyme pepsin. Vitamin B_6, an essential nutrient, must be replaced daily because it is water soluble and is not absorbed in the stomach or gastrointestinal tract but eliminated in urine. Bile is the substance secreted from the gallbladder to emulsify fats as they are consumed.

Test-taking strategy: Analyze to determine what information the question asks for, which is actions associated with gastric contents. Recall the action of the stomach and needs for digestion. Review the anatomy and physiology of the GI system if you had difficulty answering this question.

Client needs category: Physiological integrity

Client needs subcategory: Physiological adaptation

Cognitive level: Analyzing

27. The nurse is caring for a client with a ventricular septal repair receiving dopamine postoperatively. Which response **best** indicates a therapeutic response of the medication?

- ☐ **1.** Increased respiratory rate
- ☐ **2.** Decreased urine output
- ☐ **3.** Increased cardiac output
- ☐ **4.** Decreased cardiac contractility

Answer: 3

ⓔ Rationale: Dopamine stimulates β1- and β2-adrenergic receptors. It is a selective cardiac stimulant that increases cardiac output, heart rate, and cardiac contractility. Urine output increases in response to dilation of the blood vessels leading to the mesentery and kidneys. The respiratory rate will be impacted only as the client is able to increase activity.

Test-taking strategy: Analyze to determine what information the question asks for, which is identifying the therapeutic response of dopamine. Consider that dopamine is frequently prescribed in clients with heart surgery and heart failure to increase perfusion. Also, in analyzing the options, option 3 is the only one that is increasing cardiac, not respiratory, response rather than decreasing it. Recall the action of the medication in relation to the cardiovascular system if you had difficulty answering this question.

Client needs category: Physiological integrity

Client needs subcategory: Pharmacological and parenteral therapies

Cognitive level: Applying

28. A charge nurse is completing client assignments for the nursing staff on the pediatric unit. Which diagnosis would the nurse refrain from assigning to a pregnant staff member?

- ☐ **1.** A 6-year-old with ringworm
- ☐ **2.** A 3-month-old with roseola
- ☐ **3.** An 8-year-old with rubella
- ☐ **4.** A 2-year-old with Kawasaki's disease

Answer: 3

ⓔ Rationale: Rubella (German measles) has a teratogenic effect on the fetus. An infected child must be isolated from pregnant women. Ringworm is caused by a fungal infection on the skin. Standard hand hygiene is necessary. Kawasaki's disease is an autoimmune disease in which blood vessels become inflamed. Roseola is a virus transferred by oral secretions.

Test-taking strategy: Analyze to determine what information the question asks for, which is diagnosis that would not be assigned to a pregnant staff member. Consider each option for disease process with a threat to pregnancy or the fetus. Eliminate options 1, 2, and 4 as having limited or no infectious nature or spreading of symptoms. Review communicable diseases with teratogenic effects if you had difficulty answering this question.

Client needs category: Safe and effective care environment

Client needs subcategory: Safety and infection control

Cognitive level: Analyzing

29. The nurse is performing Leopold's maneuver on a woman who is at 37 weeks' gestation and finds the fetus in the following position. Which action by the nurse is anticipated?

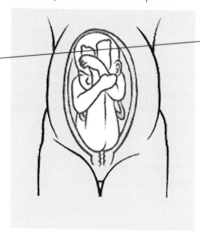

☐ **1.** Support the client while the health care provider performs external cephalic version.

☐ **2.** Instruct the client to lie on the left side to encourage independent fetal turn.

☐ **3.** Have the client report to the obstetric department for an immediate cesarean section.

☐ **4.** Encourage the client to be on bed rest for the remainder of the pregnancy.

Answer: 1

Ⓜ **Rationale:** The picture denotes a fetus in the frank breech presentation. A frank breech means that the fetus's bottom is down and feet are extended upward next to the face. The best position for a fetus to be in prior to the initiation of the labor process is the head down or vertex position. Because of the late stage of pregnancy (37 weeks), the health care provider most often performs external cephalic version in an attempt to turn the fetus to the preferable position. Neither bed rest nor lying on the left side will cause the turn of the fetus. The fetus can turn to a vertex position independently, but the client is entering a late stage of pregnancy. A cesarean section may be the chosen birth method if the external cephalic version is unsuccessful. As the client is not in active labor, the client does not need the cesarean section immediately.

Test-taking strategy: Analyze to determine what information the question asks for, which is nursing action when caring for the pictured client. The key words are "37 weeks' gestation." Analyze the picture to identify that the fetus is in a poor position for childbirth. Next, consider each option to, if possible, change the position. Fetal safety is always a priority. Review health care options for childbirth if you had difficulty answering this question.

Client needs category: Health promotion and maintenance

Client needs subcategory: None

Cognitive level: Analyzing

---

30. A child with status asthmaticus is admitted to the pediatric unit and begins to receive intermittent treatment with albuterol, given by nebulizer. When assessing the effects of the medication, which adverse effect is anticipated?

☐ **1.** Bradycardia

☐ **2.** Lethargy

☐ **3.** Tachycardia

☐ **4.** Tachypnea

Answer: 3

Ⓔ **Rationale:** Albuterol is a rapid-acting bronchodilator. Common adverse effects include tachycardia, nervousness, tremors, insomnia, irritability, and headache.

Test-taking strategy: Analyze to determine what information the question asks for, which is an adverse effect from an albuterol nebulizer treatment. Consider the type of medication and common side effects. Review the action and adverse effects of albuterol if you had difficulty answering this question.

Client needs category: Physiological integrity

Client needs subcategory: Pharmacological and parenteral therapies

Cognitive level: Applying

31. A nurse encounters a motor vehicle accident while driving from the hospital. The nurse calls 911 and assesses the most seriously injured, a 12-year-old with a suspected femur fracture. Once the scene has been determined as safe, which nursing action to this client is **most** appropriate?

☐ **1.** Avoid moving the child.

☐ **2.** Sit the child up to facilitate breathing.

☐ **3.** Move the child to the back seat where there is more room.

☐ **4.** Immobilize the extremity and wait for emergency services.

Answer: 4

Ⓔ Rationale: At the scene of a trauma, the nurse would immobilize the extremity of a child with a suspected fracture and wait for emergency services. If the child is already in a safe place, do not attempt to move the child in the vehicle. Never try to sit the child up; this could worsen the fracture.

Test-taking strategy: Analyze to determine what information the question asks for, which is nursing care for a suspected fracture. Consider that fractures are interrupted bone segments with tissues, ligaments, or tendons attached. By immobilizing, it decreases movement of the fracture and can prevent further damage. Review the care of a fractured extremity if you had difficulty answering this question.

Client needs category: Safe and effective care environment

Client needs subcategory: Safety and infection control

Cognitive level: Applying

---

32. The nurse is reviewing the following worksheet when prioritizing afternoon nursing care. Which order for administering client care at 1:00 PM (13:00 hours) is **best?**

Nurse Worksheet	
Client 1	1300 – After lunch toileting
Client 2	1300 – Dressing change to left heel wound
Client 3	1300 – Intravenous piggyback (100cc) every 6 hours
Client 4	1300 – Soonest time for requested post-operative pain medication

☐ **1.** Client 4, Client 3, Client 2, Client 1

☐ **2.** Client 4, Client 1, Client 3, Client 2

☐ **3.** Client 3, Client 1, Client 2, Client 4

☐ **4.** Client 2, Client 1, Client 3, Client 4

Answer: 2

Ⓜ Rationale: It is important for the nurse to prioritize care in an efficient manner. The highest priority for the afternoon is administering requested pain medication for a postoperative client. Next, a client on a toileting schedule would be taken to the restroom. The intravenous piggyback would be initiated, and while infusing, the wound dressing would be changed.

Test-taking strategy: Analyze to determine what information the question asks for, which is priority action for multiple clients needing care. Begin with Maslow's hierarchy of needs making a client in pain the highest priority. Consider how the nurse could efficiently accomplish tasks. Review priorities of care and time management if you had difficulty answering this question.

Client needs category: Safe and effective care environment

Client needs subcategory: Management of care

Cognitive level: Analyzing

33. The school nurse is assessing the type 1 diabetic status of a 15-year-old athlete. Which physiologic change would the nurse anticipate as the teenager becomes more physically active during the day?

☐ **1.** Increased need for food

☐ **2.** Decreased need for food

☐ **3.** Decreased risk of insulin shock

☐ **4.** Increased risk of hyperglycemia

Answer: 1

Ⓔ Rationale: If a child is more active at one time of the day than another, food intake or insulin can be adjusted to meet this increased activity pattern. Ideally in type 1 diabetes, food intake would be increased, typically with a snack, when the teen is more physically active. The child would have an increased risk of insulin shock and a decreased risk of hyperglycemia when more physically active.

Test-taking strategy: Analyze to determine what information the question asks for, which are anticipated changes as a teen with type 1 diabetes becomes more active throughout the day. Consider the relationship between blood glucose, calories, and exercise. Recall that food is the source of energy that needs to be metabolized to be available in the teen's system. Review diabetic management throughout the day if you had difficulty answering this question.

Client needs category: Safe and effective care environment

Client needs subcategory: Management of care

Cognitive level: Applying

---

34. The nurse is providing discharge instructions to the parents of a child with a hypospadias repair. Which instruction would be stressed?

☐ **1.** Care of the circumcision

☐ **2.** Techniques for providing tub baths

☐ **3.** Care for the indwelling catheter or stent

☐ **4.** Encouragement of voiding every 2 hours

Answer: 3

Ⓜ Rationale: The parents would be taught to care for the indwelling catheter or stent and irrigation techniques, if indicated. The child with hypospadias would not be circumcised because the foreskin may be needed during surgical repair. To prevent infection, tub baths would be avoided until the stent has been removed. Following surgical repair, the child will have an indwelling urinary catheter, so encouraging the child to void is not appropriate.

Test-taking strategy: Analyze to determine what information the question asks for, which is essential discharge teaching following a hypospadias repair. Consider that hypospadias repair involves lengthening the urethra to bring urine to the tip of the penis. Recall that an indwelling catheter or stent remains in place for 1 to 2 weeks as healing occurs. Review postoperative hypospadias repair care if you had difficulty answering this question.

Client needs category: Safe and effective care environment

Client needs subcategory: Management of care

Cognitive level: Analyzing

---

35. A teenager asks advice from a nurse about getting a tattoo. When the nurse is providing education, which statement about tattoos is a common misconception?

☐ **1.** Human immunodeficiency syndrome (HIV) is a possible risk factor.

☐ **2.** Hepatitis B is a possible risk factor.

☐ **3.** Tattoos are easily removed with laser surgery.

☐ **4.** Allergic response to pigments is a possible risk factor.

🅔 **Rationale:** A common misconception regarding tattoos is that tattoos can be removed. Removing a tattoo is not an easy process, and most people are left with a significant scar. Also, the cost is expensive and not covered by insurance. Because of the moderate amount of bleeding with a tattoo, both hepatitis B and HIV are potential risks if proper techniques are not followed. Allergic reactions are possible when establishments do not use Food and Drug Administration–approved pigments for tattoo coloring. Reactions can also occur in clients who are hypersensitive to the pigments or tools used.

Test-taking strategy: Analyze to determine what information the question asks for, which is a common misconception regarding tattoo use. The key word is "misconception," meaning that the statement is inaccurate. Review facts about tattoos if you had difficulty answering this question.

Client needs category: Health promotion and maintenance

Client needs subcategory: Safety and infection control

Cognitive level: Understanding

---

36. The nurse is performing a newborn assessment on a neonate in the childbirth suite. The nurse notes epispadias. Which documentation of the defect would the nurse note?

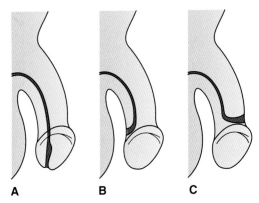

A　　　　**B**　　　　**C**

From Bulock BA, Henze RL. *Focus on Pathophysiology*. Philadelphia, PA: Lippincott Williams & Wilkins, 2000.

🅔 **Rationale:** Epispadias is characterized by the urethral opening at the top (dorsal) aspect of the penis. Though the child will be able to urinate, surgical repair will be completed. Option A is the normal opening of the urethra at the tip of the penis. Option B documents hypospadias with the urethral opening at the underside (ventral) aspect of the penis.

Test-taking strategy: Analyze to determine what information the question asks for, which is correct documentation showing epispadias. Recall that penis abnormalities include epispadias and hypospadias. Discriminate "epi" being above and "hypo" being below. Review the placement of the urethral opening in a client with epispadias if you had difficulty answering this question.

Client needs category: Physiological integrity

Client needs subcategory: Physiological adaptation

Cognitive level: Applying

37. The nurse is teaching a client about the pathophysiology of asthma. Place in chronological order the sequence of an asthma attack. All options must be used.

1. Inflammation

2. Mucus production

3. Trigger by stimulus

4. Airflow limitation

5. Acute asthma attack

6. Breathlessness

Answer: 3, 1, 2, 4, 6, 5

Ⓜ **Rationale:** Asthma is triggered by a stimulus. The stimulus may be environmental, stress related, or medication related. Inflammation in the airways occurs as a response to the stimulus, followed by an increase in mucus production. The presence of inflammation and mucus narrow the bronchi, causing limited airflow. At this point, the client experiences breathlessness, chest tightness, and wheezing—all symptoms of an acute asthma attack.

Test-taking strategy: Analyze to determine what information the question asks for, which is sequence of an asthma attack. First, place option 4 (trigger) and option 5 (attack) as the first and last in the sequence. Next, take the remaining four and place them in order moving from the beginning symptoms present until option 6 (breathlessness) occurs. Review the causes and pathophysiology of asthma if you had difficulty answering this question.

Client needs category: Physiological integrity

Client needs subcategory: Physiological adaptation

Cognitive level: Analyzing

---

38. The nurse manager of a 20-bed coronary care unit is not on duty when a staff nurse makes a serious medication error that results in a client's overdose. The client nearly dies. Which statement accurately reflects the accountability of the nurse manager?

☐ **1.** The nurse manager would receive a call at home from the on-duty nursing supervisor, apprising him/her of the problem as soon as possible.

☐ **2.** Because the nurse manager is off duty and not accountable for incidents that occur in his/her absence, he/she need not be notified.

☐ **3.** The nurse manager only needs to be informed of the incident when he/she reports to work on the next scheduled day.

☐ **4.** Although the nurse manager is off duty and not responsible for what happened, the nursing supervisor would call the nurse manager only if time permits.

Answer: 1

Ⓜ **Rationale:** The nurse manager is accountable for what happens on the unit 24 hours per day, 7 days per week. If a serious problem occurs, the nurse manager would be notified as soon as possible. None of the other choices accurately reflect the nurse manager's accountability in this situation.

Test-taking strategy: Analyze to determine what information the question asks for, which is accountability of the nurse manager when a medication error occurs. Recall that the nurse manager is not liable for the specific error by the nurse, but the nurse manager is accountable to the unit around the clock. The nurse manager needs to be informed of the status of a client, staff, or visitor to that unit. Review leadership responsibilities on the clinical unit if you had difficulty answering this question.

Client needs category: Safe and effective care environment

Client needs subcategory: Safety and infection control

Cognitive level: Analyzing

39. The nurse is caring for an elderly man who walks 2 miles every morning. The nurse notes that during his morning walk, he called his daughter and stated that he thought that he was having a "heart attack." Which symptom, identified by the client, is the **most** common and consistent with that of a heart attack (myocardial infarction)?

☐ **1.** Sternal pain

☐ **2.** Dyspnea

☐ **3.** Edema

☐ **4.** Palpitations

Answer: 1

Ⓔ Rationale: The most common symptom in a male with a myocardial infarction is crushing sternal pain, resulting from deprivation of oxygen to the heart. Dyspnea is the second most common symptom, related to an increase in metabolic needs of the body. Edema is a later sign of heart failure, commonly seen later as the body tries to recover from the tissue damage. Palpitations may result from reduced cardiac output, producing arrhythmias.

Test-taking strategy: Analyze to determine what information the question asks for, which is most common symptom of a heart attack. Recall that, in males, oxygen deprivation typically produces a crushing sternal pain that radiates into the jaw and down the left arm. It is important to note that symptoms in women may be different. Review the pathophysiology and symptoms of a myocardial infarction if you had difficulty answering this question.

Client needs category: Safe and effective care environment

Client needs subcategory: Management of care

Cognitive level: Analyzing

---

40. A nurse is reviewing diagnostic information on a newly admitted client. A chest x-ray shows a client's lungs to be clear. The Mantoux test is positive, with 10 mm of induration. The previous test was negative. Upon analysis of the data, the nurse is able to provide which information on shift handoff regarding tuberculosis (TB) status?

☐ **1.** The client had TB in the past and no longer has it.

☐ **2.** The client was successfully treated for TB, but skin tests always stay positive.

☐ **3.** The client is a seroconverter, meaning the TB has gotten to the bloodstream.

☐ **4.** The client is a tuberculin converter, meaning the client has been exposed to TB since the last skin test.

Answer: 4

Ⓜ Rationale: A tuberculin converter's skin test will be positive, meaning the client has been exposed to and infected with TB and now has a cell-mediated immune response to the skin test. The client's blood and x-ray results may stay negative. It does not mean the infection has advanced to the active stage. Because the x-ray is negative, he/she should be monitored every 6 months to see if he/she develops changes in the chest x-ray or pulmonary examination. Being a seroconverter does not mean the TB has gotten into the bloodstream; it means it can be detected by a blood test.

Test-taking strategy: Analyze to determine what information the question asks for, which is the correct analysis of a diagnostic test. Eliminate options 1 (client has had TB), 2 (treated for TB), and 3 (TB in bloodstream) as all stating that the client has had TB. Review the purpose of the Mantoux test and the disease course following exposure to TB if you had difficulty answering this question.

Client needs category: Physiological integrity

Client needs subcategory: Physiological adaptation

Cognitive level: Analyzing

41. A client at the eye clinic is newly diagnosed with glaucoma. The nurse would stress the need to take medication as prescribed because non-compliance may lead to which condition?

☐ **1.** Diplopia

☐ **2.** Permanent vision loss

☐ **3.** Intense eye pain

☐ **4.** Pupillary constriction

Answer: 2

🅒 **Rationale:** Without treatment, glaucoma may progress to irreversible blindness. Treatment will not restore visual damage but will halt disease progression. Blurred or foggy vision, not diplopia, is typical in glaucoma. Central vision loss is typical in glaucoma. Miotics, which constrict the pupil, are used in the treatment of glaucoma to permit the outflow of aqueous humor. Vision difficulty, not pain, is the main characteristic.

Test-taking strategy: Analyze to determine what information the question asks for, which is consequence of noncompliance with glaucoma treatment. Focus on the pathophysiology of glaucoma (increased pressure) as the deterioration will continue without treatment. Review signs and treatment options of glaucoma if you had difficulty answering this question.

Client needs category: Physiological integrity

Client needs subcategory: Pharmacological and parenteral therapies

Cognitive level: Applying

---

42. A client with newly diagnosed chronic obstructive pulmonary disease (COPD) comes to the clinic for a routine examination. The nurse teaches the client strategies for preventing airway irritation and infection. Which statement by the client **best** indicates that teaching was successful?

☐ **1.** "I should avoid enclosed, crowded areas during the summer."

☐ **2.** "I'm glad I only need to get the flu vaccine to prevent illnesses."

☐ **3.** "I should use products with aerosol sprays."

☐ **4.** "I should avoid using powders."

Answer: 4

🅒 **Rationale:** A client with COPD should avoid exposure to powders, dust, and smoke from cigarettes, pipes, and cigars. The client should stay indoors when the humidity, temperature, and pollen counts are high and should avoid aerosol sprays. The client should also obtain immunizations against pneumococcal pneumonia as well as influenza. A combination of measures is needed to maintain the client's highest level of respiratory function.

Test-taking strategy: Analyze to determine what information the question asks for, which is correct statement regarding exacerbation of COPD symptoms. The key words are "successful teaching," indicating that the client statement is correct. Analyze each option for accuracy. Review essential teaching for a client newly diagnosed with COPD if you had difficulty answering this question.

Client needs category: Health promotion and maintenance

Client needs subcategory: None

Cognitive level: Analyzing

43. The nurse has positioned the client on the right side (see figure). Which areas will the nurse assess for pressure when repositioning 2 hours later? Select all that apply.

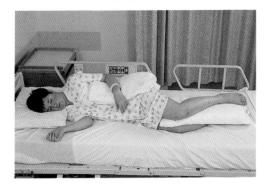

From Smeltzer SC, Bare BG. *Brunner & Suddarth's Textbook of Medical-Surgical Nursing*. 9th ed. Philadelphia, PA: Lippincott Williams & Wilkins, 2000.

☐ **1.** Auricle

☐ **2.** Clavicle

☐ **3.** Ankle

☐ **4.** Greater trochanter

☐ **5.** Coccyx

☐ **6.** Heels

Answer: 1, 2, 3, 4

Ⓓ Rationale: The nurse must access pressure points from the side-lying position every 2 hours. These points include the auricle (ears), shoulders, ribs, greater trochanter, medial and lateral condyles, and ankles. Structures to the midline of the body such as the coccyx and heels would not experience pressure when in the side-lying position.

Test-taking strategy: Analyze to determine what information the question asks for, which is pressure areas when in the side-lying position. Analyze the picture, and complete a head-to-toe assessment of the bony prominences and protuberances, which may break down if the client has pressure to the area. Review areas of highest pressure ulcers and skin breakdown if you had difficulty answering this question.

Client needs category: Physiological integrity

Client needs subcategory: Basic care and comfort

Cognitive level: Applying

---

44. The home health nurse is instructing a client and spouse on helpful recommendations to manage symptoms of multiple sclerosis (MS). Which measure would be included in teaching to avoid exacerbation of the disease?

☐ **1.** Patching the affected eye

☐ **2.** Sleeping 8 hours each night

☐ **3.** Taking hot baths for relaxation

☐ **4.** Drinking 1½ to 2 qt (1.5 to 2 L) of fluid daily

Answer: 2

Ⓔ Rationale: MS is exacerbated by exposure to stress, fatigue, and heat. Clients should balance activity with rest. Patching the affected eye may result in improvement in vision and balance but will not prevent exacerbation of the disease. Adequate hydration will help prevent UTIs secondary to a neurogenic bladder.

Test-taking strategy: Analyze to determine what information the question asks for, which is measure to prevent exacerbation of the disease. Always answer what the question is asking or an option related to exacerbation of the disease. Note that only option 2 is preventative. Review the pathophysiology of MS if you had difficulty answering this question.

Client needs category: Physiological integrity

Client needs subcategory: Reduction of risk potential

Cognitive level: Applying

45. During a multidisciplinary team conference, a nurse and dietitian discuss the best diet for a client recovering from a fracture. A high-protein diet was recommended to the health care provider for which reason?

☐ **1.** Protein promotes gluconeogenesis.

☐ **2.** Protein has anti-inflammatory properties.

☐ **3.** Protein promotes cell growth and bone union.

☐ **4.** Protein decreases pain medication requirements.

Answer: 3

Ⓔ Rationale: High-protein intake promotes cell growth and bone union. Protein does not promote gluconeogenesis, exert anti-inflammatory properties, or decrease pain medication requirements.

Test-taking strategy: Analyze to determine what information the question asks for, which is rationale to recommend a high-protein diet for a client with a fracture. Recall that protein, along with calcium and vitamin D, is an important nutrient in the formation of bone tissue. Review the benefits of protein in the diet if you had difficulty answering this question.

Client needs category: Physiological integrity

Client needs subcategory: Basic care and comfort

Cognitive level: Applying

---

46. The nurse assesses the client's pain level as a 9 on 0-to-10 pain scale and notifies the health care provider, who orders *morphine sulfate gr ½ I.M. stat.* The only available morphine is morphine sulfate in a 20-ml vial, labeled 15 mg/ml. How many milliliters of pain medication would the nurse administer? Record your answer using a whole number.

_____ ml

Answer: 2

Ⓜ Rationale: Calculate the dosage by converting grains to milligrams:

$$1 \text{ gr} : 60 \text{ mg} :: \tfrac{1}{2} \text{ gr} : X \text{ mg} = 30 \text{ mg}.$$

Then, use the ratio-and-proportion method to determine the amount of milliliters to administer:

$$15 \text{ mg} : 1 \text{ ml} :: 30 \text{ mg} : X \text{ ml}$$

$$\frac{15X \text{ ml/mg}}{15 \text{ mg}} = \frac{30 \text{ ml/mg}}{15 \text{ mg}}$$

$$X \text{ ml} = 2$$

Test-taking strategy: Analyze to determine what information the question asks for, which is how many milliliters of pain medications would be administered. Use the above formula entering known data and solving for *X*. Proofread the math calculation. Review dosage calculations using ratios and proportions, and review equivalents for the apothecaries' system if you had difficulty answering this question.

Client needs category: Physiological integrity

Client needs subcategory: Pharmacological and parenteral therapies

Cognitive level: Applying

47. A nurse is working in the office of a gastro-enterologist. When reviewing the list of clients to be seen for the day, the nurse notes the following disease processes. With which client would the nurse provide special emphasis on signs of rectal cancer when completing cancer prevention instruction?

- ☐ **1.** Adenomatous polyps
- ☐ **2.** Diverticulitis
- ☐ **3.** Hemorrhoids
- ☐ **4.** Peptic ulcer disease

Answer: 1

Ⓔ **Rationale:** A client with adenomatous polyps has a higher risk for developing rectal cancer than others do. Clients with diverticulitis are more likely to develop colon cancer. Hemorrhoids do not increase the chance of any type of cancer. Clients with peptic ulcer disease have a higher incidence of gastric cancer.

Test-taking strategy: Analyze to determine what information the question asks for, which is disease process that contains a risk of rectal cancer. Recall the adenomatous polyps (benign) can signal a potential for cancer throughout the colon to the rectum, thus the term colorectal cancer. Screening with a colonoscopy is essential. Review the signs of rectal cancer if you had difficulty answering this question.

Client needs category: Health promotion and maintenance

Client needs subcategory: None

Cognitive level: Analyzing

---

48. The nurse is caring for a client with poly-dipsia and large amounts of urine with a specific gravity of 1.003. Which disorder is anticipated?

- ☐ **1.** Diabetes mellitus
- ☐ **2.** Diabetes insipidus
- ☐ **3.** Diabetic ketoacidosis
- ☐ **4.** SIADH secretion

Answer: 2

Ⓜ **Rationale:** Diabetes insipidus is characterized by a great thirst (polydipsia) and large amounts of dilute, waterlike urine with a specific gravity of 1.001 to 1.005. Diabetes mellitus presents with polydipsia, polyuria, and polyphagia, but the client also has hyperglycemia. Diabetic ketoacidosis presents with weight loss, polyuria, and polydipsia, and the client has severe acidosis. A client with SIADH cannot excrete dilute urine; the client retains fluid and develops a sodium deficiency.

Test-taking strategy: Analyze to determine what information the question asks for, which is disease disorder with polydipsia and waterlike urine. The key is the excessive thirst coupled with urine with a specific gravity of 1.001 to 1.005 as it is a classic symptom due to the kidneys' inability to conserve water. Review the characteristic symptoms of diabetes insipidus if you had difficulty answering this question.

Client needs category: Physiological integrity

Client needs subcategory: Physiological adaptation

Cognitive level: Analyzing

49. The enterostomal therapy nurse is caring for a client with a newly placed ileal conduit. Which instruction about skin care at the stoma site would be given?

☐ **1.** Change the appliance at bedtime.

☐ **2.** Leave the stoma open to air while changing the appliance.

☐ **3.** Clean the skin around the stoma with mild soap and water, and dry it thoroughly.

☐ **4.** Cut the faceplate or wafer of the appliance no more than 4 mm larger than the stoma.

Answer: 3

Ⓔ Rationale: Cleaning the skin around the stoma with mild soap and water and drying it thoroughly helps keep the area clean from urine, which can irritate the skin. The appliance would be changed early in the morning, when urine output is less, to decrease the amount of urine in contact with the skin. The stoma would be covered with a gauze pad when changing the appliance to prevent seepage of urine onto the skin. The faceplate or wafer of the appliance would not be more than 3 mm larger than the stoma to reduce the skin area in contact with urine.

Test-taking strategy: Analyze to determine what information the question asks for, which is instruction regarding ileal conduit stoma care. Consider that the stoma is new and the surrounding skin needs meticulous care as it heals. Urine on the sensitive skin can cause breakdown. Simple soap and water care is effective in cleansing the area. Review care of an ileal conduit, stoma, and surrounding skin if you had difficulty answering this question.

Client needs category: Physiological integrity

Client needs subcategory: Basic care and comfort

Cognitive level: Applying

---

50. A client with facial lacerations requires wound care, intravenous antibiotics, and hospitalization for 1 week. During the assessment on the third admission day, the nurse notes scabs on the wounds. This finding corresponds to which phase of normal wound healing process?

☐ **1.** Contraction phase

☐ **2.** Inflammatory phase

☐ **3.** Proliferative phase

☐ **4.** Remodeling phase

Answer: 3

Ⓒ Rationale: During the proliferative phase of wound healing, which lasts from the 4th to 21st day after injury, granulation tissue appears (scabs form) and the wound edges start to pull together. Contraction, the third phase of wound healing, may begin around the 7th day and involves a significant decrease in the wound surface. The inflammatory phase, the first healing phase, immediately follows the injury and lasts 4 to 6 days; it involves control of bleeding and release of chemicals needed for healing. The remodeling phase, the final phase, may lead to scar flattening and correction of any deformities that occurred during the third phase.

Test-taking strategy: Analyze to determine what information the question asks for, which is the phase of wound healing with scab formation. Recall what occurs during the different phases of wound healing. If unsure, consider that proliferative comes from proliferation, meaning the growth or production of cells. Review the phases of wound healing if you had difficulty answering this question.

Client needs category: Physiological integrity

Client needs subcategory: Basic care and comfort

Cognitive level: Applying

51. The nurse is documenting a prenatal history of *gravida 4, para 2* on the woman's clinic electronic medical record. The information is sent to the birthing center for review. Upon the expectant mother's admission to the birthing center, the admission nurse is most correct to confirm which prenatal history?

☐ **1.** A client has been pregnant four times and had two miscarriages.

☐ **2.** A client has been pregnant four times and had two children born after 20 weeks of gestation.

☐ **3.** A client has been pregnant four times and had two cesarean deliveries.

☐ **4.** A client has been pregnant four times and had two spontaneous abortions.

Answer: 2

🅔 **Rationale:** *Gravida* refers to the number of times a client had been pregnant; *para* refers to the number of viable children born after 20 weeks of gestation. Therefore, the client who is *gravida 4, para 2* has been pregnant four times and had two live-born children.

Test-taking strategy: Analyze to determine what information the question asks for, which is specific prenatal history. Focus on the meaning of the terms *gravida* and *para* as noted above. Review documentation of prenatal history using the terms *gravida* and *para* if you had difficulty answering this question.

Client needs category: Health promotion and maintenance

Client needs subcategory: None

Cognitive level: Understanding

---

52. The nurse is caring for a client on a second course of antibiotics to eliminate osteomyelitis. It is most essential for the nurse to instruct on which aspect of daily care?

☐ **1.** Use of opioid therapy for pain management

☐ **2.** A diet high in protein and nutrients

☐ **3.** Use of assistive devices for ambulation

☐ **4.** Limited exercise to only bathroom privileges

Answer: 2

🅔 **Rationale:** It is essential for the nurse to instruct on a diet that is high in protein and nutrients to increase healing and strengthen the immune system. This, in addition to the second course of antibiotics, may be sufficient to eliminate the osteomyelitis. Opioids may be needed for pain management, but this is not most essential. Bed rest is not common in care, and assistive devices are used only in the acute period.

Test-taking strategy: Analyze to determine what information the question asks for, which is instruction for daily care. Consider the priority of care as elimination of the osteomyelitis. Review priority instruction for osteomyelitis if you had difficulty answering this question.

Client needs category: Physiological integrity

Client needs subcategory: Basic care and comfort

Cognitive level: Analyzing

53. The nurse is caring for a client in labor. The client's labor has progressed to 70% effaced and 4 cm dilated. The client has requested an epidural. Which nursing action is required before receiving an epidural?

☐ **1.** Give a fluid bolus of 500 ml.

☐ **2.** Check for maternal pupil dilation.

☐ **3.** Assess maternal reflexes.

☐ **4.** Assess maternal gait.

Ⓜ **Rationale:** One of the major adverse effects of epidural administration is hypotension. Therefore, a 500-ml fluid bolus is usually administered to help prevent hypotension in the client who wishes to receive an epidural for pain relief. Assessments of maternal reflexes, pupil response, and gait are not necessary.

Test-taking strategy: Analyze to determine what information the question asks for, which is what needs to be completed prior to an epidural. Focus on the adverse effects of epidural administration and ways to counteract. Review epidural administration if you had difficulty answering this question.

Client needs category: Physiological integrity

Client needs subcategory: Reduction of risk potential

Cognitive level: Analyzing

---

54. The nurse is assigned to the postpartum unit caring for a breast-feeding client who gave birth by cesarean section. The client asks advice on breast-feeding. Which instruction on breast-feeding is **most** helpful at this time?

☐ **1.** Delay breast-feeding until 24 hours after child birth.

☐ **2.** Breast-feed frequently during the day and every 4 to 6 hours at night.

☐ **3.** Use the cradle-hold position to avoid incisional discomfort.

☐ **4.** Use the football-hold position to avoid incisional discomfort.

Ⓔ **Rationale:** When breast-feeding after a cesarean birth, the client would be encouraged to hold her neonate in a football-holding position to avoid incisional discomfort. Breast-feeding would be initiated as soon after birth as possible. The mother would be encouraged to breast-feed her infant every 2 to 3 hours throughout the night as well as during the day to increase her milk supply.

Test-taking strategy: Analyze to determine what information the question asks for, which is breast-feeding instructions following cesarean birth. The key word is "at this time" referring to after a cesarean section and considering the incision. Consider comfort measures following surgery when breast-feeding and holding the neonate. Review breast-feeding following a cesarean if you had difficulty answering this question.

Client needs category: Physiological integrity

Client needs subcategory: Basic care and comfort

Cognitive level: Analyzing

55. The health care provider prescribes furosemide 40 mg intravenous push daily. The medication comes in a vial of 50 mg/ml. Mark on the syringe the dosage of medication the nurse would give.

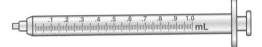

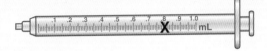

E **Rationale:** Analyze to determine what information the question asks for, which is dose of furosemide to be given intravenously. Calculate the dosage in the following way:

50 mg : 1 ml :: 40 mg : X ml Using ratio proportion

$$\frac{50 \text{ mg}/X \text{ ml}}{50 \text{ mg}} = \frac{40 \text{ mg/ml}}{50 \text{ mg}}$$

$$X \text{ ml} = 0.8 \text{ ml}$$

Test-taking strategy: Analyze to determine what information the question asks for, which is dosage of medication that is marked on the syringe. First, calculate dose (see above). See that it is a 1-mL syringe, realizing that the answer is less than 1 ml. Review medication calculations if you had difficulty answering this question.

Client needs category: Physiological integrity

Client needs subcategory: Pharmacological and parenteral therapies

Cognitive level: Applying

---

56. A nurse is caring for a 14-year-old client in skeletal traction to the left leg. The client is reporting pain on the 0 to 10 pain scale of 8. Which action would the nurse take **first?**

☐ **1.** Assess the client's pin site.

☐ **2.** Medicate for pain.

☐ **3.** Realign the client in bed.

☐ **4.** Call the health care provider.

Answer: 3

C **Rationale:** The client who reports moderate-to-severe pain may need realignment in bed. This also requires assessment of the client, which is completed prior to all other options. Assessment of the pin site is completed if the client has drainage or discomfort in that area.

Test-taking strategy: Analyze to determine what information the question asks for, which is nursing action when a client experiences pain while in skeletal traction. The key word is "first." First, the nurse must assess and analyze potential causes of the pain. Begin nursing actions with those interventions that can relieve the pain through nonpharmacological means such as reposition. Review care of the client in skeletal traction if you had difficulty answering this question.

Client needs category: Physiological integrity

Client needs subcategory: Reduction of risk potential

Cognitive level: Analyzing

57. The nurse assists the client to the operating room table and supervises the operating room technician in preparing the sterile field. Which action, completed by the surgical technician, indicates to the nurse that a sterile field has been contaminated?

☐ **1.** Sterile objects are held above the waist of the technician.

☐ **2.** Sterile packages are opened with the first edge away from the technician.

☐ **3.** The outer inch of the sterile towel hangs over the side of the table.

☐ **4.** Wetness in the sterile cloth on top of the nonsterile table has been noted.

Answer: 4

Ⓜ Rationale: Moisture outside the sterile package contaminates the sterile field because fluid can be wicked into the sterile field. Bacteria tend to settle, so there is less contamination above waist level and away from the technician. The outer inch of the drape is considered contaminated but does not indicate that the sterile field itself has been contaminated.

Test-taking strategy: Analyze to determine what information the question asks for, which is contamination of the sterile field. The key word is "contamination," indicating that there is a break in procedure with the sterile field preparation. Eliminate options 1, 2, and 3 as proper procedure for sterile fields. Review the basics of infection control and sterile field procedures if you had difficulty answering this question.

Client needs category: Safe and effective care environment

Client needs subcategory: Management of care

Cognitive level: Applying

---

58. Which intervention would be the nurse's **priority** when treating a client currently experiencing chest pain while walking?

☐ **1.** Have the client sit down.

☐ **2.** Get the client back to bed.

☐ **3.** Obtain an ECG.

☐ **4.** Administer sublingual nitroglycerin.

Answer: 1

Ⓔ Rationale: The priority intervention is to decrease the client's oxygen consumption; this would be accomplished by having the client sit down. When the client's condition is stabilized, the client can be returned to bed. An ECG can be obtained after the client is sitting down. After the ECG, sublingual nitroglycerin would be administered.

Test-taking strategy: Analyze to determine what information the question asks for, which is priority intervention when a client experiences chest pain while walking. Recall the pathophysiology of chest pain as related to the symptom of cardiac muscle not getting enough oxygen through the blood supply. Select the option that would increase blood supply to the tissues most quickly. Review the importance of preserving cardiac tissue when prioritizing interventions if you had difficulty answering this question.

Client needs category: Physiological integrity

Client needs subcategory: Basic care and comfort

Cognitive level: Analyzing

---

59. The nurse is assessing a client brought to the emergency department following a motorcycle accident. Which sign or symptom of increased intracranial pressure (ICP) after head trauma would the nurse expect to appear **first?**

☐ **1.** Bradycardia

☐ **2.** Large amounts of very dilute urine

☐ **3.** Restlessness and confusion

☐ **4.** Widened pulse pressure

Answer: 3

(E) Rationale: The earliest symptom of increased ICP is a change in mental status. Bradycardia, widened pulse pressure, and bradypnea occur later. The client may void large amounts of very dilute urine if there is damage to the posterior pituitary.

Test-taking strategy: Analyze to determine what information the question asks for, which is first sign of increased ICP. The key word is "first," indicating that there are further signs observed later. Recall that mental status changes occur first at the site of the injury. Review the signs and symptoms of increased ICP in relation to their timing if you had difficulty answering this question.

Client needs category: Physiological integrity

Client needs subcategory: Physiological adaptation

Cognitive level: Analyzing

---

60. An obese male client with history of heart failure is prescribed a beta-blocker. Which of the following is important to teach regarding home drug therapy? Select all that apply.

☐ **1.** "Take your medication at the same time daily."

☐ **2.** "Contact the health care provider if you have difficulty getting or maintaining an erection."

☐ **3.** "Weigh yourself weekly with the same amount of clothes on as the previous time."

☐ **4.** "Change positions between sitting and standing carefully."

☐ **5.** "Check your pulse for a full minute before administering your medication."

☐ **6.** "Monitor blood glucose readings every morning."

Answer: 1, 2, 4, 5

(D) Rationale: Beta-blockers treat a variety of conditions including hypertension, heart failure, glaucoma, and migraines. Beta-blockers are used to slow down the heartbeat, to reduce the force of the heart's contractions, and to reduce blood vessel contraction. Important client instructions include taking the medication at the same time daily, daily weights, changing positions daily because of hypotension, and apical pulses for a full minute. A side effect of the medication is sexual difficulties, such as difficulty getting an erection. Monitor the blood pressure, not blood glucose, each morning.

Test-taking strategy: Analyze to determine what information the question asks for, which is teaching considerations for home maintenance of beta-blockers. Consider the action of the medication (decrease heart rate and blood pressure) and then relate to possible related effects for client instruction. Review the action and side effects of beta-blockers if you had difficulty answering this question.

Client needs category: Physiological integrity

Client needs subcategory: Pharmacological and parenteral therapies

Cognitive level: Applying

61. The nurse is caring for a client on the orthopedic unit. Which discharge instructions would be given to a client after surgical repair of a hip fracture?

☐ **1.** "Do not flex the hip more than 30°, do not cross your legs, and get help putting on your shoes."

☐ **2.** "Do not flex the hip more than 60°, do not cross your legs, and get help putting on your shoes."

☐ **3.** "Do not flex the hip more than 90°, do not cross your legs, and get help putting on your shoes."

☐ **4.** "Do not flex the hip more than 120°, do not cross your legs, and get help putting on your shoes."

Answer: 3

Ⓜ Rationale: Discharge instructions would include not flexing the hip more than 90°, not crossing the legs, and getting help to put on shoes. These restrictions prevent dislocation of the new prosthesis.

Test-taking strategy: Analyze to determine what information the question asks for, which is which angle the client should not progress past when flexing at the hip. Note that each option is the same except for the hip flexion. Recall the angle of 90° is in the midposition or a high Fowler's position with the head raised. Thus, the client would not bend forward. Review postsurgical flexion restrictions if you had difficulty answering this question.

Client needs category: Safe and effective care environment

Client needs subcategory: Management of care

Cognitive level: Applying

---

62. A client is admitted with an infectious wound. Contact precautions are initiated. To help the client cope with staff using isolation procedures, which nursing action is **most** helpful?

☐ **1.** Speak to the client from the doorway unless needing close contact.

☐ **2.** Put stickers on the face mask to increase conversation.

☐ **3.** Don gloves when providing all client care.

☐ **4.** Discuss the rationale for contact precautions.

Answer: 4

Ⓔ Rationale: When assisting the client cope with contact precautions, it is most helpful to understand the client's perspective of how the use of the precautions makes him or her feel. When discussing, the nurse can explain the importance of the measures and the concerns of the client. Speaking from the door violates confidentiality. Putting stickers on the mask does not help the client cope. While it is necessary to wear gloves, it does not assist in client coping.

Test-taking strategy: Analyze to determine what information the question asks for, which is nursing action to help client cope with isolation precautions. Explanations support client understanding and acceptance. This decreases fear and anxiety and promotes support. Review therapeutic communication and isolation precaution requirements if you had difficulty answering this question.

Client needs category: Psychosocial integrity

Client needs subcategory: None

Cognitive level: Applying

63. The nurse is instructing a client on different types of medications to treat peptic ulcer disease. Which process **best** describes the mechanism of action of medications used to treat peptic ulcer disease, such as ranitidine?

☐ **1.** Neutralize acid

☐ **2.** Reduce acid secretions

☐ **3.** Stimulate gastrin release

☐ **4.** Protect the mucosal barrier

Answer: 2

Ⓜ **Rationale:** Peptic ulcer disease refers to painful sores or ulcers on the lining of the stomach or duodenum. Ranitidine is a histamine-2 receptor antagonist that reduces acid secretion by inhibiting gastrin secretion. Antacids neutralize acid, and mucosal barrier fortifiers protect the mucosal barrier.

Test-taking strategy: Analyze to determine what information the question asks for, which is the mechanism of actions of medications to treat peptic ulcer disease. Recall the pathophysiology of peptic ulcer disease and that ulcer formation results in the imbalance in the digestive fluids in the stomach. Reducing the acidity may be helpful in healing the ulcer formation. Review peptic ulcer formation and medication treatment if you had difficulty answering this question.

Client needs category: Physiological integrity

Client needs subcategory: Pharmacological and parenteral therapies

Cognitive level: Applying

64. Which nursing action is **most** beneficial to prevent fungal infections in hospitalized clients?

☐ **1.** Keep the client's skin moisturized.

☐ **2.** Bathe the client daily.

☐ **3.** Dry all skin folds thoroughly.

☐ **4.** Ensure air movement with a fan.

Answer: 3

Ⓔ **Rationale:** Fungus spreads in warm, moist environments. The nurse must keep all skin folds on the warm body dry. Moisturization is needed for dry skin but does not prevent fungal infections. Bathing is appropriate, but drying is key. Environmental air movement is not necessarily helpful.

Test-taking strategy: Analyze to determine what information the question asks for, which is prevention of fungal infection. The key word is "fungal" infections. Relate warm and moist environments. Review the favorable environment for fungal infections if you had difficulty answering this question.

Client needs category: Safe and effective care environment

Client needs subcategory: Safety and infection control

Cognitive level: Applying

65. While performing a cervical examination on a pregnant client, a nurse's fingertips feel pulsating tissue. Identify the **most** appropriate nursing intervention.

☐ **1.** Secure the client, and call the health care provider.

☐ **2.** Place the client in a semi-Fowler's position.

☐ **3.** Ask the client to push with the next contraction.

☐ **4.** Leave the fingers in place, and press the nurse's call light.

Answer: 4

🄴 **Rationale:** When the umbilical cord precedes the fetal presenting part, it is known as a prolapsed cord. Leaving the fingers in place and calling for assistance is the safest intervention for the fetus because it keeps the fetus off the cord, thereby reducing cord compression. The nursing staff can contact the health care provider to alert him/her of the situation. The client will probably need a cesarean birth because of the risk of fetal demise from the fetus's pressing against the cord during birth. Placing the client in semi-Fowler's position would increase fetal pressure on the umbilical cord. Asking the client to push with the next contraction is contraindicated because it would also force the presenting part against the cord, causing severe bradycardia and possible fetal demise.

Test-taking strategy: Analyze to determine what information the question asks for, which is nursing intervention when the nurse feels pulsating tissue on internal evaluation. Recall that the fetal head is the most appropriate presenting part descending through the birth canal. A pulsating part indicates blood flow that is essential to maintain for the fetus. Focus on the safety of the fetus when having a prolapsed umbilical cord if you had difficulty answering this question.

Client needs category: Physiological integrity

Client needs subcategory: Reduction of risk potential

Cognitive level: Applying

---

66. The nurse is instructing young mothers of infants at a community health clinic. When instructing on mealtime activity, which activity is recommended to prevent foreign body aspiration in children during meals?

☐ **1.** Insist that children are seated.

☐ **2.** Give children toys to play with.

☐ **3.** Allow children to watch television.

☐ **4.** Allow children to eat in a separate room.

Answer: 1

🄴 **Rationale:** Children should remain seated while eating. The risk of aspiration increases if a child is running, jumping, or talking with food in the mouth. Television and toys are a dangerous distraction to toddlers and young children and would be avoided. Children need constant supervision and would be monitored while eating snacks and meals.

Test-taking strategy: Analyze to determine what information the question asks for, which is safety tips for mealtime. Review activities that can lead to aspiration of food if you had difficulty answering this question.

Client needs category: Safe and effective care environment

Client needs subcategory: Safety and infection control

Cognitive level: Applying

67. The nurse is caring for a client in the intensive care unit. Which drug is **most** commonly used to treat cardiogenic shock?

☐ **1.** Dopamine

☐ **2.** Enalapril

☐ **3.** Furosemide

☐ **4.** Metoprolol

E Rationale: Cardiogenic shock is when the heart has been significantly damaged and is unable to supply enough blood to the organs of the body. Dopamine, a sympathomimetic drug, improves myocardial contractility and blood flow through vital organs by increasing perfusion pressure. Enalapril is an angiotensin-converting enzyme inhibitor that directly lowers blood pressure. Furosemide is a diuretic and does not have a direct effect on contractility or tissue perfusion. Metoprolol is an adrenergic blocker that slows heart rate and lowers blood pressure; neither is a desired effect in the treatment of cardiogenic shock.

Test-taking strategy: Analyze to determine what information the question asks for, which is medication used to treat cardiogenic shock. Consider the pathophysiology of cardiogenic shock and related medications to increase the function of the heart. Analyze the options identifying the action of the medications. Review the classifications of the listed medications and review the pathophysiology of cardiogenic shock if you had difficulty answering this question.

Client needs category: Physiological integrity

Client needs subcategory: Pharmacological and parenteral therapies

Cognitive level: Analyzing

68. The nurse is assisting a health care provider who is debriding a necrotic skin wound. The health care provider is placing bloody supplies in an emesis basin for disposal. When cleaning the basin, which nursing action is done after placing the supplies in a hazardous material bag?

☐ **1.** Wash the basin in hot, soapy water.

☐ **2.** Rinse the basin with the sprayer in the dirty utility room.

☐ **3.** Spray the basin with a disinfectant agent.

☐ **4.** Clean the basin with an antiseptic agent.

M Rationale: The basin would be taken to the dirty utility room where a sprayer would use cool/cold water to remove any protein or organic material from the basin. Hot water causes the protein of the organic material to stick to the surface of the basin. The basin does not need to be disinfected. An antiseptic is used to limit bacteria on the skin.

Test-taking strategy: Analyze to determine what information the question asks for, which is nursing action to clean the basin. Consider the use of the basin and the material left inside the basin to be cleaned. The basin is nonsterile and must be free of the organic material previously inside. Review cleaning techniques if you had difficulty answering this question.

Client needs category: Safe and effective care environment

Client needs subcategory: Safety and infection control

Cognitive level: Applying

69. The home health nurse is assisting the client and family to transition from rehabilitation unit to home. Which preventative nursing instruction for a client with quadriplegia takes **priority?**

☐ **1.** Forcing fluids to prevent renal calculi

☐ **2.** Providing daily massage to maintaining skin integrity

☐ **3.** Obtaining adaptive devices for more independence

☐ **4.** Encouraging deep breathing to prevent atelectasis

Answer: 4

ⓒ Rationale: Clients with quadriplegia have paralysis or weakness of the diaphragm and the abdominal or intercostal muscles. Maintenance of airway and breathing takes top priority. Although forcing fluids, maintaining skin integrity, and obtaining adaptive devices for more independence are all important interventions, preventing atelectasis has more priority.

Test-taking strategy: Analyze to determine what information the question asks for, which is priority instructions for the quadriplegic client. Consider the limitations of the disease process, and focus on the ABCs when prioritizing nursing instructions. Review the care of the client with quadriplegia if you had difficulty answering this question.

Client needs category: Physiological integrity

Client needs subcategory: Reduction of risk potential

Cognitive level: Applying

70. A client is being discharged from the emergency department after cast application for a tibial fracture. When instructing on the potential for a fat embolism, which instruction would the nurse provide?

☐ **1.** "Cough and deep-breathe at least every 2 hours."

☐ **2.** "Keep your leg elevated, and apply ice for the first 24 to 48 hours."

☐ **3.** "Call the health care provider at once if you experience apprehensiveness, shortness of breath, fever, or palpitations."

☐ **4.** "Restrict your fluid intake to 1 L/day."

Answer: 3

ⓔ Rationale: Fat embolism is a complication of a long bone fracture. Signs and symptoms include apprehension, altered mental status, respiratory distress, tachycardia, tachypnea, fever, and petechiae over the neck, upper arms, and chest. Coughing and deep-breathing exercises can help prevent other complications of a long bone fracture but have no effect on fat emboli. The client would also be instructed to drink plenty of fluids to stay well hydrated; this will help prevent embolic complications.

Test-taking strategy: Analyze to determine what information the question asks for, which is instruction regarding a serious complication of the long bone fracture: fat embolism. First, recall the nature of the fat embolism being small, multiple embolisms, which can have widespread effects. Consider safety, airway first, in providing nursing instruction of signs and symptoms that need immediate medical attention. If unsure, patient agitation or apprehension is typically a cardinal sign of an emergency because of the difficulty breathing or pain. Review the signs and symptoms of fat embolism and priority instruction if you had difficulty answering this question.

Client needs category: Physiological integrity

Client needs subcategory: Reduction of risk potential

Cognitive level: Applying

71. A client comes to the clinic for a follow-up appointment after diagnostic tests show gastroesophageal reflux disease. Which instruction would the nurse provide?

☐ **1.** "Lie down and rest after each meal."

☐ **2.** "Avoid alcohol and caffeine."

☐ **3.** "Drink 16 ounces of water with each meal."

☐ **4.** "Eat three well-balanced meals every day."

Answer: 2

ⓔ Rationale: A client with gastroesophageal reflux disease would avoid alcohol, caffeine, and foods that increase acidity, all of which can cause epigastric pain. To further prevent reflux, the client would remain upright for 2 to 3 hours after eating; avoid eating for 2 to 3 hours before bedtime; avoid bending and wearing tight clothing; avoid drinking large fluid volumes with meals; and eat small, frequent meals to help reduce gastric acid secretion.

Test-taking strategy: Analyze to determine what information the question asks for, which is nursing instructions for a client with gastroesophageal reflux disease. Consider the disease process, including (1) acidity of the stomach and (2) reflux of stomach contents. Eliminate options that do not address these concerns. Eliminate options 1 and 3 as inappropriate for the disease process. Discriminate between the remaining options, selecting option 2 as reducing stomach acidity. Review the nursing instructions for a client with gastroesophageal reflux disease if you had difficulty answering this question.

Client needs category: Physiological integrity

Client needs subcategory: Reduction of risk potential

Cognitive level: Applying

---

72. The nurse is caring for a client in the medical unit. The nurse receives a health care provider's order for hydrocortisone 100 mg intravenously at a rate of 10 ml/hour for a client in acute adrenal crisis. The nurse is most correct to understand that this treatment is common in clients with which disease process?

☐ **1.** Addison's disease

☐ **2.** Cushing's syndrome

☐ **3.** Hyperthyroidism

☐ **4.** Hypoparathyroidism

Answer: 1

ⓔ Rationale: Intravenous hydrocortisone for clients in acute adrenal crisis is the proper treatment for individuals with Addison's disease. Cushing's syndrome is associated with excessive amounts of glucocorticoids. Hyperthyroidism and hypoparathyroidism are not treated with hydrocortisone.

Test-taking strategy: Analyze to determine what information the question asks for, which is relating treatment associated with acute adrenal crisis to the underlying cause of Addison's disease. Recall that individuals with Addison's disease are at risk for an acute adrenal crisis because of gastric infections, diabetes, or asthma, which provides stress to the body. Review the pathophysiology of the diseases listed in relation to hydrocortisone use and adrenal crisis if you had difficulty answering this question.

Client needs category: Physiological integrity

Client needs subcategory: Pharmacological and parenteral therapies

Cognitive level: Applying

73. The nurse is irrigating a draining wound prior to packing with gauze. Which nursing actions are appropriate? Select all that apply.

☐ **1.** Washing the hands immediately after removing the sterile gloves

☐ **2.** Removing the dressing with nonsterile gloves

☐ **3.** Donning sterile gloves for the irrigation

☐ **4.** Wearing a face shield during the irrigation

☐ **5.** Obtaining a respirator mask

☐ **6.** Using clean technique for the procedure

Answer: 1, 2, 3, 4

Ⓜ **Rationale:** Because of the fact that the client's wound needs to be irrigated and packed, certain precautions are initiated, namely, wearing a gown, gloves, and a face shield. The procedure begins with removing the dressing with nonsterile gloves. Next, the nurse dons sterile gloves and, with packages open and ready, initiates the irrigation and wound packing. The nurse does not need a respirator mask for the procedure. Sterile technique is used for the procedure.

Test-taking strategy: Analyze to determine what information the question asks for, which is procedure for irrigating and packing a draining wound. Consider that contact precautions would be required because of the draining status of the wound and irrigation needed. Hands are washed before and immediately after glove use, which is a standard. While clean technique is used to remove soiled dressings, irrigation and packing are typically a sterile procedure with sterile supplies. Review standards of care when irrigating and packing a wound if you had difficulty answering this question.

Client needs category: Safe and effective care environment

Client needs subcategory: Safety and infection control

Cognitive level: Applying

---

74. A nurse is caring for a pediatric client with central diabetes insipidus. Which in-home management instruction for a child receiving DDAVP for symptomatic control of diabetes insipidus is **most** appropriate?

☐ **1.** Give DDAVP only when urine output begins to decrease.

☐ **2.** Clean the skin with alcohol before applying a DDAVP dermal patch.

☐ **3.** Increase the DDAVP dose if polyuria occurs just before the next scheduled dose.

☐ **4.** Call the health care provider for an alternate route for administering DDAVP when the child has an upper respiratory tract infection or allergic rhinitis.

Answer: 4

Ⓜ **Rationale:** Clients with central diabetes insipidus have a lack of the antidiuretic hormone (ADH). Treatment includes a synthetic hormone desmopressin administered intranasally. Excessive nasal mucus associated with an upper respiratory tract infection or allergic rhinitis may interfere with DDAVP absorption. Use only clear water to clean the skin. Soaps, oils, lotions, alcohol, or other products may irritate the skin under the patch. Parents would be instructed to contact the health care provider for advice in changing the administration route during times when nasal mucus may be increased. The DDAVP dose would remain unchanged, even if the child has polyuria just before the next dose. This is to avoid overmedicating the child.

Test-taking strategy: Analyze to determine what information the question asks for, which is "in-home" management of DDAVP. The key word is "in-home" management or daily management. Select an option that provides correct guidance on regular use. Review the rationale for administration and the routes for DDAVP if you had difficulty answering this question.

Client needs category: Safe and effective care environment

Client needs subcategory: Management of care

Cognitive level: Applying

75. A 22-year-old client reports substernal chest pain and states that his/her heart feels like "it's racing out of my chest." The client reports no history of cardiac disorders. The nurse attaches him/her to a cardiac monitor and notes sinus tachycardia with a rate of 136 beats/minute. Breath sounds are clear, and the respiratory rate is 26 breaths/minute. When a cardiorespiratory basis is eliminated, which drug would the nurse question about usage?

☐ **1.** Barbiturates

☐ **2.** Opioids

☐ **3.** Cocaine

☐ **4.** Benzodiazepines

Answer: 3

🄔 **Rationale:** Because of the client's age and negative medical history, the nurse would question about cocaine use. Barbiturate overdose may trigger respiratory depression and a slow pulse. Opioids can cause marked respiratory depression, while benzodiazepines can cause drowsiness and confusion. Cocaine increases myocardial oxygen consumption and can cause coronary artery spasm, leading to tachycardia, ventricular fibrillation, myocardial ischemia, and MI.

Test-taking strategy: Analyze to determine what information the question asks for, which is drug usage causing clinical symptoms. Focus on client symptoms and the adverse effects of the medication listed. Note that option 3 is the only option causing an increase in vital signs. Review symptoms of drug use if you had difficulty answering this question.

Client needs category: Physiological integrity

Client needs subcategory: Physiological adaptation

Cognitive level: Analyzing

76. A home health nurse is providing care to a palliative care client with liver cancer. Which classifications of medications are anticipated on the medication administration record? Select all that apply.

☐ **1.** Chemotherapeutics

☐ **2.** Narcotics

☐ **3.** Depressants

☐ **4.** Stool softeners

☐ **5.** Antiemetic

Answer: 2, 4, 5

🄜 **Rationale:** The client with liver cancer who is also a palliative care client has decided to focus on quality of life and symptom management instead of curative treatment. Narcotics for pain relief, stool softeners to maintain a bowel regimen in light of narcotic use, and antiemetics to control nausea and vomiting all assist the client to meet their goals. Chemotherapeutic agents are aggressive therapy to kill liver cancer cells. Antidepressants are used for symptoms of depression.

Test-taking strategy: Analyze to determine what information the question asks for, which is medication classifications typically seen in palliative care. Analyze each option for symptom relief, not curative focus. Review palliative care treatments if you had difficulty answering this question.

Client needs category: Physiological integrity

Client needs subcategory: Pharmacological and parenteral therapies

Cognitive level: Analyzing

77. The nurse is reading the progress notes for a client who has a pressure ulcer. Based on the nurse's note in the chart below, what stage of pressure ulcer does this client have?

Progress notes	
7/9/15 0800	Client admitted to unit from long-term care facility with a pressure ulcer on coccyx approximately 2 cm × 1 cm × 0.5 cm. No drainage noted. Base has deep pink granulation tissue without visible subcutaneous tissue. Skin surrounding ulcer pink, with intact, well-defined edges. ———————— Rebecca Stellato, RN

☐ **1.** Stage I

☐ **2.** Stage II

☐ **3.** Suspected deep tissue injury

☐ **4.** Unstageable

Answer: 2

Ⓜ **Rationale:** A stage II pressure ulcer has visible skin breaks and possible discoloration. Penetrating to the subcutaneous fat layer, the sore is painful and visibly swollen. The ulcer may be characterized as an abrasion, blister, or shallow crater. In a stage I pressure ulcer, the skin is red and intact and does not blanch with external pressure; it feels warm and firm. In suspected deep tissue injury, the skin is purple or maroon but intact; a blood-filled blister may be present. In an unstageable pressure ulcer, the ulcer destroys tissue from the skin to possibly the bone; the base of the ulcer is covered by slough, eschar, or both.

Test-taking strategy: Analyze to determine what information the question asks for, which is stage of a pressure ulcer noted in nursing documentation. Use key words in documentation of "deep pink granulation tissue," "intact well-defined edges," and "no visible subcutaneous tissue" to determine staging. Consider that this ulcer is under the skin. Review the signs and symptoms and pathophysiology of pressure ulcers, anatomy of skin, and stages of pressure ulcers if you had difficulty answering this question.

Client needs category: Physiological integrity

Client needs subcategory: Physiological adaptation

Cognitive level: Analyzing

---

78. The nurse is instructing a client's parent on care related to a 200-ml emesis from a viral illness. This is the third emesis of the day. Which instruction is stressed **first?**

☐ **1.** Give nothing by mouth for 24 hours.

☐ **2.** Brush teeth or rinse mouth after vomiting.

☐ **3.** Establish a rehydration plan.

☐ **4.** Provide sips of water.

Answer: 2

Ⓒ **Rationale:** After vomiting, it is important to brush the teeth or rinse the mouth. Stomach acid encounters the teeth during emesis. Depending upon the status of the client, a rehydration plan with sips of water may be established.

Test-taking strategy: Analyze to determine what information the question asks for, which is instruction provided first after an emesis. The key word is first. Oral care is a must to prevent problems from a stomach acid. Review immediate and follow-up care after an emesis if you had difficulty answering this question.

Client needs category: Physiological integrity

Client needs subcategory: Reduction of risk potential

Cognitive level: Applying

79. The nurse is caring for a client being discharged following kidney transplantation. The client is ordered mofetil to prevent organ rejection. Which nursing instruction is essential regarding medication use?

☐ **1.** Administer medication following breakfast daily.

☐ **2.** Contact the health care provider at first signs of an infection.

☐ **3.** Sprinkle the contents of the capsule on food.

☐ **4.** Administer the medication with an antacid to prevent stomach upset.

Answer: 2

🅔 **Rationale:** Mofetil is an organ rejection medication that diminishes the body's ability to identify and eliminate pathogens (immunosuppressant). Identifying symptoms of infection at an early state is helpful in treating the infection. This medication is administered on an empty stomach. Typically, capsules would not be opened dispensing medication at one time. Antacids may decrease the absorption of the medication.

Test-taking strategy: Analyze to determine what information the question asks for, which is nursing instruction essential to medication use. Recall that neutropenia can occur with organ rejection medications and this leads to the correct answer. Review organ transplantation medications if you had difficulty answering this question.

Client needs category: Physiological integrity

Client needs subcategory: Pharmacological and parenteral therapies

Cognitive level: Applying

---

80. A client in skeletal traction states pain 1 hour after receiving an analgesic. The nurse offers an alternative pain management measure. Which measure can be implemented within the nursing scope of practice?

☐ **1.** Acupressure and shiatsu

☐ **2.** Hypnosis and therapeutic touch

☐ **3.** Relaxation and imagery

☐ **4.** Swedish massage and the Feldenkrais method

Answer: 3

🅔 **Rationale:** Relaxation and imagery are effective adjuncts to pharmacologic pain management that the nurse can implement without a health care provider's order. Although the other therapies may promote pain management, they require special training or certification.

Test-taking strategy: Analyze to determine what information the question asks for, which is complementary therapy for pain management within the nursing scope of practice. Consider which of the answers may require special training, and eliminate them as possibilities. Review complementary treatments for pain management if you had difficulty answering this question.

Client needs category: Physiological integrity

Client needs subcategory: Basic care and comfort

Cognitive level: Applying

81. A 30-year-old client experiences weight loss, abdominal distention, crampy abdominal pain, and intermittent diarrhea after the birth of her second child. Diagnostic tests reveal gluten-induced enteropathy. Which foods would the nurse instruct that she eliminate from her diet permanently?

☐ **1.** Milk and dairy products

☐ **2.** Protein-containing foods

☐ **3.** Cereal grains (except rice and corn)

☐ **4.** Carbohydrates

Answer: 3

Ⓔ **Rationale:** To manage gluten-induced enteropathy, the client must eliminate gluten, which means avoiding all cereal grains except rice and corn. In initial disease management, clients eat a high-calorie, high-protein diet with mineral and vitamin supplements to help normalize the nutritional status. Lactose intolerance is sometimes an associated problem, so milk and dairy products are limited until improvement occurs. Cereal grains are the only carbohydrates this client must eliminate.

Test-taking strategy: Analyze to determine what information the question asks for, which is foods that must be eliminated to manage gluten-induced enteropathy. Focus on which food group contains gluten, which is a protein composite found in foods processed from wheat and related grains such as rye and barley. Review dietary management of gluten-induced enteropathy and the gluten-free diet if you had difficulty answering this question.

Client needs category: Physiological integrity

Client needs subcategory: Basic care and comfort

Cognitive level: Applying

---

82. When reviewing an elderly client's care and treatment plan, which physiological changes does the nurse evaluate as a concern for medication management because of a prolonged drug half-life? Select all that apply.

☐ **1.** Decreased hydrochloric acid production

☐ **2.** Decreased liver mass

☐ **3.** Increased fat layer

☐ **4.** Decreased kidney function

☐ **5.** Decrease in liver perfusion

☐ **6.** Increased thirst

Answer: 2, 3, 4, 5

Ⓒ **Rationale:** The nurse must understand the aging body when managing care and particularly when managing medications. With aging, body fat increases and total body water as well as lean body mass decrease affecting drug half-life. Also, hepatic and renal changes reduce biotransformation of medications and glomerular filtration. Decreased hydrochloric acid function does not provide the opportunity for a prolonged drug-half life. Thirst is not increased in the elderly.

Test-taking strategy: Analyze to determine what information the question asks for, which is medication management with focus on prolonged drug half-life in the elderly. Recall that drug half-life focuses on absorption, metabolism, and excretion. Common occurrences are a decrease in metabolism and excretion. Review the physiological changes of aging and medication management if you had difficulty answering this question.

Client needs category: Safe and effective care environment

Client needs subcategory: Management of care

Cognitive level: Analyzing

83. A nurse is reviewing the laboratory reports prior to health care provider rounds. The serum calcium level of a client with hyperthyroidism is 14.6 mg/dl (3.65 mmol/L). Which treatment would the nurse anticipate?

☐ **1.** Withholding fluids

☐ **2.** Starting oral calcium supplements

☐ **3.** Giving vitamin D supplements

☐ **4.** Administering intravenous fluids at 200 ml/hour

Answer: 4

M **Rationale:** Normal calcium levels are 8.2 to 10.2 mg/dl (2.05-2.55 mmol/L), so a level of 14.6 mg/dl (3.65 mmol/L) is dangerously high. To decrease the calcium level, intake of calcium would be reduced and calcium excretion would be promoted by administering intravenous and oral fluids and diuretics. Giving vitamin D would increase the calcium level.

Test-taking strategy: Analyze to determine what information the question asks for, which is anticipated treatment for a client with hypercalcemia. First, identify that calcium level is above normal limits. Next, analyze each option for the impact of decreasing calcium levels. Review normal values for serum calcium and treatments for hypercalcemia if you had difficulty answering this question.

Client needs category: Physiological integrity

Client needs subcategory: Physiological adaptation

Cognitive level: Analyzing

---

84. The nurse is caring for a 5-year-old who had surgery 12 hours ago. The child tells the nurse that she does not have pain, but a few minutes later tells her parent that she does. Which would the nurse consider when interpreting this?

☐ **1.** Truthful reporting of pain should occur by this age.

☐ **2.** Inconsistency in pain reporting suggests that pain is not present.

☐ **3.** Children use pain experiences to manipulate their parents.

☐ **4.** Children may be experiencing pain even though they deny it to the nurse.

Answer: 4

E **Rationale:** The preschool or young school-aged children feels afraid of further treatments if they state pain; thus, they tell the nurse that everything is fine. Children at this age can have magical thinking or feel that they are sick because of something that they did. Age-appropriate instruction is needed.

Test-taking strategy: Analyze to determine what information the question asks for, which is interpretation of client statement of pain. Consider developmental age and motivation of client statement. Review pain management considerations of the preschool/young school-aged client if you had difficulty answering this question.

Client needs category: Physiological integrity

Client needs subcategory: Basic care and comfort

Cognitive level: Analyzing

85. A 10-year-old child monitors and adjusts insulin dosage independently. Which response reflects an understanding of appropriate adjustment of insulin dosage when the child has the flu?

☐ **1.** "I won't take my insulin because I'm too sick to eat right now."

☐ **2.** "I'll take my usual dose of regular and NPH insulin."

☐ **3.** "I'll check my capillary blood glucose first and then figure out how much insulin to take."

☐ **4.** "I'll check my capillary blood glucose and record the results."

Answer: 3

Ⓔ Rationale: Because of the stress of illness, serum glucose will likely be elevated during an episode of the flu. Appropriate adjustment of insulin dosage based on a capillary blood glucose reading will help prevent the child from becoming hypoglycemic or ketoacidotic.

Test-taking strategy: Analyze to determine what information the question asks for, which is correct management of diabetes and insulin dosage in times of illness. Consider the effect illness has on serum glucose levels. Recall that any stress on body systems raises blood sugars. Review management of diabetes in times of illness if you had difficulty answering this question.

Client needs category: Physiological integrity

Client needs subcategory: Physiological adaptation

Cognitive level: Analyzing

---

86. The selection of a nursing care delivery system (NCDS) is critical to the success of client care in a nursing area. Which factor is essential to the evaluation of an NCDS?

☐ **1.** Determining how planned absences, such as vacation time, will be scheduled so that all staff are treated fairly

☐ **2.** Identifying who will be responsible for making client care decisions

☐ **3.** Deciding what type of dress code will be implemented

☐ **4.** Identifying salary ranges for various types of staff

---

Answer: 2

Ⓔ Rationale: Determining who has responsibility for making decisions regarding client care is an essential element of all client care delivery systems. Dress code, salary, and scheduling planned staff absences are important to any organizations, but they are not actually determined by the NCDS.

Test-taking strategy: Analyze to determine what information the question asks for, which is evaluation of the components of an NCDS. Note the words in the title "nursing care delivery," indicating the focus on nursing care eliminating dress code, salary, and scheduling. Focus on the definition of type of delivery system discussed if you had difficulty answering this question.

Client needs category: Safe and effective care environment

Client needs subcategory: Management of care

Cognitive level: Applying

---

87. Which action associated with restraint use on a confused client can be delegated to an unlicensed health care worker/nursing assistant?

☐ **1.** Assessment of client restraint location in relation to mental status

☐ **2.** Evaluation of client response to restraint type

☐ **3.** Completion of range of motion on limbs restrained

☐ **4.** Release of restraints as client symptoms improve

Answer: 3

Ⓔ **Rationale:** Any client assessment and subsequent decision making/judgment is in the scope of practice of the nurse. The unlicensed health care worker (UHW)/ nursing assistant (NA) is able to complete the task of range of motion.

Test-taking strategy: Analyze to determine what information the question asks for, which is delegated action when caring for a client in restraints. Recall the UHW/NA practice guidelines and relate to the actions needed with restraints. Remember that assessment is always the responsibility of the nurse. Review delegation opportunities for the client in restraints if you had difficulty answering this question.

Client needs category: Safe and effective care environment

Client needs subcategory: Management of care

Cognitive level: Applying

---

88. During the postpartum period, the nurse documents that the client's fundus is firm to palpation. Which client status does a firm fundus indicate?

☐ **1.** A firm tumor at the top of the uterus

☐ **2.** Contraction of the uterus

☐ **3.** Continuing labor contractions

☐ **4.** Bladder distention

Answer: 2

Ⓔ **Rationale:** A firm postpartum fundus indicates that the uterus has contracted and is constricting blood vessels, thereby decreasing lochial flow. A uterine tumor does not necessarily cause a firm fundus. The client would not experience labor contractions during the postpartum period. Bladder distention restricts the uterus from contracting downward, resulting in a soft, boggy uterus and increased vaginal bleeding.

Test-taking strategy: Analyze to determine what information the question asks for, which is status indicating a firm fundus. Focus on the term *postpartum* in relation to the condition of the fundus, and relate that a firm fundus is progressing in the involution process. Review nursing assessment of the fundus in the postpartum period if you had difficulty answering this question.

Client needs category: Physiological integrity

Client needs subcategory: Physiological adaptation

Cognitive level: Applying

89. The nurse is teaching the family of a client diagnosed with leukemia about ways to prevent infection. Which instruction has the **most** impact?

☐ **1.** Bathing the client daily

☐ **2.** Covering the client's mouth when coughing

☐ **3.** Maintaining an intact skin integrity

☐ **4.** Ingesting a plant-based diet

Answer: 3

ⓔ Rationale: A client with leukemia has a compromised immune system. Maintaining skin integrity is a priority as the skin is a barrier to pathogens. If a pathogen enters the client's system, the client may not be able to fight off the bacteria, and it will multiply and spread. Bathing daily can decrease bacteria on the skin, but unless there is a break in the skin, the bacteria will remain on the skin. Covering the mouth when coughing protects others but does not have an impact on the client. Ingesting a plant-based diet may be nutritious, which helps the immune system, but this does not have the most impact.

Test-taking strategy: Analyze to determine what information the question asks for, which is infection control for a client with a compromised immune system. Discriminate through each option, and consider the impact on keeping the client free of infection. Review infection control practices if you had difficulty answering this question.

Client needs category: Safe and effective care environment

Client needs subcategory: Safety and infection control

Cognitive level: Analyzing

---

90. A client with a subarachnoid hemorrhage is prescribed a 1,000-mg loading dose of phenytoin intravenously. Which consideration is **most** important when administering this dose?

☐ **1.** Therapeutic drug levels would be maintained between 20 and 30 mg/ml.

☐ **2.** Rapid phenytoin administration can cause cardiac arrhythmias.

☐ **3.** Phenytoin would be mixed with dextrose in water before administration.

☐ **4.** Phenytoin would be administered through an intravenous catheter in the client's hand.

Answer: 2

ⓔ Rationale: Phenytoin intravenously would not be given at a rate exceeding 50 mg/minute because rapid administration can depress the myocardium, causing arrhythmias. Therapeutic drug levels range from 10 to 20 mg/ml. Phenytoin would not be mixed in solution for administration. However, because it is compatible with normal saline solution, it can be injected through an intravenous line containing normal saline solution. When given through an intravenous catheter in the hand, phenytoin may cause purple glove syndrome.

Test-taking strategy: Analyze to determine what information the question asks for, which is considerations when administering phenytoin. Knowledge of phenytoin and adverse effects are essential in answering this question. If unsure, note that cardiac arrhythmias are the most dangerous outcomes of therapy and the only outcome noted in the options. Review the adverse effects of this medication on various body systems if you had difficulty answering this question.

Client needs category: Physiological integrity

Client needs subcategory: Pharmacological and parenteral therapies

Cognitive level: Applying

91. A client arrives at the emergency department confused and disoriented. The client does not have anyone else present to provide information. Which route of communication used by the nurse is **most** effective?

☐ **1.** Therapeutic touch

☐ **2.** Speaking slowly and enunciating words

☐ **3.** Writing down the nurse's questions

☐ **4.** Speaking loud and clear to maintain client focus

🄲 **Rationale:** Option 1 is the only option that does not require being oriented. Therapeutic touch can calm the client while the nurse is assessing client symptoms. The client is not hard of hearing to need to speak slowly and enunciate or need a loud tone. Writing down the questions requires that the client is oriented enough to answer them.

Test-taking strategy: Analyze to determine what information the question asks for, which is most effective route of communication. Consider which route would provide the nurse with information on client status. Review communication techniques when caring for a disoriented client if you had difficulty answering this question.

Client needs category: Psychosocial integrity

Client needs subcategory: None

Cognitive level: Applying

---

92. A client has a percutaneous endoscopic gastrostomy tube in place for tube feedings. Before starting a continuous feeding, the nurse would place the client in which position?

☐ **1.** Semi-Fowler's

☐ **2.** Supine

☐ **3.** Reverse Trendelenburg's

☐ **4.** High Fowler's

🄲 **Rationale:** To prevent aspiration of stomach contents, the nurse would place the client in a semi-Fowler position. The supine and reverse Trendelenburg positions may cause aspiration. High Fowler's position is not necessary and may not be as well tolerated as semi-Fowler's in this situation.

Test-taking strategy: Analyze to determine what information the question asks for, which is position of client when administering a continuous tube feeding. Recall that common protocols state that the client's head be elevated to prevent aspiration of stomach contents. If unsure, consider appropriate oral feeding positions. Also, focus on the importance of maintaining the airway during a tube feeding. Review nursing protocol for maintaining a continuous tube feeding if you had difficulty answering this question.

Client needs category: Physiological integrity

Client needs subcategory: Reduction of risk potential

Cognitive level: Applying

93. A client calls the nurse to his room, stating he is experiencing substernal chest pain that radiates to his jaw. The nurse records a rhythm strip and monitors the client's vital signs. Which graphic highlights the portion of the client's ECG complex that may become elevated above the baseline, indicating myocardial infarction (MI)?

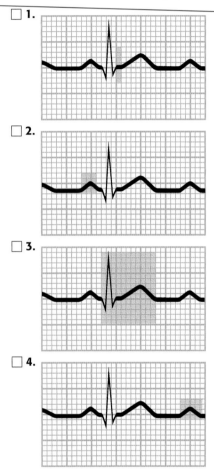

☐ **1.**

☐ **2.**

☐ **3.**

☐ **4.**

Ⓜ Rationale: A change in the ST segment (option 1) may indicate myocardial damage. The ST segment typically elevates at the onset of an MI, indicating myocardial injury is occurring. Option 2 is highlighting the PR interval, option 3 is highlighting the QT interval, and option 4 is highlighting a U wave. These components do not elevate above the baseline with an MI.

Test-taking strategy: Analyze to determine what information the question asks for, which is elements of an ECG indicating an MI. Recall that the ST segment is sensitive to myocardial tissue damage and assists to determine medical treatment options. Review the components of an ECG rhythm and focus on the characteristic changes seen with an MI if you had difficulty answering this question.

Client needs category: Physiological integrity

Client needs subcategory: Physiological adaptation

Cognitive level: Analyzing

94. The nurse is caring for a client who is experiencing increasing shortness of breath. The client is pale, and slight circumoral cyanosis is developing. Which laboratory test **best** measures the adequacy of tissue oxygenation?

- ☐ **1.** Arterial blood gases
- ☐ **2.** Red blood cell count
- ☐ **3.** Pulmonary function test
- ☐ **4.** Hemoglobin level

Ⓔ Rationale: Arterial blood levels include levels of oxygen in the body and determine the adequacy of alveolar gas exchange. Red blood cell count provides information on the quantity of red blood cells in the system. Pulmonary function tests measure lung volume and capacity. Although hemoglobin is the red pigment in the red blood cells that carries oxygen, it is not the best measurement of tissue oxygenation.

Test-taking strategy: Analyze to determine what information the question asks for, which is the laboratory test that best measures tissue oxygenation. Eliminate option 3 as a diagnostic, not a laboratory, test, which requires the client to be in a stable state to complete. Of the 3 remaining blood tests, eliminate option 2 as providing information on the blood count but not as pertinent information on tissue oxygenation. Of the remaining two options, the arterial (oxygenated) blood gas lab work provides data on the amount of oxygen to the tissue. Review the components of arterial blood gases if you had difficulty answering this question.

Client needs category: Physiological integrity

Client needs subcategory: Physiological adaptation

Cognitive level: Applying

95. Which nursing instruction is **most** applicable to a client who is newly diagnosed with chronic pyelonephritis?

- ☐ **1.** Remain on bed rest for up to 2 weeks.
- ☐ **2.** Expect to take an analgesic on a regular basis for the next 6 months.
- ☐ **3.** Expect to provide a urine specimen for culturing every 2 weeks for up to 6 months.
- ☐ **4.** Expect to be on an antibiotic for several weeks or even months.

Ⓔ Rationale: Chronic pyelonephritis is a long-term condition, often requiring antibiotic treatment for several weeks or months and close monitoring to prevent permanent kidney damage. Bed rest and analgesics may be prescribed during the acute stage, but they are not usually required long term. A urine culture is typically ordered 2 weeks after stopping antibiotics to ensure that the infection has been eradicated.

Test-taking strategy: Analyze to determine what information the question asks for, which is nursing instruction for a client with chronic pyelonephritis. The key term is "chronic" as options 1, 2, and 3 are unrealistic expectations of client care. Review treatment modalities related to long-term inflammatory conditions such as chronic pyelonephritis if you had difficulty answering this question.

Client needs category: Physiological integrity

Client needs subcategory: Reduction of risk potential

Cognitive level: Applying

96. A client receiving chemotherapy is nauseated and has lost 15 lb (6.8 kg) in 1 month. Which nutritional instruction would the nurse include in the plan of care?

☐ **1.** Encourage fluids with meals.

☐ **2.** Eat 2 large meals per day.

☐ **3.** Eat hot or cold foods.

☐ **4.** Eat frequent but small meals.

Answer: 4

ⓔ Rationale: Small quantities of food offered frequently allow the client to ingest food with the best chance of not having nausea. Large quantities of food, although only having 2 meals per day, overwhelm the stomach, causing nausea. Fluids take room in the stomach and can cause nausea. Extremes in temperature can precipitate nausea.

Test-taking strategy: Analyze to determine what information the question asks for, which is nutritional instruction for a client nauseated from chemotherapy treatment. The goal of the plan of care is to provide nutrition so that weight loss stops and weight maintenance or gain occurs. Select the option that provides the opportunity to limit nausea and retain food. Review nutritional considerations when on chemotherapy if you had difficulty answering this question.

Client needs category: Physiological integrity

Client needs subcategory: Basic care and comfort

Cognitive level: Applying

---

97. A nurse completes the discharge teaching for a client being treated for a sexually transmitted infection (STI) and provides him a copy of written instructions. Which comment would indicate that the client has understood the instructions?

☐ **1.** "I don't need to use a condom unless I have a temperature or signs of infection."

☐ **2.** "I'll notify my sex partners and avoid having unprotected sex from now on."

☐ **3.** "I'll just be careful not to have intercourse with someone who has an STI."

☐ **4.** "I guess there's not much anyone can do to prevent it. If you're going to get it, you're going to get it."

Answer: 2

ⓔ Rationale: The nurse would know that the client understands the teaching when he/she can describe preventive behaviors and good, safe health practices. The other options indicate that the client does not understand the need to take preventive measures.

Test-taking strategy: Analyze to determine what information the question asks for, which is client statement indicating an understanding of discharge instructions. The key word is "understanding," suggesting a correct client statement. Analyze each option for a correct statement regarding STIs. Review the pathophysiology of STIs and how they are transmitted if you had difficulty answering this question.

Client needs category: Safe and effective care environment

Client needs subcategory: Safety and infection control

Cognitive level: Analyzing

98. The nurse is working in the emergency room and is assigned to a neonatal client with necrotizing enterocolitis. When assessing the client, the nurse would expect which finding?

☐ **1.** Abdominal distention and paralytic ileus

☐ **2.** Gastric retention and guaiac-negative stools

☐ **3.** Metabolic alkalosis and abdominal distention

☐ **4.** Guaiac-negative stools and metabolic alkalosis

Answer: 1

Ⓔ **Rationale:** Necrotizing enterocolitis is an ischemic disorder of the gut. The cause is unknown, but it is more common in preterm neonates who have had a hypoxic episode. The neonate's intestines become dilated and necrotic, and the abdomen becomes extremely distended. Paralytic ileus develops, causing gastric retention. These retained gastric contents, along with any passed stool, will be guaiac positive. The neonate also develops metabolic acidosis, not metabolic alkalosis.

Test-taking strategy: Analyze to determine what information the question asks for, which is symptoms a client experiences when diagnosed with necrotizing enterocolitis. Use knowledge of medical terminology to link necrosis and colon. Eliminate options 2 and 4 when having no blood in the stools (negative guaiac). Review the pathophysiology of necrotizing enterocolitis and symptoms that present if you had difficulty answering this question.

Client needs category: Physiological integrity

Client needs subcategory: Physiological adaptation

Cognitive level: Understanding

---

99. The nurse is having difficulty communicating with a hospitalized 6-year-old child. What technique is **most** helpful?

☐ **1.** Suggest that the child keep a diary.

☐ **2.** Suggest that the parent read fairy tales to the child.

☐ **3.** Ask the parent if the child is always uncommunicative.

☐ **4.** Ask the child to draw a picture.

Answer: 4

Ⓔ **Rationale:** The 6-year-old is a school-aged child. The client at this age is creative and can express self with art easier than with oral communication. A diary is best for adolescents who are able to express themselves with the written word. Reading to the client does not give the child the opportunity to express his or her feelings. Asking the parent if the client does not speak is not a communication technique.

Test-taking strategy: Analyze to determine what information the question asks for, which is communication strategies for a 6-year-old. Consider his/her developmental level and anxiety when in the hospital. Provide an opportunity, at the appropriate level, for the child to express self. Review developmental level and communication strategies for the school-aged client if you had difficulty answering this question.

Client needs category: Psychosocial integrity

Client needs subcategory: None

Cognitive level: Applying

100. A child has been diagnosed with mumps, a viral infection that involves the parotid glands. Indicate on the illustration below where the nurse expects to assess swelling.

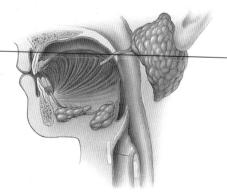

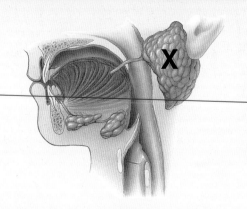

D **Rationale:** The parotid glands are one of three pair of salivary glands located below and in front of the ears.

Test-taking strategy: Analyze to determine what information the question asks for, which is location of the parotid glands. Recall that the gland is a salivary gland in close approximation to the mandible. Review the anatomy of the head and neck and the location of the salivary glands if you had difficulty answering this question.

Client needs category: Physiological integrity

Client needs subcategory: Physiological adaptation

Cognitive level: Analyzing